Oral & Maxillofacial Radiology

Radiologic/Pathologic Correlations

Dale A. Miles, B.A., D.D.S., M.S.
Director, Graduate Program
Dental Diagnostic Sciences
Indiana University School of Dentistry
1121 W. Michigan St., Rm. S110
Indianapolis, Indiana 46202

George E. Kaugars, B.S., D.D.S.
Department of Oral Pathology
Medical College of Virginia
School of Dentistry, Box 566
Richmond, Virginia 23298

Margot Van Dis, D.D.S., M.S.
Associate Professor
Dept. of Dental Diagnostic Sciences
Indiana University School of Dentistry
1121 W. Michigan St.
Indianapolis, Indiana 46202

John G. L. Lovas, B.S., D.D.S.
Division of Oral Pathology
Department of Oral Biology
Faculty of Dentistry
Dalhousie University
Halifax, Nova Scotia B3H 3J5
Canada

1991

W.B. SAUNDERS COMPANY
Harcourt Brace Jovanovich, Inc.
Philadelphia   London   Toronto   Montreal   Sydney   Tokyo

W. B. SAUNDERS COMPANY
Harcourt Brace Jovanovich, Inc.

The Curtis Center
Independence Square West
Philadelphia, PA 19106

Library of Congress Cataloging-in-Publication Data

Oral and maxillofacial radiology : radiologic/pathologic
correlations / Dale A. Miles . . . [et al.].

    p.   cm.

ISBN 0–7216–3070–7

1. Face—Radiography.   2. Maxilla–Radiography.
    3. Face—Diseases—Diagnosis.   4. Maxilla–Diseases—
Diagnosis.   I. Miles, Dale A.
[DNLM: 1. Stomatognathic Diseases—pathology.   2.
Stomatognathic Diseases—radiography. WU 140 06254]

RC936.073 1991

617.5′20757—dc20

DNLM/DLC   90–8985

Editor: John Dyson
Designer: Joan Wendt
Production Manager: Bill Preston
Manuscript Editor: Ruth Low
Illustration Coordinator: Lisa Lambert
Indexer: Kathleen Cole
Cover Designer: Michelle Maloney

Oral and Maxillofacial Radiology: Radiologic/Pathologic Correlations   ISBN 0–7216–3070–7

Last digit is the print number: 9   8   7   6   5   4   3   2   1

PREFACE

Several years ago, in Halifax, Nova Scotia, one of us (D.A.M.) was approached by several dental students just prior to their final examination in Oral Radiology, an interpretation course. They asked if they could borrow slides for several lectures to review before the examination. "There aren't enough illustrations in the book," they said. They were right. Students learning to interpret radiographs frequently ask to see more cases in order to improve their ability to "diagnose." This is not surprising because diagnostic radiology is at least partially based on pattern recognition. A deficiency of many prior dental diagnostic texts has been the use of only one radiographic example to illustrate what is considered the "classic" appearance. Although no one text can contain all possible radiographic variants, we have attempted in this book to demonstrate the remarkable range in clinicoradiographic appearance that is noted with some lesions.

In subsequent discussions, all of us felt that what students needed was a separate, interpretive radiology textbook. Such a textbook not only would be well illustrated with classic lesion appearances as well as variants but also would contain more histopathology, or "oral pathology" if you will, because **the pathologic process dictates the lesion appearance.** Recognizing the "picture" is not enough; a clinician must also understand the pathologic process that produced the image. Several of us have tried to integrate oral pathology lectures on odontogenic cysts and tumors with those of oral radiology in our dental school curricula. In this way we hope to lessen the confusion for the student, eliminate older terminology for certain disease processes, and reduce the use of contradictory terms.

We are also struck by the fact that discussions of *treatment* are missing from most radiology textbooks. All of us share the philosophy of Dr. Harold M. Worth, the grandfather of oral radiology, who stated in his 1964 textbook that "radiography comes to its greatest fruition in the hands of those who are best informed clinically." To us, this means that in order to interpret radiographs, the practitioner must master information about the clinical, radiographic, and pathologic characteristics of lesions that affect the oral and maxillofacial region. Only then can a working diagnosis be formed and the patient properly treated.

In this textbook we have adopted a format that addresses these areas. Our purpose is to present the student with a precise and complete picture of the more common disorders that he or she will encounter in dental practice, including the clinical, histopathologic, and radiologic features, and then to suggest the current accepted treatment modalities. Each chapter has a list of the most common lesions in a disease category. Each lesion is treated separately, first with a few paragraphs of introductory information and then by sections called Clinical Features, Radiographic Appearance, Histopathologic Findings, and, finally, Treatment. This information is followed by classic and current references for each lesion. We then present the reader with illustrations of each lesion, including when possible, multiple radiographic examples supported by photomicrographs. Thus, the reader does not have to flip back and forth between pages to find the illustration that matches the description. We feel this format is more efficient for learning purposes.

We have also tried to incorporate examples of lesions using advanced imaging modalities such as computed tomography (CT) and magnetic resonance imaging (MRI). This is the first oral radiology textbook to use such images in any quantity. We issue a request to our colleagues and fellow educators to share examples of odontogenic lesions, systemic diseases, and sinus, temporomandibular joint, or traumatic lesions imaged by MRI or CT. We would be most willing to consider including them in a subsequent edition. The future of oral and maxillofacial imaging—including radiologic interpretations—is in our hands. We need to bring "dental radiology" out of the dark age of film and into the electronic imaging age. This textbook may be the first small step.

DALE A. MILES
Indianapolis, Indiana
MARGOT VAN DIS
Indianapolis, Indiana
GEORGE KAUGARS
Richmond, Virginia
JOHN LOVAS
Halifax, Nova Scotia

ACKNOWLEDGMENTS

The authors wish to thank the following people for their help and perseverance with this manuscript: From Indiana University School of Dentistry, Dr. Charles E. Tomich, Professor and Chairman, Department of Oral Pathology, for his unselfish donation of multiple radiographs for illustrations; Ms. Julie R. LeHunt, Administrative Secretary, Department of Dental Diagnostic Sciences, for her expert and **patient** help with the word processing of the text; Michael Halloran and Alana Barra, Dental Illustrations, for the photographic reproductions; Ms. Susan Shafer, Department of Dental Diagnostic Sciences, for her assistance with selected tables.

Thanks also to John Dyson, Senior Medical Editor; Mimi McGinnis, Copy Editor; and Bill Preston, Production Manager—W. B. Saunders Company—very competent and understanding individuals.

Finally, we wish to thank our respective families for their patience and support throughout this project. Kathy, Kelly, Chris, Jeff, Claire, Matthew, Sandy, Michael, and David, we owe you some quality time.

Dale A. Miles

Margot L. Van Dis

George E. Kaugars

John G. Lovas

CONTENTS

T w e l v e

DENTAL ANOMALIES AND INHERITABLE DISORDERS AFFECTING TEETH

THE INTERPRETIVE METHOD

D. MILES

PATTERN MATCHING VS. HISTOPATHOLOGIC-RADIOLOGIC CORRELATION
PATTERN MATCHING

HISTOPATHOLOGIC-RADIOLOGIC CORRELATION

LESION DESCRIPTION (THE LANGUAGE OF RADIOLOGY)

PATTERN MATCHING VS. HISTOPATHOLOGIC-RADIOLOGIC CORRELATION

Radiologic interpretation of radiographic information is not an exact science. Many different and varied histopathologic processes can result in similar clinical radiographic presentations. A student of mine several years ago, following a one-semester course in radiologic interpretation, wrote on his course evaluation: "This course should be called 'the radiographic interpretation of all pathologic lesions which look the same on radiographs.' " Clearly, the student was impressed with the radiographic similarities of the pathologic processes—odontogenic and non-odontogenic cysts, tumors, and developmental lesions—and clearly just as unimpressed with any specific presentation of those lesions. The method that I chose to teach the basic information about each group of lesions was the **pattern-matching** method.

PATTERN MATCHING

This method attempts to group various distinct pathologic lesions by their most usual or customary radiographic appearance into a list of differential diagnoses. For example, a differential diagnosis for lesions that commonly present as **multilocular lesions** usually includes the ameloblastoma (an odontogenic tumor), the keratocyst (an odontogenic cyst), and the central giant cell granuloma (a vascular or reactive lesion), among others. Each lesion has a distinct histopathologic appearance and arises from completely separate etiologic processes. Yet

1

each commonly appears radiographically as a so-called multilocular lesion (Figs. 1–1 to 1–3).

The method of pattern matching is a good way to help the student to remember a short but precise list of lesions that might give rise to the particular radiographic picture discovered on examination of the patient. However, the matching of a particular or common radiographic appearance (the pattern) to the name of a lesion is only the first step toward diagnosis of that lesion. The next step assumes first that the student can recall details about the common **clinical features** of each lesion on his or her differential list and second that by relating features such as age and sex incidence, common locations of the lesion, and certain signs and symptoms to the radiographic appearance of the lesion, he or she can then select with some accuracy the name of the lesion that is most probable. That selection process further presumes that the student has mastered and can recall information about the **pathologic behavior** of all of the lesions on the differential list.

HISTOPATHOLOGIC-RADIOLOGIC CORRELATION

The pathologic process, which gives rise to the histopathologic picture from which we obtain the final diagnosis, dictates the radiographic appearance of the lesion. This is the **histopathologic-radiologic correlation** of a disease process. Thus, the pathologic process dictates both the histologic and the radiologic appearance of the lesion.

As an example, compare Figures 1–4 and 1–5. Figure 1–4A reveals a well-circumscribed, homogeneous, periapical radiolucency that is well demarcated by a sclerotic (opaque) border. It has expanded uniformly in all directions, and it appears at the apex of a tooth. The periodontal ligament space is continuous with the periapical radiolucency. The tooth reveals evidence of a gross carious lesion. This appearance is characteristic of an apical cyst. Cysts are often fluid-filled, and one should expect a uniform expansion from such a "hydraulic" process. In contrast, Figure 1–5A depicts another periapical radiolucency, which is also rather well defined. However, it lacks a cortical or sclerotic margin, the periodontal ligament is not continuous with the periapical lucency, and the radiolucency is not homoge-

neous. In addition, there is a dense region of sclerotic bone about the radiolucent area that is diffusely radiopaque. Clearly, the pathologic process producing this periapical radiolucency must be different from that producing the lesion seen in Figure 1–4A. However, the associated tooth is also grossly carious. In fact, the etiologies of both lesions are identical. In both cases the pulp was infected, the pulp died, and the products of inflammation and necrosis, coupled with the body's immune response, produced both periapical radiolucencies. In the first case, a cyst lining consisting of epithelium was produced, and the vascular supply to the area was cut off (Fig. 1–4B). In the second case, a chronic granulomatous response ensued, which maintained a vascular connection. The bone about the lesion is reactive, but no epithelial transformation has yet occurred to "wall off" the lesion (Fig. 1–5B).

In this textbook we will attempt to teach you the basic features of various lesions that you will encounter in dental practice. We have grouped them by pathologic process for the most part, but we will summarize the information in the final chapter by regrouping them into their most common clinical radiographic appearances—that is, using the differential diagnostic approach of pattern matching. In this manner we hope to give you the tools to allow you to describe precisely the radiologic features of important lesions that you might encounter, organize them into a logical and succinct differential diagnostic list, and direct the management of the patient's lesion based on your knowledge of the pathologic behavior of a particular lesion. When you have mastered the content, the differential list or gamuts in the appendix will allow you to review your skills and will serve as a quick checklist of different pathologic lesions with similar radiographic appearances.

LESION DESCRIPTION (THE LANGUAGE OF RADIOLOGY)

One of the most important and most often overlooked aspects of radiologic interpretation is the precise description of the clinicoradiographic appearance of the presenting lesion. Words such as multilocular and pericoronal evoke specific images in the oral and maxillofacial radiologist's mind. Precise descriptions also start the diagnostic process of differentiation between lesions with similar radiographic features. Sometimes it will be a very subtle radiographic characteristic or feature that will tip the clinician to consider one lesion rather than another in his or her list of differential diagnoses.

Several questions the clinician should always ask him- or herself that will begin this process and will become second nature when posed each time he or she sees a lesion are as follows:

1. What size is the lesion? Is it large or small? (Precise measurement is often difficult, especially on extraoral views, owing to magnification.)

2. Is the border ill defined or well defined?

3. Is the border sclerotic (corticated, hyperostotic) or not?

4. Is the border continuous or interrupted?

5. Is the lesion primarily radiolucent, radiopaque, or mixed (diffuse)?

6. Is the lesion unilocular, multilocular, or multifocal (in more than one location)?

As you read through this textbook pay careful attention to the descriptions used by the authors. Most of them are commonly accepted radiographic descriptors. All have been carefully chosen to make you aware of the "language of radiology."

Table 1–1 is a scheme or approach using common radiologic descriptors that you may find useful. The left column lists words used

Table 1–1. COMMON RADIOLOGIC DESCRIPTORS

Primary Description	Secondary Features
Lesion	*Bone*
Size	Expansion or not
Small	Perforation
Medium	Erosion
Large	Remodeling
Border	*Teeth*
Ill-defined	Resorption or not
Well-defined	Displacement or not
Sclerotic or not	
Continuous or not	
Density	
Radiolucent	
Radiopaque	
Mixed	
Diffuse	
Internal structure or not	
Number	
Unilocular	
Multilocular	
Multifocal	

to describe the characteristics of the primary lesion. The right column contains words used to describe what the lesion identified has done to the surrounding or adjacent structures. These descriptors, when properly applied, also suggest useful information about the behavior and possibly the progression of the lesion.

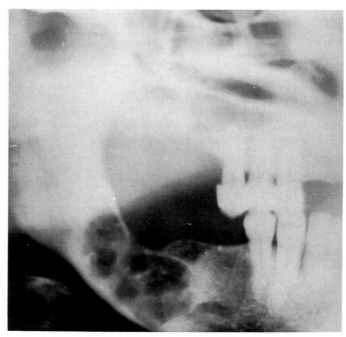

Figure 1–1. Well-defined multilocular lesion in the posterior mandible with erosion of the lower cortical border representing an ameloblastoma.

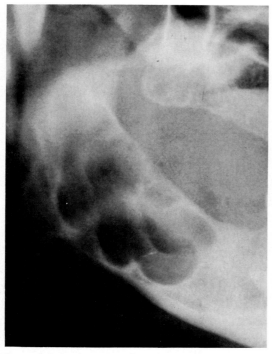

Figure 1–2. Large, expansile, soap-bubble–like multilocular radiolucency that has remodeled the lower cortical border representing an odontogenic keratocyst.

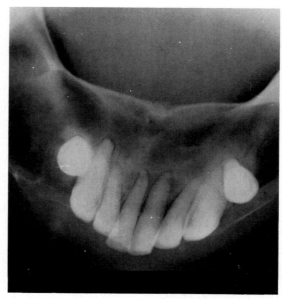

Figure 1–3. Large, expansile multilocular radiolucency crossing the midline of the mandible that has displaced teeth and expanded the inner and outer cortices without perforation representing a central giant cell granuloma.

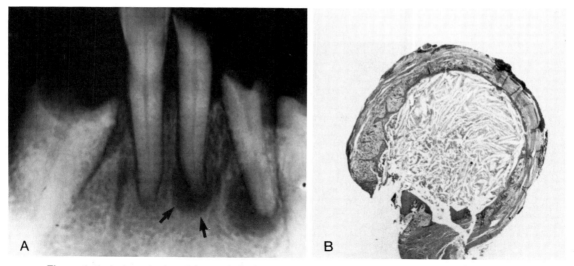

Figure 1–4. *A*, An apical cyst *(arrows)*. *B*, An epithelium-lined cavity with a central area of necrosis.

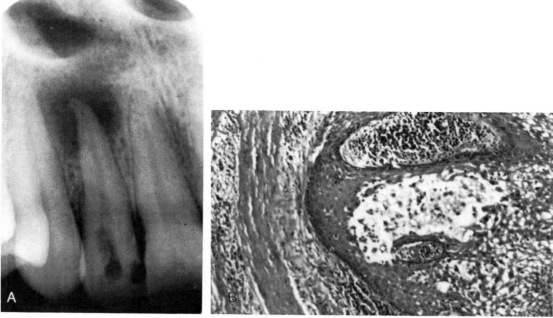

Figure 1–5. *A*, A periapical granuloma. *B*, Proliferating epithelial rests of Malassez within a periapical granuloma. High-power view showing an increased volume of epithe-lium and resultant very early cyst formation as the central cells start to undergo ischemic necrosis.

INFECTION/ INFLAMMATION

J. LOVAS

PERIAPICAL LESIONS
PERIAPICAL GRANULOMA
APICAL ABSCESS (Alveolar Abscess)

OSTEOMYELITIS
ACUTE SUPPURATIVE OSTEOMYELITIS
CHRONIC SUPPURATIVE
   OSTEOMYELITIS

CHRONIC DIFFUSE SCLEROSING
   OSTEOMYELITIS
CHRONIC FOCAL SCLEROSING
   OSTEOMYELITIS (Condensing
   Osteitis, Sclerosing Osteitis)
CHRONIC OSTEOMYELITIS WITH
   PROLIFERATIVE PERIOSTITIS
   (Garré's Osteomyelitis)

Inflammatory and infectious processes are so intimately interrelated and uncontaminated bacteriologic cultures from within jawbones are so difficult to obtain (Jacobsson et al, 1982; Krutchkoff and Runstad, 1989) that we cannot be sure whether bacteria are consistently present in this group of diseases.

Apical periodontitis is the collective term for the three closely related sequelae of irreversible pulpitis: **periapical granuloma, radicular cyst,** and **apical abscess.** Caries is by far the most common initial cause of apical periodontitis. Microscopically, and sometimes radiographically, detectable external root resorption is present in all forms of apical periodontitis.

References

Jacobsson, S., Dahlen, G., and Moller, A.J.R.: Bacteriologic and serologic investigation in diffuse sclerosing osteomyelitis (DSO) of the mandible. Oral Surg. Oral Med. Oral Pathol., 54:506–512, 1982.

Krutchkoff, D.J., and Runstad, L.: Unusually aggressive osteomyelitis of the jaws: A report of two cases. Oral Surg. Oral Med. Oral Pathol., 67:499–507, 1989.

PERIAPICAL LESIONS

PERIAPICAL GRANULOMA

The first and most common result of irreversible pulpitis, periapical granuloma, represents inflamed granulation tissue at the root apex. Periapical granulomas can give rise to radicular cysts (Figs. 2–1 and 2–2) and apical abscesses and vice versa. There is a continuous spectrum among these lesions. Even at the microscopic level, some features of all three conditions are often seen concurrently, and histopathologic diagnosis is based on the most predominant features seen in the given lesion.

Clinical Features

The tooth is often asymptomatic and has a previous history of prolonged sensitivity to heat or cold. Deep caries, a deep restoration, or a history of trauma should be evident. The tooth is often tender to pressure and percussion (because the apical periodontal ligament contains inflamed granulation tissue) and should fail to react to thermal or electrical stimulation (because the pulp is nonvital).

Radiographic Appearance

A thickened periodontal ligament space at the root apex is the earliest radiographic sign. With time, the periapical radiolucency enlarges. Large lesions are seldom well defined and even less frequently have hyperostotic borders. The lamina dura is lost between the root apex and the apical lesion. If an apical radiolucency has these features and the root canals appear to have been obturated, the radiolucency may still represent a periapical granuloma if the canals were inadequately cleaned or obturated (Fig. 2–3C) or if there is a vertical root fracture. Unless the cause was trauma, the radiograph should reveal caries or a restoration in or near the pulp. If the cause of pulp devitalization was rapid orthodontic tooth movement, shortened roots are often evident.

Histopathologic Findings

Inflamed granulation tissue, containing proliferating epithelial rests of Malassez, is found between the root apex and alveolar bone. Like granulation tissue elsewhere, this tissue is composed of plump fibroblasts and young capillaries in an edematous, sparsely collagenized stroma. Variable proportions of histiocytes, lymphocytes, plasma cells (Fig. 2–3B), neutrophils, and cholesterol clefts surrounded by foreign body giant cells are present. Often there is compressed collagen, forming a capsule at the periphery.

Treatment

Periapical granulomas resolve following removal of the necrotic pulp by means of conservative endodontic therapy or tooth extraction. Sometimes apical curettage, apicoectomy, and retrograde filling are indicated.

APICAL ABSCESS (Alveolar Abscess)

Clinical Features

The tooth is usually but not always spontaneously painful, with a previous history of prolonged sensitivity to sweets, heat, or cold. Deep caries, a deep restoration, incomplete endodontics or orthodontics, or a history of trauma should be evident. The tooth is usually very tender to pressure and percussion (because the apical periodontal ligament contains acutely inflamed granulation tissue and pus) and is tender to heat (heat causes further expansion and thus pressure in the periapex), and it should fail to react to cold or electrical stimulation (because the pulp is nonvital). There can be intraoral and extraoral soft tissue swelling, erythema, and draining fistulas. Regional lymphadenitis, fever, and malaise are also present in some cases.

Radiographic Appearance

An apical radiolucency with diffuse (poorly defined) and irregular margins is characteristic of an apical abscess. The lamina dura is lost between the root apex and the apical lesion. With time, the periapical radiolucency enlarges. Unless the cause was trauma, the radiograph should reveal caries or a restoration in or near the pulp. If the cause of pulp devitalization was rapid orthodontic tooth movement, shortened roots are often evident. If an apical radiolucency has these features and the root canals appear to have been obturated, the radiolucency may still represent an apical ab-

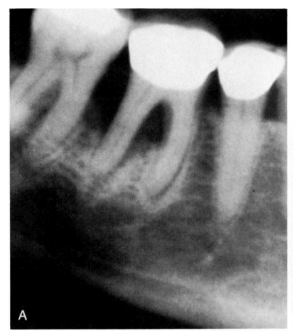

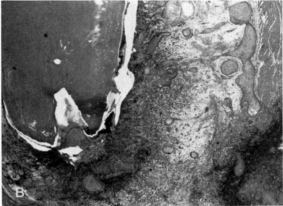

Figure 2–1. *A,* A diffuse radiolucent area at the apex of the mandibular right first molar in a patient with long-standing periodontal problems. Note the widened peri-odontal ligament spaces and thickened lamina dura or areas of hyperostosis adjacent to the periodontal liga-ment spaces. *B,* Periapical granuloma, proliferating epi-thelial rests of Malassez, and external root resorption. Low-power view of a root with microscopic external root resorption (scalloped outline on the right side). A large mass of inflamed granulation tissue has replaced normal alveolar bone about the apex. Inflammation stimulates the epithelium to proliferate.

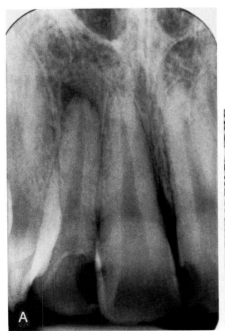

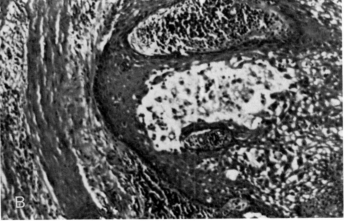

Figure 2–2. *A,* Ill-defined radiolucency at the apex of a grossly carious lateral incisor consistent with a periapical granuloma. *B,* Proliferating epithelial rests of Malassez within a periapical granuloma. High-power view showing an increased volume of epithelium and resultant very early cyst formation as the central cells start to undergo ischemic necrosis.

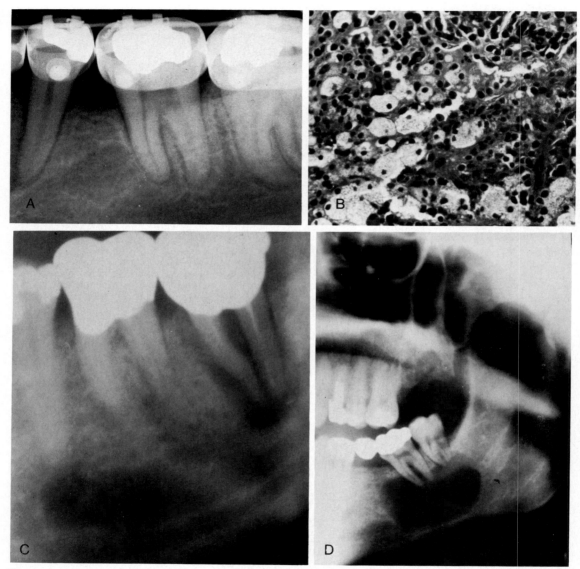

Figure 2–3. *A,* Widened periodontal ligament space about a second premolar undergoing orthodontic movement. *B,* Periapical granuloma. High-power view of chronically inflamed granulation tissue. A young blood capillary is seen at bottom right. The large cells with clear cytoplasms are "foamy" histiocytes; the rest are lymphocytes and plasma cells. *C,* Periapical granuloma of pulpal or periodontal origin. *D,* Large periapical granuloma with rather well defined borders secondary to a failed fixed prosthetic bridge.

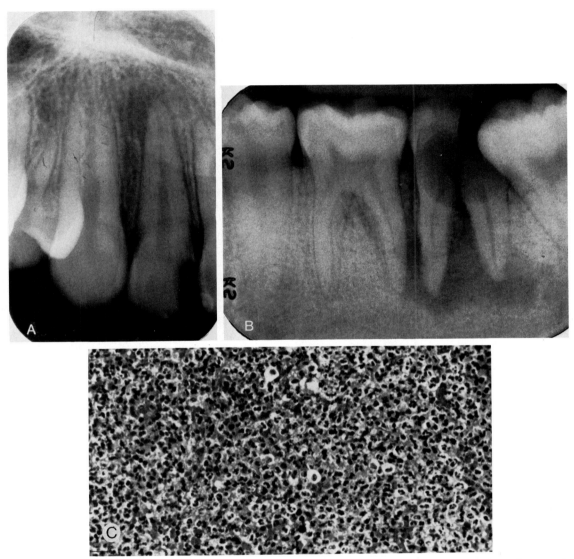

Figure 2–4. *A,* Apical lucency with diffusely defined borders. Note how the periodontal ligament space "blends" into the lesion. *B,* Long-standing caries has led to this well-defined but diffuse radiolucency. The clinical presentation involved facial swelling and a draining fistula. The histopathologic diagnosis was apical abscess. *C,* Apical abscess. Medium-power view of an acute inflammatory infiltrate containing a few foamy histiocytes but dominated by neutrophils. Typically, all other tissues in the center of the abscess have been destroyed and replaced by "a sea of neutrophils."

scess if the canals were inadequately cleaned or obturated or if there is a vertical root fracture.

Histopathologic Findings

Because this lesion represents an acute exacerbation of a preexisting periapical granuloma or radicular cyst, some of the histologic features of these are often preserved. The predominant feature, however, is that of inflammatory cells, with neutrophils dominating (Fig. 2–4C).

Treatment

Apical abscesses resolve following removal of the necrotic pulp by means of conservative endodontic therapy or tooth extraction. Systemic antibiotics and incision and drainage are sometimes indicated.

OSTEOMYELITIS

Osteomyelitis can be defined as inflammation/infection of bone and bone marrow. Most cases are caused by microorganisms (usually bacteria such as mixed normal oral flora, *Staphylococcus aureus,* or *S. albus*) that enter the bone (1) through a contiguous infection (usually an abscessed tooth), (2) from the oral mucosa or skin after direct trauma (accidental or surgical), or, least commonly, (3) hematogenously (secondary to bacteremia).

Osteomyelitis of the jaws is uncommon in places where dental health care and antibiotics are readily available (Adekeye and Cornah, 1985). When the disease does occur, it indicates that the host defenses, sometimes despite the aid of antibiotics, are incapable of completely eliminating the infection/inflammation. Systemic predisposing factors include diabetes, malnutrition, and tobacco and alcohol abuse (Calhoun et al, 1988). Local predisposing factors include the presence of necrotic bone or dentinal tubules of residual tooth fragments, which offer bacteria shelter from antibiotics and the host's immune response (Wannfors and Hammarstrom, 1985), and prior radiation therapy, which causes decreased vascularization.

The mandible is much more often involved than the maxilla because the mandible has a thicker cortical plate, making spread of infection within medullary bone easier than through the cortex, and because the mandible is not as well vascularized. The mandibular canal can act as a pathway for the spread of infection; the patient may experience paresthesia or anesthesia, and radiographically diffuse mandibular canal borders may be seen (Wannfors and Hammarstrom, 1985).

The features and clinical course of the disease are determined primarily by the shifting balance between microbial virulence and host resistance. The age of the patient is also an important determinant; young patients are capable of mounting a proliferative periosteal response, whereas older patients tend to respond with medullary sclerosis. Radiographically, early suppurative osteomyelitis is difficult to detect. Bone scintigraphy (using technetium-99m scans) permits early detection of osteomyelitis before radiographic changes become apparent (Treves et al, 1976; Calhoun et al, 1988). Well-established disease is easy to detect radiographically but can be very difficult to distinguish from malignancy because both processes are infiltrative and destructive, with ill-defined borders.

Sequestra and involucra are typical of advanced suppurative osteomyelitis. A sequestrum forms when a piece of bone, devitalized by the infectious/inflammatory process, separates from vital bone and is either resorbed by osteoclasts or rejected as if it were foreign material. When a sequestrum is large, it sometimes becomes necessary to excise it surgically (sequestrectomy). An involucrum is a sequestrum around which new, viable bone has been laid down.

References

Adekeye, E.O., and Cornah, J.: Osteomyelitis of the jaws: A review of 141 cases. Br. J. Oral Maxillofac. Surg., 23:24–35, 1985.

Calhoun, K.H., Shapiro, R.D., Stiernberg, C.M., Calhoun, J.H., and Mader, J.T.: Osteomyelitis of the mandible. Arch. Otolaryngol. Head Neck Surg., 114:1157–1162, 1988.

Treves, S., Khettry, J., Brooker, F.H., Wilkinson, R.H., and Watts, H.: Osteomyelitis: Early scintigraphic detection in children. Pediatrics 57:175–185, 1976.

Wannfors, K., and Hammarstrom, L.: Infectious foci in chronic osteomyelitis of the jaws. Int. J. Oral Surg., 14:493–503, 1985.

ACUTE SUPPURATIVE OSTEOMYELITIS

Clinical Features

The symptoms and signs of acute inflammation/infection are evident: pain, fever, lymphadenitis, and malaise. There can be intraoral and extraoral soft tissue swelling, erythema, and draining fistulas associated with an abscessed tooth, jaw fracture, or site of previous surgery. The mandible is more frequently and more extensively involved than the maxilla. Inflammation/infection can directly affect the inferior alveolar nerve, resulting in paresthesia or anesthesia of the lower lip. Teeth in the area are sore and loose.

Radiographic Appearance

The inflammation/infection spreads rapidly through the medullary bone, resulting in subtle, diffuse, lytic changes that become progressively more evident radiographically after a 1- to 2-week lag period. The trabeculae appear less radiopaque and less well defined, whereas the spaces between trabeculae enlarge.

Histopathologic Findings

Progressive loss of bone viability, characterized by loss of osteocytes from lacunae, and pus—severe inflammatory cell infiltrates composed primarily of neutrophils—are the chief histologic features. In time, fragments of necrotic bone (sequestra) or even involucra become evident (Figs. 2–5*B* and 2–6*C*).

Treatment

Parenteral antibiotics (ideally given after culture and sensitivity testing of deep bone biopsy specimens), incision and drainage, sequestrectomy, excision and grafting, dental extractions, and sometimes hyperbaric oxygen therapy can be employed (Calhoun et al, 1988; Krutchkoff and Runstad, 1989). Vital teeth that are symptomatic only because of their location in the involved segment of jaw do not require extraction (Krutchkoff and Runstad, 1989).

References

Calhoun, K.H., Shapiro, R.D., Stiernberg, C.M., Calhoun, J.H., and Mader, J.T.: Osteomyelitis of the mandible. Arch. Otolaryngol. Head Neck Surg., 114:1157–1162, 1988.

Krutchkoff, D.J., and Runstad, L.: Unusually aggressive osteomyelitis of the jaws: A report of two cases. Oral Surg. Oral Med. Oral Pathol., 67:499–507, 1989.

CHRONIC SUPPURATIVE OSTEOMYELITIS

Clinical Features

The symptoms and signs are similar to but milder than those for acute suppurative osteomyelitis. In the chronic form, the virulence of the organisms is relatively lower, and host resistance is relatively greater. Therefore, the infection is milder and better localized, and may persist for years with periodic exacerbations marked by drainage of pus and expulsion of sequestra.

Radiographic Appearance

The radiographic features are similar to those seen in the acute suppurative form, but the margins of the lesion are somewhat better defined, and, in addition, sequestra (necrotic bone fragments) exhibiting greater radiodensity can be seen as well as intervening areas of residual normal bone. Cortical discontinuities can sometimes be seen. These represent fistulous tracts between the focus of infection/inflammation in the medullary bone and the point of drainage into or through the soft tissues to the surface.

Histopathologic Findings

The histologic features are similar to those characteristic of the acute suppurative form, but the ratio of neutrophils (characteristic of acute inflammation) to lymphocytes and plasma cells (characteristic of chronic inflammation) is lower. Sequestra and involucra are also less frequent.

Treatment

The treatment is the same as that for the acute form but is less aggressive.

CHRONIC DIFFUSE SCLEROSING OSTEOMYELITIS

Although many cases previously reported under this name are more likely to be examples of florid cemento-osseous dysplasia, a "florid" form of periapical cemental dysplasia, chronic diffuse sclerosing osteomyelitis is nevertheless a true entity (Waldron, 1985).

Clinical Features

When the infecting organisms have low virulence and the host has relatively high resistance, the net result is chronic low-grade stimulation of osteoblastic activity. This is in contrast to rapid or slow but progressive bone destruction and purulence in the acute and chronic suppurative forms, respectively. Except for diffuse enlargement of the affected jaw, seen mainly in younger patients, few other signs of osteomyelitis are evident. There can be recurrent episodes of pain, swelling, low-grade fever, and trismus. Unlike the focal form of this condition, the diffuse form tends to occur in middle-aged to elderly individuals and is often associated with current or previous generalized periodontitis.

Radiographic Appearance

There are usually widespread, diffuse or multifocal, sometimes bilateral, ill-defined sclerotic changes in the mandible that mimic Paget's disease of bone. Lytic areas are usually intermingled with areas of sclerosis. Computed tomography (CT) scans reveal subperiosteal new bone formation and endosteal sclerosis (VanMerkesteyn et al, 1988).

Histopathologic Findings

The lesion contains thick, mature (lamellar) viable bone, laid down in a haphazard pattern. A scanty fibrous marrow is seen with very few, if any, chronic inflammatory cells, consisting primarily of lymphocytes (Fig. 2–7B).

Treatment

Conservative treatment consists of management of occasional exacerbations with antibiotics. A more radical approach involves surgical decortication of the involved jaw. Complete elimination of symptoms and signs is difficult to achieve (VanMerkesteyn et al, 1988).

References

VanMerkesteyn, J.P.R., Groot, R.H., Bras, J., and Bakker, D.J.: Diffuse sclerosing osteomyelitis of the man-dible: Clinical, radiographic and histologic findings in twenty-seven patients. J. Oral Maxillofac. Surg., 46:825–829, 1988.

Waldron, C.A.: Fibro-osseous lesions of the jaws. J. Oral Maxillofac. Surg., 43:249–262, 1985.

CHRONIC FOCAL SCLEROSING OSTEOMYELITIS (Condensing Osteitis, Sclerosing Osteitis)

This condition, unlike the chronic diffuse form, is quite common. It represents an endosteal reactive hyperplastic response of bone to chronic low-grade infection/inflammation of pulpal origin. The patients are usually under 30 years of age.

Clinical Features

Young people with high host resistance are usually affected. There is seldom a previous history of pain or tenderness. The associated tooth (usually a mandibular first molar) is heavily restored, carious, or both. Especially in the case of molars, the pulp is often only partially necrotic. Cortical expansion seldom if ever occurs.

Radiographic Appearance

There is a periapical radiopacity, usually with a radiolucent area, between the opacity and the apex (Fig. 2–8 A). A portion of the lesion is in intimate contact with the apex. The opacity is usually but not always well defined. Five radiographic patterns have been identified (Eversole et al, 1984). The root outline remains distinct, unlike that in benign cementoblastomas. Despite extraction or successful endodontic therapy of the associated tooth, the radiographic lesion can persist for years.

Histopathologic Findings

The histologic features are identical to those of the chronic diffuse sclerosing form of osteomyelitis (Fig. 2–8B).

Treatment

Removal of the necrotic pulp through conservative endodontic therapy or tooth extraction is indicated. Resolution of the apical lesion may occur but only after several months or years. When normal-appearing bone is seen between the lesion and the tooth apex, pulpitis cannot be documented, and when there is cortical expansion, the possibility of focal periapical osteopetrosis, osteosarcoma, or osteoblastic metastatic disease should be considered.

Reference

Eversole, L.R., Stone, C.E., and Strub, D.: Focal sclerosing osteomyelitis/focal periapical osteopetrosis: Radiographic patterns. Oral Surg. Oral Med. Oral Pathol., 58:456–460, 1984.

CHRONIC OSTEOMYELITIS WITH PROLIFERATIVE PERIOSTITIS (Garré's Osteomyelitis)

Clinical Features

This uncommon condition usually presents as an asymptomatic, unilateral, bony-hard, cortical swelling of the buccal or inferior aspect of the mandible in children or young adults. The expanded buccal or inferior cortex is usually associated with an erupted carious molar or an erupting molar with chronic pericoronitis.

Radiographic Appearance

Radiographs generally reveal cortical expansion, cortical redundancy (onion-skinning), or both (Fig. 2–9*A* and *C*). Proliferation of the periosteum at the inferior border of the mandible may also be seen in Ewing's sarcoma (see Chapter 5). Gross caries, with an associated ill-defined apical radiolucency, is usually also evident.

Histopathologic Findings

Except for more fibrous connective tissue and a lower density of bone, the histologic features of this entity are identical to those of the chronic diffuse sclerosing form of osteomyelitis (Fig. 2–9*B*).

Treatment

Endodontic therapy, extraction, or conservative management of the pericoronitis results in partial to complete resolution of the bony swelling in 2 months to as long as 6 years (Eversole et al, 1979; Lichty et al, 1980).

References

Eversole, L.R., Leider, A.S., Corwin, J.O., and Karian, B.K.: Proliferative periostitis of Garré: Its differentiation from other neoperiostoses. J. Oral Surg., 37:725–731, 1979.
Lichty, G., Langlais, R.P., and Aufdemorte, T.: Garré's osteomyelitis: Literature review and case report. Oral Surg. Oral Med. Oral Pathol., 50:309–313, 1980.

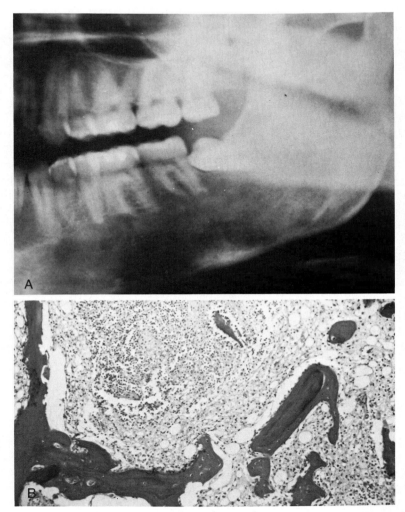

Figure 2–5. *A,* Mixed areas of diffuse radiolucency and radiopacity are seen throughout the mandibular body from the canine to the third molar region. This is an ill-defined radiolucent-radiopaque lesion. *B,* Acute suppurative osteomyelitis. Low-power view of an acute inflammatory infiltrate dominated by neutrophils that fills the marrow spaces. Because the residual bone trabeculae have empty lacunae, they are known to be necrotic.

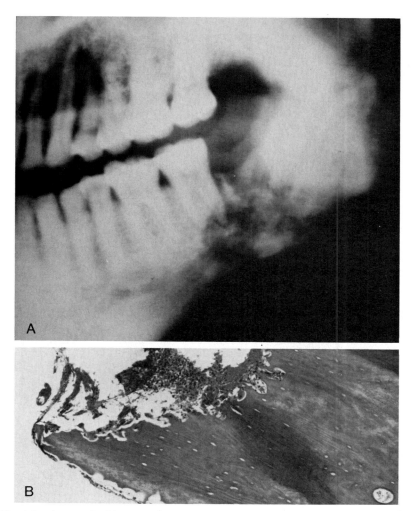

Figure 2–6. *A,* The lytic changes in this case of osteomyelitis are more apparent. Several areas of sequestra are suggested. There is also the suggestion of perforation of the inferior cortex. *B,* Sequestrum. Medium-power view of a large sequestrum exhibiting empty lacunae, scalloped borders, and an adjacent focus of inflammatory cells. The scalloped borders result from previous attempts by osteoclasts to eliminate and ''recycle'' the necrotic bone by resorption.

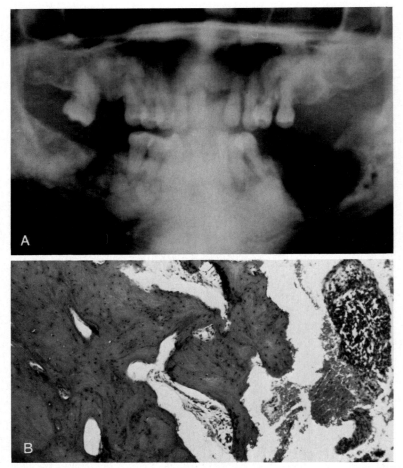

Figure 2–7. *A,* Chronic diffuse sclerosing osteomyelitis of all four quadrants. Biopsy was performed in the mandibular left region for confirmation. Note that all changes are bilateral. *B,* Chronic diffuse sclerosing osteomyelitis. Low-power view of markedly thickened, viable, lamellar bone with a rare focus of adjacent chronic inflammatory infiltrate.

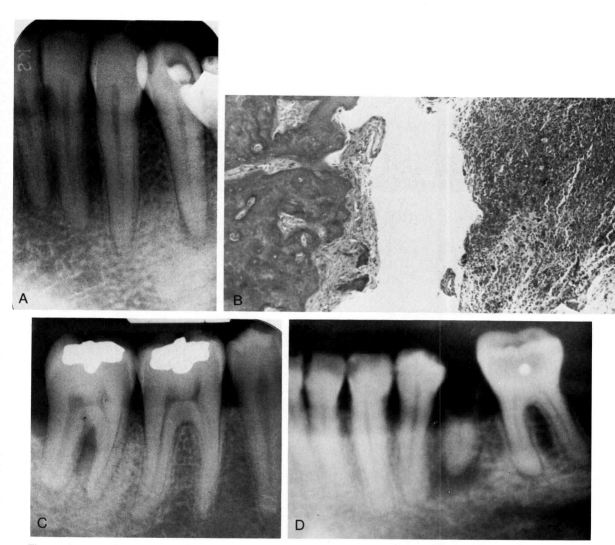

Figure 2–8. *A,* Condensing osteitis or chronic focal sclerosing osteomyelitis. The periapical opacity apical to the tooth is separated by a radiolucent area. The temporary restoration has failed. *B,* Chronic focal sclerosing osteomyelitis. Medium-power view of an area of dense, viable bone (*left*) and inflamed granulation tissue (*right*). The dense reactive bone corresponds to the apical radiopacity, whereas the granulation tissue corresponds to the radiolucency, which is often seen between the root apex and the opacity. *C,* Condensing osteitis of periodontal origin around a molar. *D,* The sclerotic or opaque changes in this patient have occurred about the mesial root of the first molar. Note the intervening radiolucency. The lesion around the premolar root tip is more suggestive of an apical periodontitis—either an abscess or a granuloma.

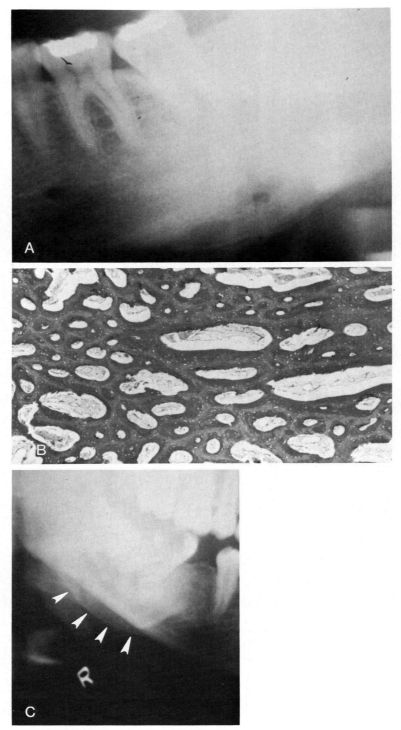

Figure 2–9. *A,* Garré's osteomyelitis. Note the proliferation of the periosteum. The typical "onion-skin" appearance of this mandibular cortex is apparent. *B,* Chronic osteomyelitis with proliferative periostitis. Low-power view of subperiosteal new bone formation peripheral to (outside of) and in addition to the normal cortical bone. Note the orderly parallel orientation of the trabeculae and marrow spaces; the normal cortex is outside the field of view at the bottom, whereas the periosteum, also out of view, is at the top. Radiographically, this formation is seen as cortical redundancy or "onion skin" appearance. *C,* Proliferative periostitis at the inferior border of the mandible (*arrowheads*) secondary to a long-standing gross carious lesion of the second molar.

CYSTS

J. LOVAS

ODONTOGENIC CYSTS
*RADICULAR CYST (Apical Periodontal
    Cyst, Periapical Cyst, Dental Cyst)
DENTIGEROUS CYST (Follicular Cyst)
Eruption Cyst
ODONTOGENIC KERATOCYST (OKC,
    "Primordial Cyst")
DEVELOPMENTAL LATERAL
    PERIODONTAL CYST*

NONODONTOGENIC CYSTS
*INCISIVE CANAL CYST (Nasopalatine
    Duct Cyst)
NASOLABIAL CYST (Nasoalveolar Cyst)*

CONTROVERSIAL CYSTS
*PRIMORDIAL CYST
GLOBULOMAXILLARY CYST
MEDIAN MANDIBULAR CYST
MEDIAN PALATAL CYST (Midpalatal
    Cyst of Infants)
MEDIAN ALVEOLAR CYST*

   A **true cyst** is a pathologic cavity lined by epithelium (Table 3–1). The lumen contains fluid or semisolid material depending on the relative proportion of plasma to necrotic cellular debris. A fibrous capsule, consisting of compressed connective tissue, separates the cystic epithelium from surrounding normal tissue.

   True cysts arise when inflammation or unknown factors stimulate epithelium within tissues to proliferate. Because epithelium is avascular, it is totally dependent on diffusion of nutrients from adjacent vascular connective tissue. As the epithelial mass enlarges, the central cells become farther and farther removed from the nutrient source. These cells become necrotic when the level of nutrients becomes inadequate. The necrotic debris creates an osmotic gradient, drawing fluid (transudate) into the center of the emerging cyst. As long as the causative stimulus persists, the epithelium continues to divide at the periphery, die near the center, and draw in more fluid. Thus, like a balloon that continues to be filled with water, the cyst continues to expand centrifugally. If the stimulus subsides, expansion stops. If, as is often the case, the stimulus is inflammation, an increase in its intensity beyond a critical point causes necrosis of the cyst lining, and an abscess, inflamed granulation tissue, or fibrous scar results.

   Odontogenic cysts are cysts derived from odontogenic epithelium during or after odontogenesis. As expected, these arise either within alveolar bone or within mucosa immediately adjacent to alveolar bone.

   A **residual cyst** is any cyst that remains after inadequate treatment of the

Table 3–1. RADIOLOGIC-PATHOLOGIC CORRELATION: TRUE CYSTS OF THE JAWS

Radiographic Appearance*	Histopathologic Correlation
Well-defined radiolucency, hyperostotic borders	Without severe inflammation
Well-defined radiolucency, without hyperostotic borders	With severe inflammation
Ill-defined radiolucency, diffuse to ragged borders	Severe inflammation; rule out malignancy

*Plain film.

original cyst; it is not a specific diagnosis. Inadequate treatment can include inadequate removal of the original cause or incomplete removal of the cyst itself. Because the radicular cyst is the most common type of jaw cyst, the residual radicular cyst is likewise the most common type of residual cyst. Although the majority of residual radicular cysts are asymptomatic and remain static, a minority exhibit pain and swelling. The source of inflammation in longstanding residual cysts is difficult to explain (High and Hirschmann, 1988). To determine the specific entity represented by a suspected residual cyst, previous history, radiographs, and pathology reports are important. Excisional biopsy is diagnostic.

Any mass of epithelium, including benign and malignant neoplasms, can undergo **cystic degeneration.** Ameloblastomas are particularly noted for containing large cystic areas (see Chapter 4).

In general, static or slowly enlarging lesions appear corticated radiographically (High and Hirschmann, 1988). This appearance is modified by an inverse relationship between the radiographic cortication of a bone lesion and the severity of acute inflammation. A well-

Table 3–2. HISTOGENIC CLASSIFICATION OF ODONTOGENIC CYSTS

(GP Wysocki)

I. Origin from rests of Malassez
   Radicular cyst
II. Origin from reduced enamel epithelium
   Dentigerous cyst
   Eruption cyst
III. Origin from rests of (Serres) dental lamina
   Odontogenic keratocyst
   Developmental lateral periodontal cyst
   Gingival cyst of the adult
   Dental lamina cyst of the newborn

defined, circular, radiolucent lesion with hyperostotic (corticated) borders is strongly suggestive of a cyst and can be referred to as a cyst-like radiolucency. Similarly, a fluid-filled soft tissue "sac" curetted from the jaws can be called cyst-like, but only histologic examination can determine whether a lesion is a true cyst and what specific type it is (Table 3–2).

Reference

High, A.S., and Hirschmann, P.N.: Symptomatic residual radicular cysts. J. Oral Pathol., 17:70–72, 1988.

ODONTOGENIC CYSTS

RADICULAR CYST (Apical Periodontal Cyst, Periapical Cyst, Dental Cyst)

By far the most common cyst of the jaws, this inflammatory odontogenic cyst arises as a result of pulpal necrosis secondary to caries or other injury. Mediators of inflammation exist through the root apex or lateral canals, stimulating the epithelial rests of Malassez to proliferate. These rests, within the periodontal ligament, normally surround the roots of teeth like fishnet stockings. Radicular cysts arise in periapical granulomas, and either lesion can become an apical abscess if the intensity of inflammation increases sufficiently. When the inflammation in an apical abscess decreases, a renewed attempt at healing will give rise to another periapical granuloma (inflamed granulation tissue). **Apical periodontitis is the collective term for periapical granuloma, radicular cyst, and apical abscess** (see Chapter 2). The specific type of apical periodontitis that results from pulp necrosis is therefore determined by the intensity of inflammation and the presence or absence of epithelial rests of Malassez.

Clinical Features

The patient usually but not always has had previous symptoms of irreversible pulpitis or pulpal abscess such as spontaneous pain or prolonged tenderness to heat, cold, or pressure. Unless they are acutely inflamed, radicular cysts are usually asymptomatic. The associated tooth is carious, heavily restored, or previously traumatized. There can be cortical expansion, thinning, or even perforation if the cyst is of sufficient size. Any tooth can be involved, but the first permanent molar is most commonly affected. Deciduous teeth are rarely associated with radicular cysts.

Radiographic Appearance

A well-defined, circular radiolucency with hyperostotic borders at the apex of a grossly carious or heavily restored tooth is highly characteristic. The periodontal ligament space is typically continuous with the apical radiolucency. The cyst may also be located on the lateral **(inflammatory lateral periodontal cyst)** aspect of the root in association with a lateral canal. It is not possible to distinguish the three types of apical periodontitis radiographically.

Histopathologic Findings

A lumen filled with necrotic cellular debris is surrounded by nonkeratinized stratified squamous epithelium. The epithelium exhibits reactive proliferation (irregularly acanthotic rete ridges but no evidence of dysplasia) in response to the inflammatory cell infiltrate in the connective tissue capsule. The inflammatory cells usually include lymphocytes, plasma cells, foamy histiocytes, neutrophils, and foreign body giant cells surrounding cholesterol clefts (Figs. 3–1 to 3–3). **Residual radicular cysts** frequently have thin, nonkeratinized stratified squamous epithelial linings with minimal or no inflammatory cell infiltrate, presumably because the cause (necrotic pulp tissue) has long since been removed.

Hyaline (Rushton) bodies are sometimes seen within the epithelium of radicular cysts (and less frequently in dentigerous and odontogenic keratocysts) (Chen et al, 1981).

Portions of the epithelial lining are often destroyed by the inflammatory cells and replaced by inflamed granulation tissue (periapical granuloma). The pathologic diagnosis in such cases is based on the predominant form of apical periodontitis observed histologically.

Treatment

Treatment is predicated on removal of the cause (i.e., the necrotic pulp) by means of conservative endodontic therapy. Apicoectomy, apical curettage, and root-end amalgam are performed if conservative endodontic therapy fails. Dental extraction and curettage of the socket are also effective.

Loss of pulp vitality must be documented prior to and during endodontic therapy. Should vital pulp tissue be found in a tooth with presumed apical periodontitis, further work-up, including biopsy by means of apical curettage, is immediately required. Whenever soft tissue is excised, histopathologic confirmation of the preoperative diagnosis is advisable professionally and medicolegally (Lovas and Loyens, 1985).

Radicular cysts do not give rise to odontogenic tumors, and their malignant potential is extremely low.

References

Chen, S.-Y., Fantasia, J.E., and Miller, A.S.: Hyaline bodies in the connective tissue wall of odontogenic cysts. J. Oral Pathol., 10:147–157, 1981.
Lovas, J.G.L., and Loyens, S.: The dentist, the biopsy, and the law. J. Can. Dent. Assoc., 51:29–31, 1985.

DENTIGEROUS CYST
(Follicular Cyst)

Although it is the most common developmental odontogenic cyst, the dentigerous cyst nevertheless has a low incidence—on the order of 0.0002 to 0.001% (Shear and Singh, 1978). The stimulus that induces reduced enamel epithelium (of the dental follicle) around the crown of an embedded or impacted tooth to proliferate and form a cyst is unknown. Cyst formation begins after the crown is fully formed but before root formation has started.

The dentigerous cyst is a specific disease entity. **The word dentigerous should therefore no longer be used in a nonspecific, descriptive fashion to denote a pericoronal relationship.**

Dentigerous cysts have considerable growth potential, sometimes resulting in replacement of large portions of normal jawbone by the lesion. Coexistence with clinically more significant lesions such as ameloblastoma and carcinoma is rare. The combined incidence of all types of ameloblastoma is only 0.00025 to 0.00003% (Shear and Singh, 1978), and less than 5% of ameloblastomas are associated with dentigerous cysts (Shteyer et al, 1978). It is debatable whether dentigerous cysts actually "give rise to" ameloblastoma, squamous cell carcinoma, or mucoepidermoid carcinoma. There is, however, general agreement that the malignant potential of dentigerous cysts is extremely low (Stephens et al, 1989).

Clinical Features

Dentigerous cysts are usually asymptomatic unless they are inflamed, infected, or associated with a pathologic fracture. Cortical expansion and erosion can occur with large cysts, sometimes giving the overlying mucosa a bluish appearance. Paresthesia, in the absence of secondary infection, is uncommon. Permanent teeth are much more frequently involved than deciduous teeth. Third molars and canines are most often affected. The cyst is fluid-filled and situated pericoronally.

Radiographic Appearance

Dentigerous cysts usually appear as well-defined, unilocular or multilocular, pericoronal radiolucencies with hyperostotic borders around the crowns of embedded or impacted teeth (especially third molars and maxillary canines) and, much less frequently, in association with odontomas. The radiolucency typically starts at the cervical line. The associated tooth may be displaced, and adjacent roots may be resorbed. However, unlike odontogenic keratocysts or ameloblastomas, which frequently expand the mandible, dentigerous cysts remodel the cancellous portion of the mandible but spare the cortical bone. Nevertheless, they often extend well up into the ramus without concurrent expansion.

There is no scientific basis for assuming that a pericoronal radiolucency of 2.5 mm or greater represents a dentigerous cyst although this figure is often quoted (Stephens et al, 1989). Many small pericoronal radiolucencies represent normal or hyperplastic dental follicles, the size of which has been artifactually magnified on the panoramic radiograph. Little is known about the relationship between hyperplastic dental follicles (dental follicles exhibiting a thickened, glycosaminoglycan-rich, connective tissue capsule) and dentigerous cysts.

In general, the larger the pericoronal radiolucency, the more likely the existence of a pathologic condition, and the most common of these conditions is the dentigerous cyst.

Histopathologic Findings

A uniformly thin layer of nonkeratinized (infrequently orthokeratinized) stratified squamous epithelium with occasional areas of mucous cell prosoplasia lines the fibrous connective tissue capsule (Figs. 3–4 and 3–5).

Evidence of inflammation is usually minimal or absent. When there is inflammation, it is secondary to pericoronitis or periodontitis of an adjacent erupted tooth. An inflamed dentigerous cyst can be histologically indistinguishable from a radicular cysts.

Treatment

An embedded or impacted tooth associated with a pericoronal radiolucent lesion should be extracted, and the pericoronal soft tissue should be thoroughly curetted and submitted for histopathologic examination.

Eruption Cyst

An eruption cyst is a fairly common, bluish, soft tissue swelling that is located pericoronal to an erupting deciduous or permanent tooth. For unknown reasons, transudate (or blood, in which case the lesion is called an **eruption hematoma**) accumulates beneath the dental follicle. The lesion usually ruptures spontaneously, but if eruption is delayed, conservative excision of the soft tissue should be performed.

References

Shear, M., and Singh, S.: Age-standardized incidence rates of ameloblastoma and dentigerous cyst on the Witwaterstrand, South Africa, community. Dent. Oral Epidemiol., 6:195–199, 1978.

Shteyer, A., Lustman, J., and Lewin-Epstein, J.: The mural ameloblastoma: A review of the literature. J. Oral Surg., 36:866–872, 1978.

Stephens, R.G., Kogon, S.L., and Reid, J.A.: The unerupted or impacted third molar: A critical appraisal of its pathologic potential. J. Can. Dent. Assoc., 55:201–207, 1989.

ODONTOGENIC KERATOCYST
(OKC, "Primordial Cyst")

This is a relatively uncommon developmental cyst that arises from rests of dental lamina owing to unknown stimuli. After tooth germs are formed, the dental lamina is fragmented into numerous epithelial islands (rests of Serres) in both the jawbone and the overlying alveolar ridge mucosa. The OKC is clinically important because of its destructive potential, high recurrence rate following curettage, and occasional association with the basal cell nevus syndrome.

At one time, all odontogenic cysts that exhibited some form of keratinization were called keratocysts. We now know that although a number of odontogenic and nonodontogenic cysts exhibit varying degrees and types of keratinization, only lesions that satisfy specific histologic criteria (see later under Histopathologic Findings) have the natural history and prognosis of the OKC. Keratinization per se in a cyst suggests neither an increased recurrence rate nor an increased malignant potential (Anneroth and Hansen, 1982).

Clinical Features

The posterior mandible is the most common site of an OKC, often in a pericoronal relationship with impacted or embedded third molars. The peak incidence occurs in the second and third decades. In the absence of secondary inflammation/infection or pathologic fracture, OKCs are asymptomatic. Large lesions can expand and erode cortical bone.

Aspiration of the luminal contents yields thick, semisolid material with silvery flecks (desquamated keratin) and a low soluble protein content (Toller, 1972; Kramer and Toller, 1973). Such an aspirate is suggestive but not diagnostic of an OKC.

At surgery, OKCs are described as being "cigarette paper thin." The thinness of the walls, the difficulty in curetting multilocular lesions, the weak bond between the epithelium and the connective tissue capsule, and the presence of daughter cysts are all factors contributing to a high recurrence rate. It is also feasible that new OKCs can arise from other rests of dental lamina following surgery. One theory suggests that OKCs recur because they actually originate from alveolar mucosal epithelium. To avoid recurrence, it is recommended that the mucosa overlying the OKC be excised along with the lesion itself (Stoelinga and Peters, 1973).

An increased epithelial turnover rate (Toller, 1972) has been demonstrated in OKCs, suggesting that their growth may be more similar to that of neoplasms than that of cysts. The malignant potential of OKCs is extremely low.

Occurrence of an OKC at an early age, multifocality, and a family history of OKCs are suggestive of the basal cell nevus syndrome (see Chapter 12). This disorder comprises multiple odontogenic keratocysts and is also called the Gorlin-Goltz syndrome or the nevoid basal cell carcinoma syndrome. Also characteristic of the disorder are bifid ribs, calcified falx cerebri, and skin lesions including multiple basal cell carcinomas, multiple milia, and keratotic pitting of the palms of the hands (palmar) and soles of the feet (plantar).

Radiographic Appearance

OKCs are cyst-like but otherwise have no distinctive radiographic features. They can arise anywhere there are rests of dental lamina (i.e., in alveolar bone). They can be unilocular or (especially larger lesions) multilocular and may be either associated with teeth in a pericoronal, interradicular, or periapical relationship or unrelated to teeth ("primordial"). Although OKCs often cause expansion of bone, they rarely perforate the cortex. They can resorb roots and displace teeth. Some authors believe that OKCs may be less radiolucent radiographically because some lesions produce keratin, which attenuates more x-ray photons and thus becomes diffusely radiopaque. The borders of OKCs are well defined and sclerotic and frequently appear thinned.

Histopathologic Findings

The histology of OKCs is pathognomonic. Surrounding a lumen containing parakeratin squames is a "corrugated" (wavy), parakeratinized, stratified squamous epithelium of even thickness (just six to eight cells thick). The basal epithelial cells are cuboidal to columnar with hyperchromatic, palisaded (evenly aligned) nuclei. Usually the epithelial–connective tissue junction is flat, with areas of separation suggestive of weak adherence. Occasionally the epithelial lining exhibits "budding" downgrowth, which can be mistaken for dysplasia or ameloblastoma. There can be additional tiny "daughter cysts" in the adjacent connective tissue (Figs. 3–6 to 3–9). The connective tissue wall, like the epithelium, is very thin. Secondary inflammation can obscure the diagnostic features.

An uncommon **orthokeratinized variant** of the OKC has been reported (Wright, 1981). It tends to be unilocular, most often in a pericoronal relationship to impacted mandibular third molars, is not associated with the basal cell nevus syndrome, is of limited growth potential, and infrequently recurs after curettage.

Text continued on page 41

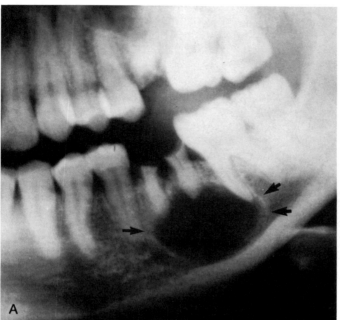

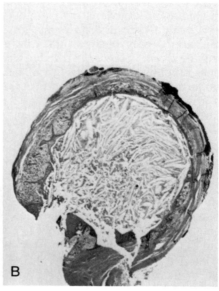

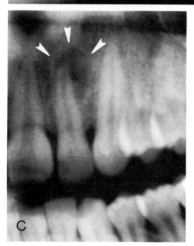

Figure 3–1. *A,* This well-defined unilocular radiolucency, apical to the grossly carious root tips of the lower first permanent molar, represents a radicular cyst. Hyperostotic borders may be seen along the anterior and posterior aspects of the lesion *(arrows). B,* Radicular cyst. Low-power view of an almost intact cyst. *C,* A radicular cyst about the apex of a permanent maxillary lateral incisor. Note the areas of cortication *(arrowheads)* surrounding the uniform radiolucency.

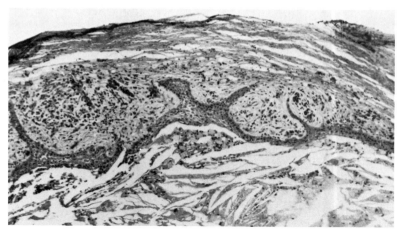

Figure 3–2. Radicular cyst. Higher-power view of a portion of the cyst seen in Figure 3–1B. From top to bottom are seen the condensed fibrous connective tissue wall, exhibiting an inflammatory cell infiltrate immediately above the lining epithelium; the nonkeratinized stratified squamous epithelium, showing a mild, reactive proliferation secondary to the inflammation; and, at bottom, the necrotic epithelial cell debris within the lumen.

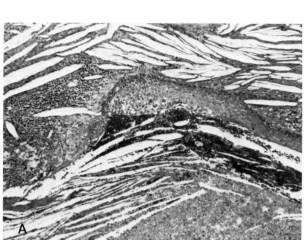

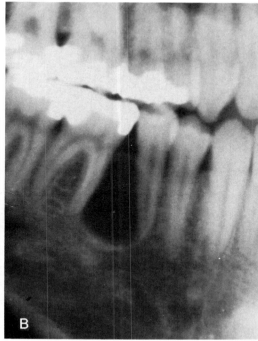

Figure 3–3. *A,* Radicular cyst with cholesterol granuloma. High-power view of another area of the same cyst, exhibiting cholesterol clefts (pointy, clear spaces at top) in the cyst wall. Long-standing cellular necrosis results in accumulation of membrane lipids. These are thought to form crystalline deposits that elicit a granulomatous inflammatory reaction. Cholesterol granulomas are also found in periapical granulomas. *B,* A possible inflammatory lateral periodontal cyst. Note the well-defined cortical outline and "hydraulic" appearance of the radiolucency.

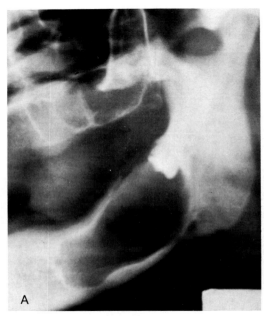

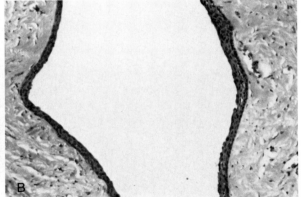

Figure 3–4. *A,* A dentigerous cyst about the crown of an unerupted and displaced lower third molar. Note the well-defined cortical outline and the remodeling of the inferior cortical border. Despite the large size, there is little expansion except perhaps along the superior aspect. *B,* Dentigerous cyst. Medium-power view of a cyst with a densely collagenized wall with no evidence of inflammation. The epithelial lining is nonkeratinized and has a very uniform thickness.

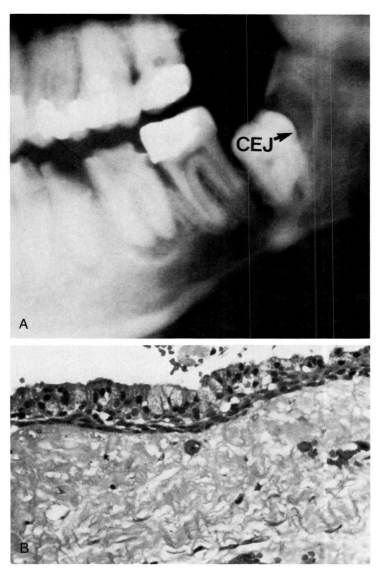

Figure 3–5. *A,* A dentigerous cyst about an impacted third molar. Note that the cystic change is lateral to the coronal portion of the tooth. The attachment of the cortical outline of the cyst below the cementoenamel junction *(arrow)* suggests that there has been cystic degeneration of the follicle and that the size and location are not normal. *B,* Dentigerous cyst with mucous cells. High-power view of the cyst lining, exhibiting mucous cell prosoplasia, an uncommon finding. Such mucous cells are considered to be a possible source of origin for the rare, central mucoepidermoid carcinoma.

Illustration continued on following page

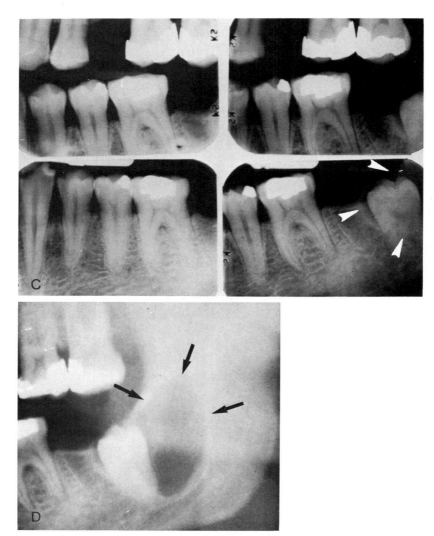

Figure 3–5 *Continued C,* This figure shows two posterior bitewing and two posterior periapical films. The only suggestion of an abnormality appears on the lower molar periapically around the crown of the impacted third molar *(arrowheads).* (Courtesy of Dr. B. Glass, University of Texas, San Antonio.) *D,* Dentigerous cyst about crown of impacted third molar. This panoramic film reveals the cystic lesion *(arrows).* (Courtesy of Dr. B. Glass, University of Texas, San Antonio.)

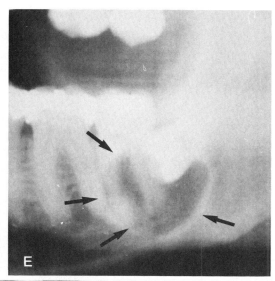

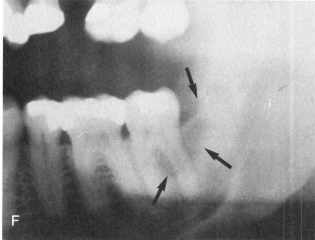

Figure 3–5 *Continued E*, Well-defined radiolucent lesion with corticated or hyperostotic border *(arrows)*. This pericoronal radiolucency is consistent with a dentigerous cyst. *F*, This film shows the healed surgical site *(arrows)* after the removal of the impacted tooth and dentigerous cyst seen in *C*.

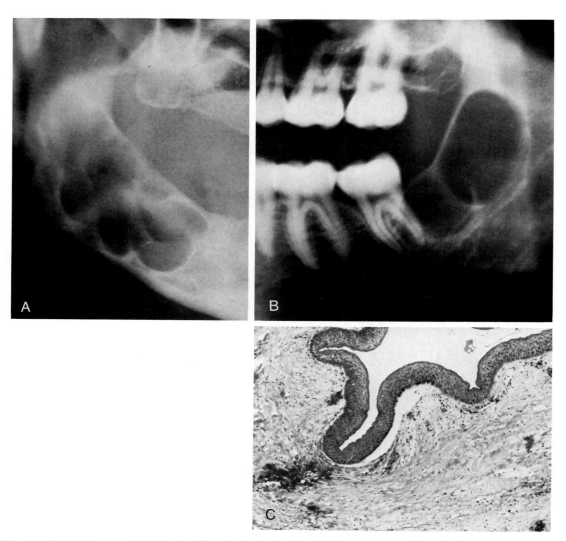

Figure 3–6. *A,* A large, well-defined multilocular lesion in the right posterior mandible. There is the suggestion of remodeling of the external oblique ridge and some expansion along the superior aspect. This was an odontogenic keratocyst. *B,* A large, well-defined multilocular radiolucency in the posterior left mandible. Note the thinning and expansion of the ascending ramus. Two large locules are apparent in this odontogenic keratocyst. (Courtesy of Dr. C. Tomich, Indiana University School of Dentistry, Indianapolis, Indiana.) *C,* Odontogenic keratocyst. Medium-power view of a cyst with a uniform thickness of epithelial lining. The split (seen in the center of the picture) demonstrates the fragile epithelial–connective tissue adherence.

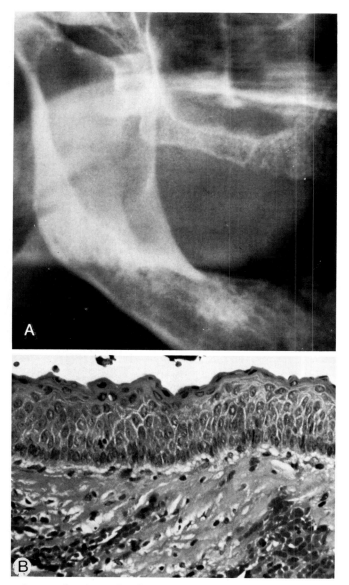

Figure 3–7. *A,* This large, almost unilocular, well-defined radiolucency extends from the external oblique ridge up to the condyle and sigmoid notch area. Some extension is probable into the coronoid process as well. The central portion of this lesion is gray rather than totally radiolucent. Although part of this appearance may be due to soft tissue shadows from the panoramic technique, it may also be due to the presence of keratin within the odontogenic keratocyst. *B,* Odontogenic keratocyst. High-power view of the "corrugated" parakeratin surface. The stratified squamous epithelial lining is uniformly six to eight cell layers thick, and the nuclei of the basal cells are hyperchromatic (more densely staining) and palisaded.

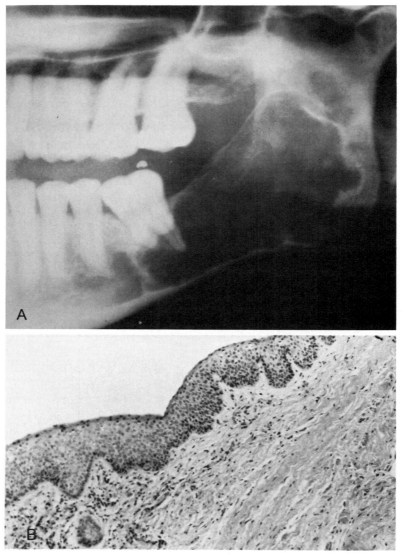

Figure 3–8. *A,* This large, well-defined expansile radiolucency shows areas of "budding" or outpouching along the inferior aspect. These may be representative of the "daughter cysts" that are present in an odontogenic keratocyst. The posterior aspect of this lesion shows the hyperostotic corticated borders. The inferior border of the mandible has been remodeled and appears thin. *B,* "Budding" in the lining of an odontogenic keratocyst. High-power view of this unusual pattern of rete ridge formation, sometimes seen in odontogenic keratocysts. This phenomenon should not be interpreted as histologic evidence of precancer (epithelial dysplasia). A small daughter cyst is visible at bottom left.

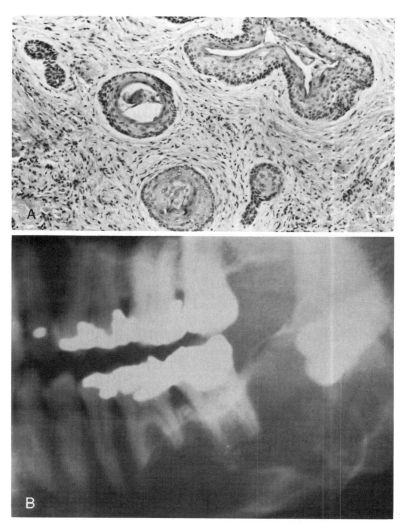

Figure 3–9. *A,* Daughter cysts in an odontogenic keratocyst. Medium-power view of numerous smaller odontogenic keratocysts ("daughters") within the connective tissue wall of a large odontogenic keratocyst. *B,* This large, multilocular expansile radiolucency appears to be in a pericoronal position with respect to the impacted third molar. The second most common radiographic presentation for an odontogenic keratocyst is one of a pericoronal radiolucency.

Illustration continued on following page

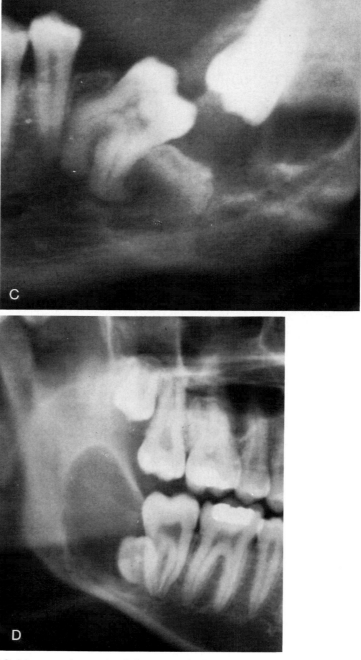

Figure 3–9 *Continued C,* A large, pericoronal radiolucent lesion associated with the impaction of two permanent molars. This is another odontogenic keratocyst that appears somewhat like a pericoronal lesion (Courtesy of Dr. C. Tomich, Indiana University School of Dentistry, Indianapolis, Indiana.) *D,* A unilocular, pericoronal radiolucency in the posterior mandible. This is an odontogenic keratocyst. (Courtesy of Dr. C. Tomich, Indiana University School of Dentistry, Indianapolis, Indiana.)

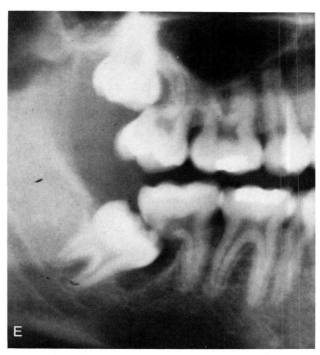

Figure 3–9 *Continued E,* A small, well-defined pericoronal radiolucency associated with an impacted third molar. Note the complete resorption of the distal root of the second permanent molar. A lesion such as an ameloblastoma or an odontogenic keratocyst may have the potential to cause such resorption.

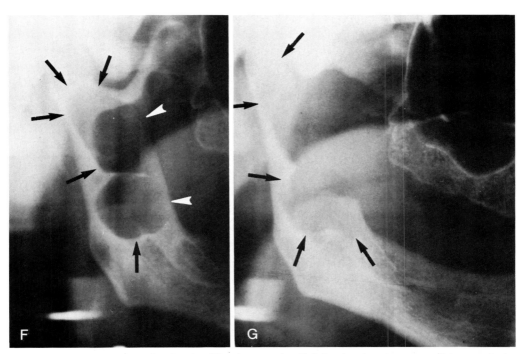

Figure 3–9 *Continued F,* A large, well-defined multilocular lesion *(arrows* and *arrowheads)* in the posterior ramus consistent with an odontogenic keratocyst. *G,* A somewhat ill-defined and moth-eaten radiolucency in the same location of the mandible as the lesion seen in *F* represents an occurrence of an odontogenic keratocyst after 2 years.
Illustration continued on following page

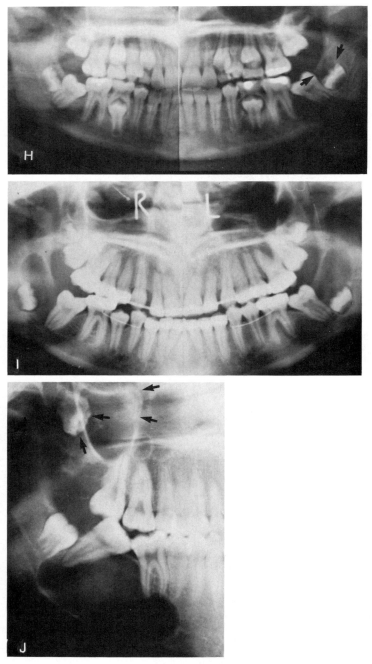

Figure 3–9 *Continued H,* A small, pericoronal radiolucency around the developing third molar in the patient's left quadrant (*arrows*). In *I* two large, well-defined pericoronal radiolucencies are associated with the developing third molars. These figures represent odontogenic keratocysts in a patient with nevoid basal cell carcinoma syndrome. There is a difference of 18 months between the films seen in *H* and *I. I,* An odontogenic keratocyst with a pericoronal radiographic presentation. *J,* This is also a film in a patient with the nevoid basal cell carcinoma syndrome. One lesion is very apparent in the posterior mandible as a large, well-defined expansile unilocular radiolucency. The second lesion is less apparent and is situated in the right maxillary sinus associated with an impacted developing third molar (*arrows*).

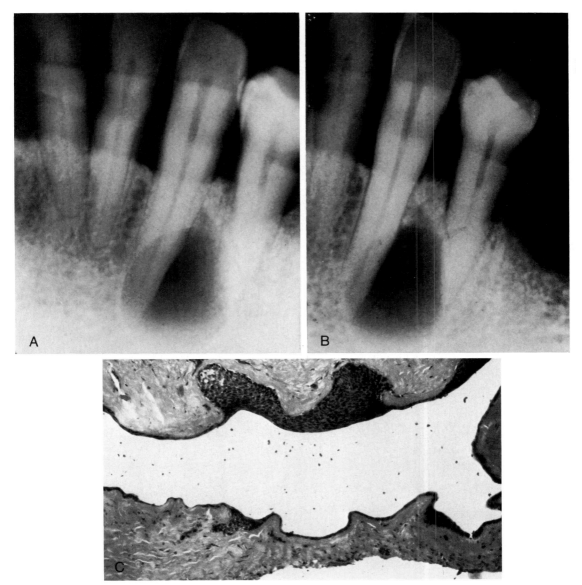

Figure 3–10. *A*, A unilocular, well-defined radiolucency between the roots of the canine and the first premolar in the left mandibular arch. Both teeth tested vital. *B*, The radiolucency seen in *A* is still situated in between the roots of the canine and the first premolar. This was found to be a lateral periodontal cyst. *C*, Developmental lateral periodontal cyst. Medium-power view of a cyst with a thin, nonkeratinized epithelial lining, exhibiting characteristic focal areas of thickening "plaques."

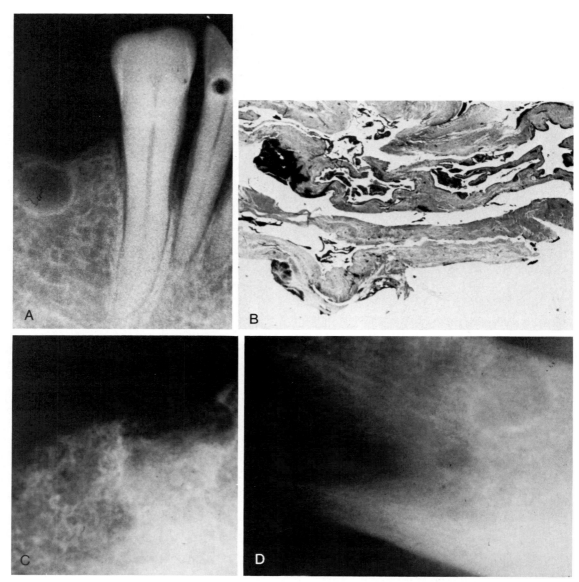

Figure 3–11. *A,* This small, well-defined, unilocular, corticated lesion was proved histopathologically to be a botryoid cyst. Notice that it is not multilocular. *B,* Botryoid variant of the developmental lateral periodontal cyst. Low-power view, in cross section, of a large, radiographically multilocular cyst. The apparently multiple luminal spaces are actually interconnected. *C,* Periapical radiograph of a small botryoid cyst with a suggestion of multilocularity. *D,* Panoramic view of the lesion seen in *C.* This was a botryoid cyst in a 49-year-old man.

Treatment

Cyst-like jaw lesions are generally treated by curettage, definitive diagnosis being made postoperatively by a pathologist. The recurrence rate following curettage of OKCs is 27%, and the mean time elapsed between treatment and first recurrence is 5 years (Ahlfors et al, 1984). Large size, multilocularity, multifocality, thinness of the cyst, association with the basal cell nevus syndrome, and daughter cyst formation have all been suspected to increase the probability of recurrence, but the inherent proliferative capacity of the epithelial lining may be the most significant factor (Ahlfors et al, 1984). Preoperative biopsy, marginal resection with a rim of uninvolved bone, and possibly excision of the overlying alveolar mucosa have been recommended to decrease the probability of recurrence (Stoelinga and Peters, 1973; Ahlfors et al, 1984).

References

Ahlfors, E., Larsson, A., and Sjögren, S.: The odontogenic keratocyst: A benign tumor? J. Oral Maxillofac. Surg., 42:10–19, 1984.

Anneroth, G., and Hansen, L.S.: Variations in keratinizing odontogenic cysts and tumors. Oral Surg. Oral Med. Oral Pathol., 54:530–546, 1982.

Kramer, I.R.H., and Toller, P.A.: The use of exfoliative cytology and protein estimations in preoperative diagnosis of odontogenic keratocysts. Int. J. Oral Surg., 2:143–151, 1973.

Stoelinga, P.J.W., and Peters, J.H.: A note on the origin of keratocysts of the jaws. Int. J. Oral Surg., 2:37–44, 1973.

Toller, P.A.: Newer concepts of odontogenic cysts. Int. J. Oral Surg., 1:3–16, 1972.

Wright, J.M.: The odontogenic keratocyst: Orthokeratinized variant. Oral Surg. Oral Med. Oral Pathol., 51:609–618, 1981.

DEVELOPMENTAL LATERAL PERIODONTAL CYST

Clinical Features

As the name suggests, this is a developmental cyst arising from rests of dental lamina (Wysocki et al, 1980). Unlike with the inflammatory lateral periodontal cyst, there is no causal relationship between this lesion and pulpal necrosis. The mandibular premolar and maxillary lateral incisor areas are most frequently involved. These lesions are asymptomatic, have a limited growth potential (seldom exceeding 1 cm in diameter), and do not tend to recur following curettage.

The **botryoid odontogenic cyst** appears to be simply a larger, multilocular variant of the developmental lateral periodontal cyst.

Radiographic Appearance

The developmental lateral periodontal cyst usually presents as a small, well-defined, circular, interradicular, unilocular (multilocular for the botryoid variant) radiolucency with hyperostotic borders. Typically, it is found between the roots of mandibular premolars or between a maxillary canine and a lateral incisor.

Histopathologic Findings

The lumen of developmental lateral periodontal cysts is lined by a thin layer of nonkeratinized stratified squamous epithelium, often exhibiting focal areas of clear cells. Inflammatory cells are seldom seen (Figs. 3–10 and 3–11).

Treatment

Treatment of the developmental lateral periodontal cyst consists of conservative curettage, but because these lesions are often very close to the mental foramen, there is a risk of temporary if not permanent paresthesia. Although this lesion has a limited growth potential, without a biopsy a definitive diagnosis cannot be made. The risk-benefit ratio must therefore be carefully considered prior to treatment.

Reference

Wysocki, G.P., Brannon, R.B., Gardner, D.G., and Sapp, P.: Histogenesis of the lateral periodontal cyst and the gingival cyst of the adult. Oral Surg. Oral Med. Oral Pathol. 50:327–334, 1980.

NONODONTOGENIC CYSTS

INCISIVE CANAL CYST
(Nasopalatine Duct Cyst)

This is a developmental nonodontogenic cyst arising from vestigial bilateral oronasal ducts or vomeronasal organs of Jacobson (Stam et al, 1979) joining the floor of the nose with the midline of the anterior hard palate. Although inflammation and mild symptoms are common features of these lesions, the stimulus for cyst formation is unknown. The lesion may be completely within bone, completely within soft tissue (then called a **cyst of the incisive papilla**), or partially in both.

Clinical Features

The anterior palate is sometimes swollen, tender, or even painful, and patients sometimes complain about a salty-tasting fluid exudate. Occasionally these lesions are discovered when drainage of a straw-colored fluid occurs immediately following injection of local anesthetic into the incisive canal. There is no direct relationship between this lesion and pulpal necrosis of the maxillary central incisors.

Radiographic Appearance

A well-circumscribed, circular, oval, or heart-shaped radiolucency with hyperostotic borders that is greater than 6 mm across in the area of the incisive foramen is typical. Two radiographs taken at different angles help to differentiate this lesion from apical periodontitis of the maxillary central incisors. The heart shape is an "apparent" shape caused by using a steep vertical angulation of the x-ray tube, which superimposes the anterior nasal spine over the superior portion of the cyst.

Histopathologic Findings

These cysts are lined by a thin, nonkeratinized layer of stratified squamous or respiratory epithelium of relatively uniform thickness. The connective tissue wall often contains inflammatory cells as well as fairly large neurovascular bundles (incisive nerves and vessels) (Figs. 3–12 and 3–13). Lobules of minor salivary glands and hamartomatous cartilaginous rests are also seen occasionally.

Treatment

These lesions are removed by curettage, using a palatal approach. Recurrence is rare.

Reference

Stam, F.C., van der Waal, I., and van der Kwast, W.A.M.: Pigment in the lining of nasopalatine duct cysts: Report of two cases. J. Oral Pathol., 8:170–175, 1979.

NASOLABIAL CYST
(Nasoalveolar Cyst)

This is a rare developmental nonodontogenic cyst that occurs in the soft tissues between the nose and the upper lip. It is thought to arise from epithelium of the nasolacrimal or nasopalatine duct.

Clinical Features

A soft, mobile, soft tissue mass that obliterates the nasolabial fold extraorally and the labial vestibule intraorally is the typical clinical finding.

Radiographic Appearance

Pressure from this soft tissue cyst may cause a "cupped-out" resorption of the anterior maxilla.

Histopathologic Findings

The cyst lining is composed of one or more pseudostratified columnar, cuboidal, or stratified squamous epithelia. The connective tissue is frequently inflamed and sometimes hyalinized (Fig. 3–14).

Treatment

The lesion is excised through an intraoral approach. Recurrence is rare.

CONTROVERSIAL CYSTS

"Fissural" cysts were formerly thought to arise from entrapment of surface epithelium along lines of fusion of embryonic processes. The fissural epithelial entrapment theory, however, is (with one exception: see later under Median Palatal Cyst) no longer accepted (Christ, 1970). Lesions previously considered to be fissural include globulomaxillary, median mandibular, median palatal, and median alveolar cysts.

PRIMORDIAL CYST

This lesion was thought to arise instead of a tooth owing to degeneration of epithelium of the enamel organ before hard tissue formation had started. The histology was usually that of an odontogenic keratocyst. Such a developmental concept depended on finding a cyst in place of a missing tooth. Because "missing" supernumerary and third molar teeth are very common, when a cyst with the histologic features of an odontogenic keratocyst is found in the position of such a missing tooth, it is now simply diagnosed as an OKC (Fig. 3–15).

GLOBULOMAXILLARY CYST

An inverted pear-shaped radiolucent lesion causing divergence of the roots of a maxillary cuspid and lateral incisor was previously considered to represent a fissural cyst—the "globulomaxillary cyst." Most (25 of 37) of the lesions with these radiographic features are in fact examples of apical periodontitis, and the rest represent various other specific defined entities (Wysocki, 1981). Accordingly, continued use of the term is inappropriate (Fig. 3–16).

MEDIAN MANDIBULAR CYST

This is a questionable, rare entity defined as a noninflammatory, nonkeratinizing epithelial cyst in the midline of the mandible, with no direct contact with overlying vital teeth (Main, 1985).

MEDIAN PALATAL CYST
(Midpalatal Cyst of Infants)

This lesion is rare and controversial. Most authors consider it to represent a posteriorly displaced nasopalatine duct cyst or cyst of the incisive papilla (Gardner et al, 1978). In the jaws, the only site at which true fusion of embryologic processes occurs is the midline of the palate (Ten Cate, 1980). Therefore, if this lesion exists as a distinct entity, it represents the only example of a true fissural developmental cyst of the jaws (Main, 1985). Figure 3–17 shows an example of a median palatal cyst.

MEDIAN ALVEOLAR CYST

This rare lesion was once thought to be a "primordial cyst" arising from a mesiodens. It often had the histologic features of an odontogenic keratocyst. Like other cysts with histologic features of an odontogenic keratocyst regardless of site or relationship to teeth, or lack thereof, it is now simply called an odontogenic keratocyst.

Note. Calcifying odontogenic cysts are classified as odontogenic tumors (Main, 1985) (see Chapter 4).

References

Christ, T.F.: The globulomaxillary cyst: An embryologic misconception. Oral Surg. Oral Med. Oral Pathol., 30:515–526, 1970.

Gardner, D.G., Sapp, J.P., and Wysocki, G.P.: Odontogenic and "fissural" cysts of the jaws. Pathol. Annu., 13(I):177–200, 1978.

Main, D.M.G.: Epithelial cysts of the jaws: 10 years of the WHO classification. J. Oral Pathol., 14:1–7, 1985.

Ten Cate, A.R.: Oral Histology: Development, Structure, and Function. St. Louis: C.V. Mosby, 1980, p. 22.

Wysocki, G.P.: The differential diagnosis of globulomaxillary radiolucencies. Oral Surg. Oral Med. Oral Pathol., 51:281–286, 1981.

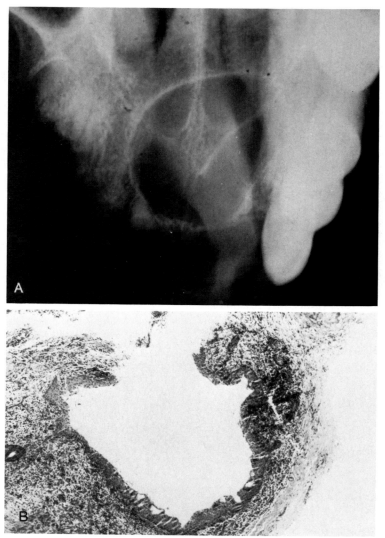

Figure 3–12. *A,* A large, well-defined unilocular lesion with hyperostotic borders in the midline of the maxilla consistent with an incisive canal cyst. *B,* Incisive canal cyst. Medium-power view of a large cyst, lined by respi- ratory epithelium. The epithelial lining retains a relatively uniform thickness despite the marked inflammatory cell infiltrate commonly seen in these cysts.

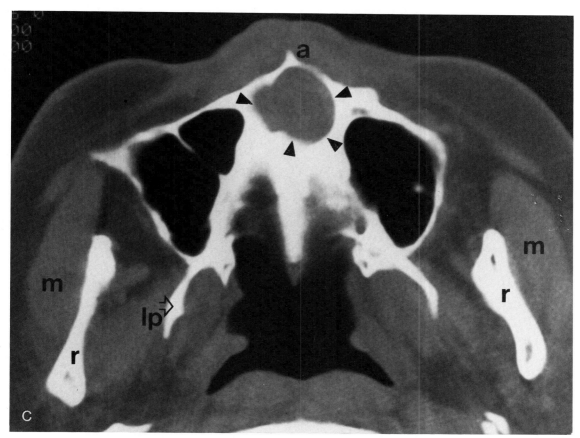

Figure 3–12 *Continued C,* A CT image of an incisive canal cyst (*arrowheads*). a = anterior nasal spine; r = ramus of mandible; lp = lateral pterygoid plate; m = masseter muscle (soft tissue). (From Pollei S, Harnsberger HR: The radiologic evaluation of the sinonasal region. Postgrad Radiol 9[4]: 242, 1989.)

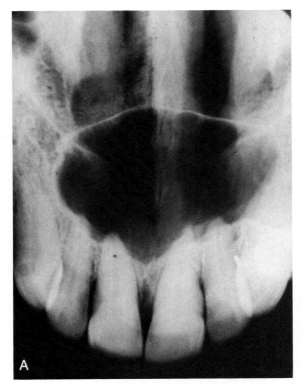

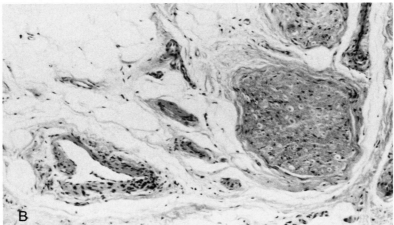

Figure 3–13. *A,* An incisive canal (nasopalatine duct) cyst. *B,* Large blood vessels and peripheral nerves near an incisive canal cyst. Characteristic histologic findings adjacent to these cysts are branches of the nasopalatine arteries, veins, and nerves.

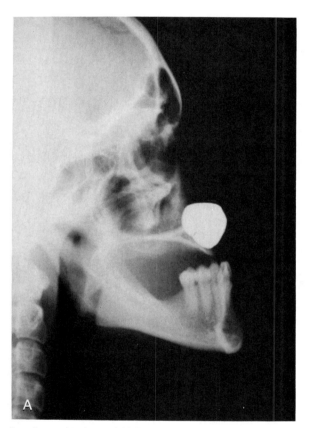

Figure 3–14. *A,* Lateral skull radiograph of nasolabial cyst with contrast medium injected into the area to delineate the lesion. (Courtesy of Dr. R. Langlais, University of Texas, San Antonio.)

Illustration continued on following page

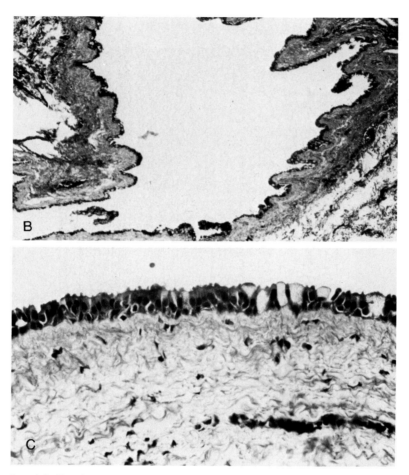

Figure 3–14 *Continued B,* Nasolabial cyst. Low-power view of a cyst lined by a thin, pseudostratified columnar epithelium. The underlying connective tissue wall appears hyalinized (amorphous, glassy, pink). *C,* Nasolabial cyst. High-power view of the cyst lining exhibiting a uniformly thin layer of pseudostratified columnar epithelium and occasional mucous ("goblet") cells.

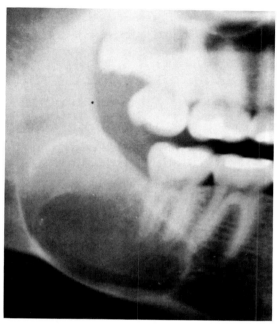

Figure 3–15. A large, expansile, well-defined radiolucency in the posterior mandible. The lesion has hyperostotic borders but is not resorbing adjacent teeth. It occurs in a region of the usual development of the lower third molar. This was termed a primordial cyst. (Courtesy of Dr. C. Tomich, Indiana University School of Dentistry, Indianapolis, Indiana.)

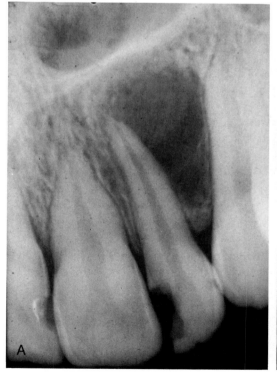

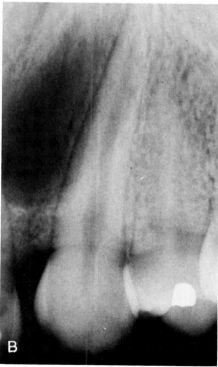

Figure 3–16. *A,* Such large, inverted, pear-shaped radiolucencies in the past have been called globulomaxillary cysts. This lesion is related to the nonvital pulp of the carious lateral incisor. *B,* This classic globulomaxillary cyst, more appropriately termed a globulomaxillary radiolucency, is actually just a periapical cyst located in the lateral fossa. The etiology for the lesion is simply dental caries.

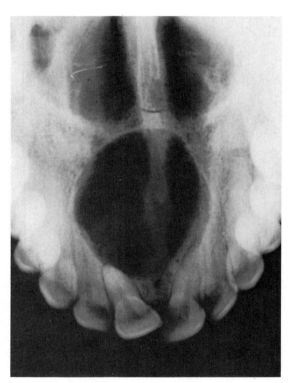

Figure 3–17. Large, expansile median palatal cyst displacing apices of maxillary central incisors.

ODONTOGENIC TUMORS

G. KAUGARS

AMELOBLASTOMA

CALCIFYING EPITHELIAL ODONTOGENIC TUMOR

SQUAMOUS ODONTOGENIC TUMOR

ADENOMATOID ODONTOGENIC TUMOR

CENTRAL ODONTOGENIC FIBROMA

ODONTOGENIC MYXOMA

BENIGN CEMENTOBLASTOMA

AMELOBLASTIC FIBROMA

ODONTOMA

AMELOBLASTIC FIBRO-ODONTOMA

AMELOBLASTIC ODONTOMA

CALCIFYING ODONTOGENIC CYST

Odontogenic tumors are a diagnostic challenge because of their many clinical, radiographic, and histologic similarities, but at the same time they are characterized by a remarkable diversity. These seemingly paradoxical statements are related to the multiple tissues of origin of odontogenic tumors:

ECTODERMAL TISSUES

Dental lamina
Outer enamel epithelium
Stellate reticulum
Stratum intermedium
Inner enamel epithelium
Ameloblasts
Reduced enamel epithelium
Cervical loop
Hertwig's epithelial root sheath
Cell rests of Malassez
Surface epithelium

CONNECTIVE TISSUES

Dental papilla
Dental sac
Odontoblasts
Cementoblasts

You can see from this list that it is possible to have tumors that differ considerably from each other in histologic appearance but are still closely related. The nomenclature and classification of odontogenic tumors are controversial because of the many overlapping features and the relatively small numbers of reported cases. As larger series are published, it is anticipated that the relationships among these tumors will be clarified.

AMELOBLASTOMA

The ameloblastoma (Fig. 4–1 *A–U*) has received more attention than any other odontogenic tumor. The reason for this is not entirely clear but may be related to the fact that it was one of the first to be described and is relatively common compared with other odontogenic tumors. Initially, some other tumors that are similar in appearance were misdiagnosed as ameloblastoma, but subsequently these were identified as separate entities. This early confusion is understandable because the histologic appearance of many odontogenic tumors mimics various stages of tooth development.

Clinical Features

The reported mean age of patients is about 35 years, but this figure is meaningless because the wide age range indicates occurrence in every decade of life. Only about 12% of ameloblastomas occur in patients under the age of 20 years. A definite predilection (85%) for the mandible has been noted. Most (70%) of the mandibular lesions are located in the molar-ramus region, and likewise, maxillary lesions are more commonly associated (80%) with the molars or antrum. Ameloblastomas are uncommon (8.7%) between the canines. A key point to remember is that 58.4% of all ameloblastomas occur in the posterior mandible. Many patients (80%) present with expansion of the mandible as their chief complaint. The expansion is generally painless and can become quite large before prompting the patient to seek care.

Radiographic Appearance

Although ameloblastomas are traditionally thought of as being multilocular, one study showed that only 53% were either multilocular or "soap bubble" in form, whereas the re-mainder were unilocular. The intuitive notion that ameloblastomas begin as unilocular lesions and evolve into multilocular lesions is supported by the finding that the mean age for unilocular cases is 26.4 years, whereas it is 37.5 years for multilocular ones. Approximately 75% of ameloblastomas in patients under 20 years of age are unilocular. There are no pathognomonic radiographic features for an ameloblastoma because its appearance is similar to numerous other jaw lesions. One distinguishing feature is that an ameloblastoma does not produce radiopacities within the lesion. When a lesion is multilocular, the internal margins of bone are often thickened and curved, unlike those of a central giant cell granuloma, in which the margins frequently appear thinner or even "lacy" (Poyton, 1982).

The association between dentigerous cysts or impacted teeth and ameloblastomas is well accepted, and previously published surveys have documented this in 15.1 to 68.6% of cases. Stanley and Diehl (1965) showed that ameloblastomas arising in association with a dentigerous cyst or impacted tooth occur in patients with an average age at time of diagnosis of 21 years, and less than 5% occurred in patients over 40 years. The implication of this finding is that a dentigerous cyst loses some of its ameloblastic potential after the age of 40 years.

Histopathologic Findings

The "classic" appearance of ameloblastoma is that of numerous, well-defined islands of odontogenic epithelium that contain a central portion resembling stellate reticulum surrounded by columnar peripheral cells that exhibit palisading and polarization of the nuclei toward the center of the island. The associated fibrous connective tissue is normal. Vickers and Gorlin (1970) defined the early changes in ameloblastoma as hyperchromaticity of the basal cells, palisading and polarization of the basal cell nuclei, and cytoplasmic vacuolization of basilar cells.

It is common for an ameloblastoma to display more than one histologic pattern, but one type usually predominates. The five main histologic types are **follicular, plexiform, acanthomatous, granular cell,** and **basal cell**. However, this is an artificial distinction because there is histologic overlap, and little information is available to suggest that there is any clinical significance to this classification.

The granular cell ameloblastoma, which makes up only 5 to 11% of all cases, has probably received an undeserved reputation for being most likely to metastasize and to have a high recurrence rate. One study showed a recurrence rate of 73%, but of the four cases in this study that were adequately treated, none recurred. Other authors have not felt that its prognosis is worse than that of other types, and this conclusion seems reasonable because the reported aggressive granular cell ameloblastomas had extraordinary treatments.

The unicystic ameloblastoma has a better prognosis because proliferation is limited to the cystic epithelium and lumen. It is most likely to occur in young people (mean age, 18 years), is associated with a dentigerous cyst in most cases (86.4%), occurs in the mandible in almost all cases, and has a recurrence rate of only 9.4%. Because of the low recurrence rate, it has been suggested that these lesions be treated less aggressively than a typical ameloblastoma.

Ameloblastic carcinoma is the term used to designate carcinomatous change in a preexisting ameloblastoma. Some foci of typical ameloblastoma are usually found within the specimen. These rare tumors can be expected to behave like an intraosseous carcinoma.

Treatment

Surgery is the treatment of choice, but there is considerable debate about the efficacy of various techniques. There is little justification for the use of curettage because of the excessively high recurrence rate. Small and Waldron (1955) found an overall recurrence rate of 32% in the literature but noted a large disparity when comparing cases treated with curettage (46%) with those that were resected (13%). One interesting finding in another study was that the radiographic appearance had a significant effect on the prognosis. Multilocular ameloblastomas had a recurrence rate of 73%, but unilocular ones recurred in only 20% of cases. This observation may be attributable to the greater surgical problem encountered when dealing with a large multiloculated tumor. Although most recurrences are diagnosed within 5 years after the initial surgery, a large number (21%) recur after more than 5 years. Maxillary lesions are usually more aggressive and, not surprisingly, have a higher recurrence rate. In light of this potential for recurrence, prudent clinicians should perform periodic radiographic follow-up, at least annually, for 5 or more years following excision of the lesion. The treatment for mandibular unicystic lesions can be conservative because the ameloblastic proliferation is confined to the cystic epithelium.

One study examined the treatment of ameloblastomas in children and discovered a relatively high recurrence rate (43%) despite the fact that all eight cases were well-defined, unilocular radiolucencies. The reason for the recurrence rate is unclear but might be related to reluctance by the surgeon to perform an extensive procedure in a child. Another study found a much lower recurrence rate (15%) in cases diagnosed during the first two decades of life.

Radiation therapy is usually discouraged, but one series of ten cases showed promising results. These patients were treated with curative intent by using 45 Gy of radiation fractioned over 4 weeks. Multiple chemotherapeutic agents have been tried but with no success.

The metastatic potential of ameloblastomas is low, and metastasis has been reported to occur in less than 2% of all cases. Typically, the lesions that have metastasized have been large or have been subjected to multiple surgical procedures.

References

Atkinson, C.H., Harwood, A.R., and Cummings, E.J.: Ameloblastoma of the jaw: A reappraisal of the role of megavoltage irradiation. Cancer 53:869–873, 1984.

Buff, S.J., Chen, J.T.T., Ravin, C.C., and Moore, J.D.: Pulmonary metastasis from ameloblastoma of the mandible: Report of a case and review of the literature. J. Oral Surg., 38:374, 1980.

Carr, R.F., and Halperin, V.: Malignant ameloblastoma from 1953 to 1966: Review of the literature and report of a case. Oral Surg. Oral Med. Oral Pathol., 26:514–522, 1968.

Cranin, A.N., Bennett, J., Solomon, M., and Quarcoo, S.: Massive granular cell ameloblastoma with metastasis: Report of a case. J. Oral Maxillofac. Surg., 45:800–804, 1987.

Gardner, D.G.: Plexiform unicystic ameloblastoma: A diagnostic problem in dentigerous cysts. Cancer, 47:1358–1363, 1981.

Gardner, D.G., and Corio, R.L.: Plexiform unicystic ameloblastoma: A variant of ameloblastoma with a low-recurrence rate after enucleation. Cancer, 53:1730–1735, 1984.

Gardner, D.G., and Pecak, A.M.J.: The treatment of ameloblastoma based on pathologic and anatomic principles. Cancer, 46:2514–2519, 1980.

Hartman, K.S.: Granular-cell ameloblastoma: A survey of twenty cases from the Armed Forces Institute of Pathology. Oral Surg. Oral Med. Oral Pathol., 38:241–253, 1974.

Text continued on page 63

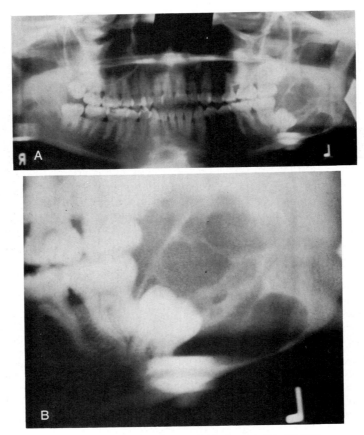

Figure 4–1. *A* and *B*, The ameloblastoma in this 29-year-old woman had a "classic" multilocular radiographic appearance and had prevented eruption of the wisdom tooth. (Courtesy of Dr. J. Julian, Virginia Beach, Virginia.)

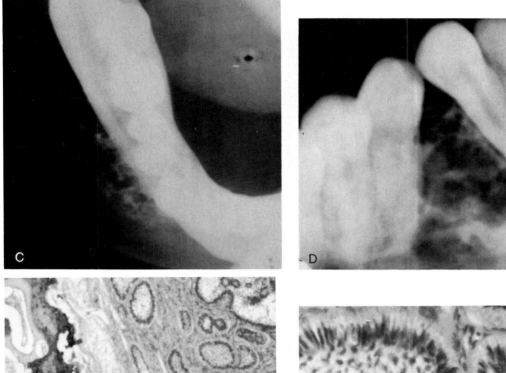

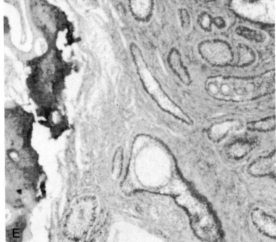

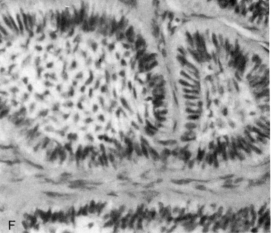

Figure 4–1 *Continued C* and *D,* A 22-year-old woman presented with buccal clinical expansion of the right mandible and some migration of the teeth. The occlusal radiograph shows a lesion that extends from the right canine to the right first molar and shows buccal expansion. The multilocular nature of the lesion is readily evident on the periapical radiograph. The multilocularity of this ameloblastoma indicates a potential for recurrence that is much higher than that for unilocular lesions. (Courtesy of Dr. P. Smith, Fairfax, Virginia.) *E,* Numerous ameloblastic islands of variable size are scattered throughout the specimen. Note that the fibrous connective tissue is normal. *F,* This high-power view demonstrates the characteristic histologic features of an ameloblastic island: palisading of the peripheral cells, polarization of the nuclei toward the center in the peripheral cells, and a stellate reticulum appearance of the cells in the central portion. Considerable variation from this classic pattern may be encountered because several different histologic types of ameloblastoma are recognized.

Illustration continued on following page

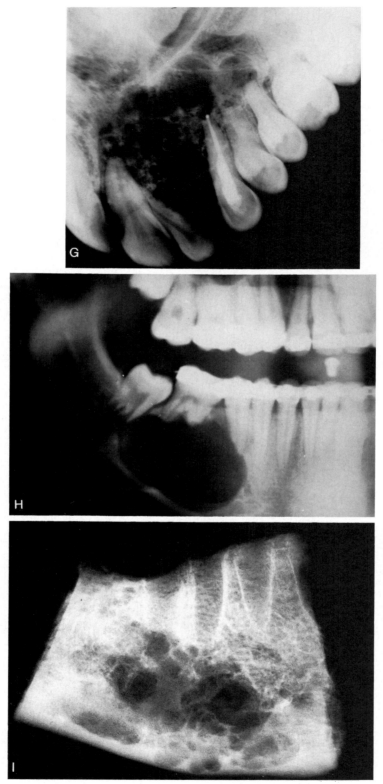

Figure 4–1 *Continued G,* This occlusal radiograph reveals a multilocular ameloblastoma in the maxilla that contains many small compartments and has caused divergence of the roots. (Courtesy of Dr. R. Whitmore, Virginia Beach, Virginia.) *H,* A unicystic ameloblastoma. Note the marked root resorption and remodeling of the lower cortical border of the mandible. *I,* A multilocular, soap-bubble appearance of the ameloblastoma. This resected specimen shows how even small tumorous projections at the edge of the lesion have the potential to resorb mandibular cortical bone.

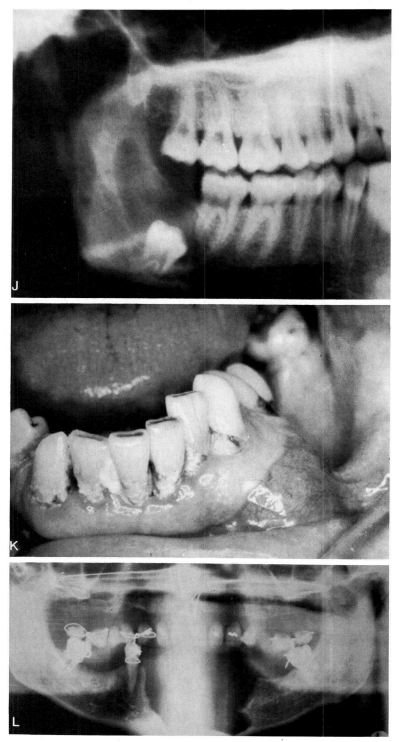

Figure 4–1 *Continued J,* An ameloblastoma that arose from the lining of a dentigerous cyst. This lesion could be described as pericoronal because it surrounds the crown of a tooth. The impaction of the third molar was most probably the result of the tumor. *K,* Expansion of buccal bone in the left mucobuccal fold area by the ameloblastoma. (Parts *K* through *P* represent a single case, courtesy of Dr. D. Precious and Dr. S. Fitch, Dalhousie University, Halifax, Nova Scotia.) *L,* Pathologic fracture secondary to surgical removal.

Illustration continued on following page

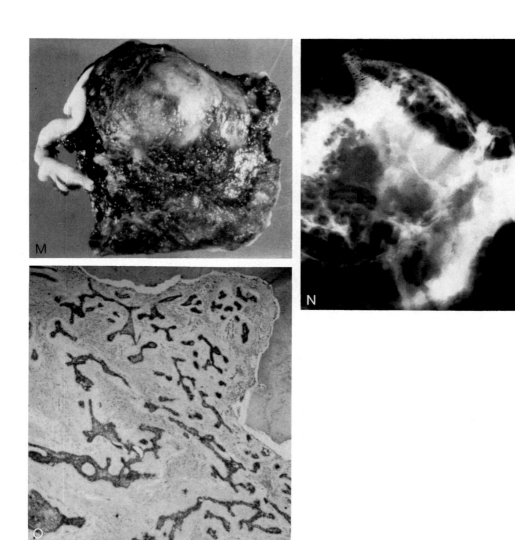

Figure 4–1 *Continued M*, Gross specimen of the tumor. *N*, Radiograph of the tumor specimen demonstrating multilocularity. *O*, Lower-power histopathologic slide showing nests and cords of odontogenic epithelium in connective tissue stroma.

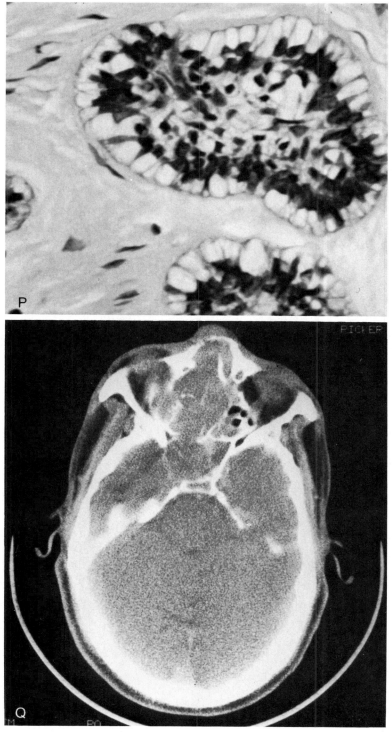

Figure 4–1 *Continued P,* Another high-power micro-scopic view of polarized nuclei and cells resembling stellate reticulum in central portion. *Q,* CT (computed tomographic) scan of a maxillary ameloblastoma invading the nasal fossae and the sphenoid and ethmoid sinuses. It has also destroyed the medial wall of the left orbit and is advancing into the middle cranial fossa. (From Bre-denkamp, J.K., Zimmerman, M.C., and Mickel, R.A.: Maxillary ameloblastoma. A potentially lethal neoplasm. Arch. Otolaryngol. Head Neck Surg., *115*:99–104, 1989, Copyright 1989, American Medical Association.)

Illustration continued on following page

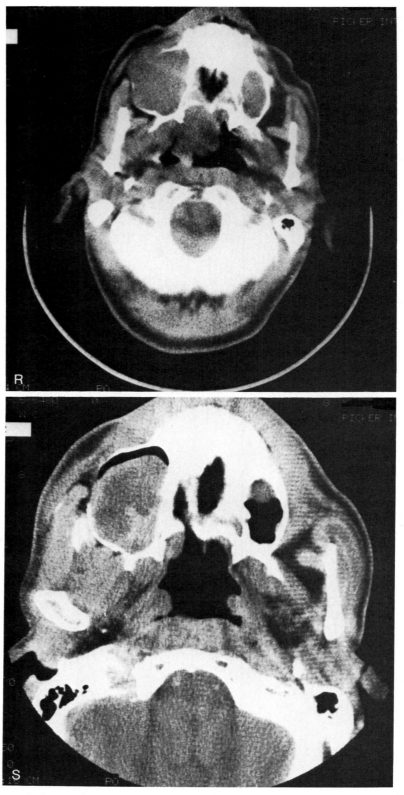

Figure 4–1 *Continued R,* Another CT scan at the level of the midmaxillary sinus. Note the destruction of the antral wall and extension of the lesion into the mucobuccal fold area. *S,* Appearance of the lesion 4½ months postoperatively at level of midsinus. Repair and remodeling of the wall are apparent.

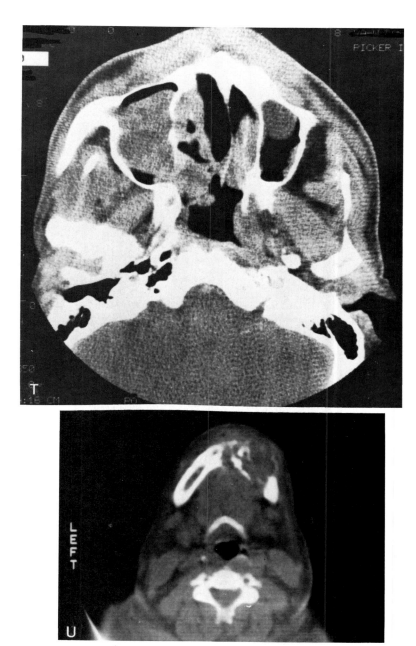

Figure 4–1 *Continued T,* Another view, slightly superior to that seen in *Q,* shows an intact lateral sinus wall. Even the medial aspect of the sinus shows some resolution. Soft tissue masses appearing within the spaces were interpreted as inflammatory sequelae of the surgical procedure. *U,* Ameloblastoma in the anterior mandible. Note the multilocular appearance on this CT scan and the expansile nature of the tumor. Many muscles of the head and neck areas are visible on this scan, which has been windowed for soft tissue.

Illustration continued on following page

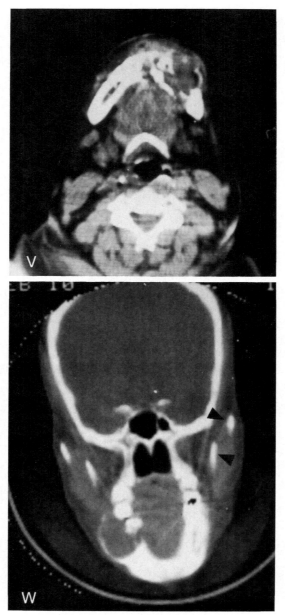

Figure 4–1 *Continued V,* This CT scan has been windowed to reveal bone in and around the tumor. *W,* A coronal section through the ameloblastoma shows an intact lateral border, at least at this anteroposterior "cut." *Arrows* point to the coronoid and condylar processes.

Kahn, M.A.: Ameloblastoma in young persons: A clinicopathologic analysis and etiologic investigation. Oral Surg. Oral Med. Oral Pathol., 67:706–715, 1989.

Keszler, A., and Dominquez, F.V.: Ameloblastoma in childhood. J. Oral Maxillofac. Surg., 44:609–613, 1986.

Lanham, R.J.: Chemotherapy of metastatic ameloblastoma: A case report and review of the literature. Oncology, 44:133–134, 1987.

Mehlisch, D.R., Dahlin, D.C., and Masson, J.K.: Ameloblastoma: A clinicopathologic report. J. Oral Surg., 30:9–22, 1972.

Muller, H., and Slootweg, P.J.: The ameloblastoma, the controversial approach to therapy. J. Oral Maxillofac. Surg., 13:79–84, 1985.

Muller, H., and Slootweg, P.J.: The growth characteristics of multilocular ameloblastomas: A histological investigation with some inferences with regard to operative procedures. J. Oral Maxillofac. Surg., 13:224–230, 1985.

Poyton, H.G.: Oral Radiology. Baltimore: Williams & Wilkins, 1982, pp. 280–296.

Robinson, L., and Martinez, M.G.: Unicystic ameloblastoma: A prognostically distinct entity. Cancer, 40:2278–2285, 1977.

Sehdev, M.K., Huvos, A.G., Strong, E.W., et al: Proceedings: Ameloblastoma of maxilla and mandible. Cancer, 33:342–333, 1974.

Shafer, W.G., Hine, M.K., and Levy, B.M.: A Textbook of Oral Pathology, 4th ed. Philadelphia: W. B. Saunders, 1983, pp. 276–285.

Slootweg, P.J., and Muller, J.: Malignant ameloblastoma or ameloblastic carcinoma. Oral Surg. Oral Med. Oral Pathol., 57:168–176, 1984.

Small, I.A., and Waldron, C.A.: Ameloblastomas of the jaws. Oral Surg. Oral Med. Oral Pathol., 8:281–297, 1955.

Stanley, H.R., and Diehl, D.L.: Ameloblastoma potential of follicular cysts. Oral Surg. Oral Med. Oral Pathol., 20:260–268, 1965.

Tsaknis, P.J., and Nelson, J.F.: The maxillary ameloblastoma: An analysis of 24 cases. J. Oral Surg., 38:336–342, 1980.

Ueda, M., Kaneda, T., Imaizumi, M., and Abe, T.: Mandibular ameloblastoma with metastasis to the lungs and lymph nodes: A case report and review of the literature. J. Oral Maxillofac. Surg., 47:623–628, 1989.

Ueno, S., Nakamura, S., Mushimoto, K., Shirasu, R.: A clinicopathologic study of ameloblastoma. J. Oral Maxillofac. Surg., 44:361–365, 1986.

Ueno, S., Mushimoto, K., and Shirasu, R.: Prognostic evaluation of ameloblastoma based on histologic and radiographic typing. J. Oral Maxillofac. Surg., 47:11–15, 1989.

Vickers, R.A., and Gorlin, R.J.: Ameloblastoma: Delineation of early histopathologic features of neoplasia. Cancer, 26:699–710, 1970.

CALCIFYING EPITHELIAL ODONTOGENIC TUMOR

The calcifying epithelial odontogenic tumor (CEOT) (Fig. 4–2) is more widely known by its eponym, the Pindborg tumor, in honor of the pathologist who first described it. Its unique histologic appearance allowed easy initial recognition of the tumor but with time came the realization that some variants are harder to diagnose. The CEOT is similar to an ameloblastoma but differs in that calcifications can be seen on the radiograph and the tumor is usually less aggressive. The ameloblastoma is much more (15 times more) common than the CEOT.

Clinical Features

The mean age of patients is 40.4 years, but the reported ages range from 8 to 92 years. Most tumors (68%) occur in the mandible, especially in the molar region.

Radiographic Appearance

A lesion may progress from a well-defined radiolucency to one that demonstrates small radiopacities and eventually to a multilocular lesion that has a considerable amount of calcification (see Fig. 4–2). The term driven snow has been applied to the streaky quality of the opacification seen on radiographs. The presence of calcification helps to separate the CEOT from an ameloblastoma. Impacted teeth are associated with a CEOT in approximately 62% of cases.

Histopathologic Findings

The CEOT contains polyhedral, eosinophilic epithelial cells with prominent intercellular bridges. The epithelial cells are usually in large sheets but can occur in small nests that resemble an adenocarcinoma. Calcifications are usually but not always present. There is great variation not only in the type but also in the amount of calcification noted in any individual tumor.

Treatment

The recommended treatment is excision with a rim of normal bone; the recurrence rate is 23%.

References

Franklin, C.D., and Pindborg, J.J.: The calcifying epithelial odontogenic tumor: Review and analysis of 113 cases. Oral Surg. Oral Med. Oral Pathol., 42:753–765, 1976.

Gargiulo, E.A., Ziter, W.D., and Mastrocola, R.: Calcifying epithelial odontogenic tumor: Report of case and review of literature. J. Oral Surg., 29:862–866, 1971.

Krolls, S.O., and Pindborg, J.J.: Calcifying epithelial odontogenic tumor: A survey of 23 cases and discussion of histomorphologic variation. Arch. Pathol., 98:206–210, 1974.

Pindborg, J.J.: Calcifying epithelial odontogenic tumors. Acta Pathol. Microbiol. Scand., 111(Suppl):71, 1956.

Shafer, W.G., Hine, M.K., and Levy, B.M.: A Textbook of Oral Pathology, 4th ed. Philadelphia: W. B. Saunders, 1983, pp. 286–289.

SQUAMOUS ODONTOGENIC TUMOR

When the squamous odontogenic tumor (SOT) was first described in 1975, it was apparent that it had been previously misdiagnosed as an ameloblastoma. It is a unique odontogenic tumor that probably arises from the rests of Malassez (Fig. 4–3).

Clinical Features

The SOT is usually diagnosed in adults but has a relatively wide age range (11 to 67 years). One unusual finding has been the high incidence of cases reported in blacks (77%). Most lesions are found in the posterior region of the jaws. Approximately 25% of patients have multiple separate foci of SOT. In about half of the cases, the patient presents with a mobile tooth or other symptom related to the loss of alveolar bone. Multicentric SOTs have been reported in three black siblings, but a genetic mode of transmission has not been established.

Radiographic Appearance

In many cases there is a triangular or semicircular radiolucency adjacent to the cervical portion of the tooth. Other tumors are located at the apex of a tooth or in association with impacted teeth. Because of these findings, an SOT can mimic either localized periodontal disease or periapical pathosis.

Histopathologic Findings

The typical SOT contains well-defined islands of epithelial cells that lack the peripheral palisading and polarization found in an ameloblastoma. The cells within the islands are uniform in appearance and rarely show keratinization. Occasionally, microcystic degeneration within the central portion of an epithelial island and small foci of calcification are present.

Treatment

Maxillary lesions are more aggressive, possibly because of the relative porosity of the maxilla. Recurrences are more common in patients with multiple lesions. Although the SOT is a benign lesion, complete surgical excision is recommended to prevent recurrence and the small possibility of malignant transformation.

References

Goldblatt, L.I., Brannon, R.B., and Ellis, G.L.: Squamous odontogenic tumor: Report of five cases and review of the literature. Oral Surg. Oral Med. Oral Pathol., 54:187–196, 1982.

Hietanen, J., Lukinmaa, P.L., Ahonen, P., Krees, R., and Calonius, P.E.: Peripheral squamous odontogenic tumor. Br. J. Oral Maxillofac. Surg., 23:362–365, 1985.

Hopper, T.L., Sadeghi, E.M., and Pricco, D.F.: Squamous odontogenic tumor: Report of a case with multiple lesions. Oral Surg. Oral Med. Oral Pathol., 50:404–410, 1980.

Leider, A.S., Jonker, A., and Cook, H.E.: Multicentric familial squamous odontogenic tumor. Oral Surg. Oral Med. Oral Pathol., 68:175–181, 1989.

Mills, E.P., Davila, M.A., Beuttenmuller, E.A., and Koudelka, B. M.: Squamous odontogenic tumor: Report of a case with lesions in three quadrants. Oral Surg. Oral Med. Oral Pathol., 61:557–563, 1986.

Norris, L.H., Baghaei-Rad, M., Maloney, P.L., Simpson, G., and Guinta, J.: Bilateral maxillary squamous odontogenic tumors and the malignant transformation of a mandibular radiolucent lesion. J. Oral Maxillofac. Surg., 42:827–834, 1984.

Pullon, P.A., Shafer, W.G., Elzay, R.P., et al: Squamous odontogenic tumor: Report of six cases of a previously undescribed lesion. Oral Surg. Oral Med. Oral Pathol., 40:616–630, 1975.

Unal, T., Gomel, M., and Gunel, O.: Squamous odontogenic tumor-like islands in a radicular cyst: Report of a case. J. Oral Maxillofac. Surg., 45:346–349, 1987.

Wright, J.M.: Squamous odontogenic tumor-like proliferations in odontogenic cysts. Oral Surg. Oral Med. Oral Pathol., 47:354–358, 1979.

ADENOMATOID ODONTOGENIC TUMOR

Since being described by Dreibaldt in 1907 as a pseudoadenoma adamantinum, the adenomatoid odontogenic tumor (AOT) (Fig. 4–4) has been burdened with inappropriate names such as adenoameloblastoma. **The discontinuation of any reference to ameloblastoma is desirable because this is a benign, self-limiting lesion that is best treated by conservative excision.**

Text continued on page 71

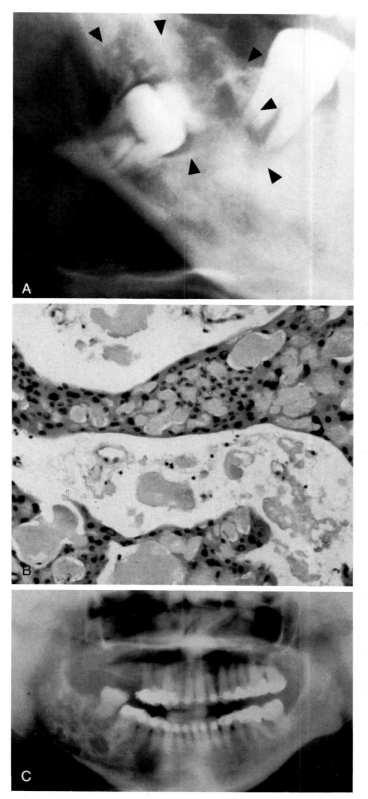

Figure 4–2. *A,* The radiopaque-radiolucent lesion (*arrows*) surrounding this impacted mandibular third molar was diagnosed as a calcifying epithelial odontogenic tumor. This lesion is typically associated with impacted teeth and demonstrates variable numbers and types of radiopacities. (Courtesy of Dr. C. Cuttino, Richmond, Virginia.) *B,* Large epithelial cells that retain a deep eosinophilic stain are a hallmark of this tumor. The cells can be found in large sheets or in smaller isolated clusters. *C,* This panoramic radiograph demonstrates a multilocular destructive radiolucency of the right posterior mandible. *Illustration continued on following page*

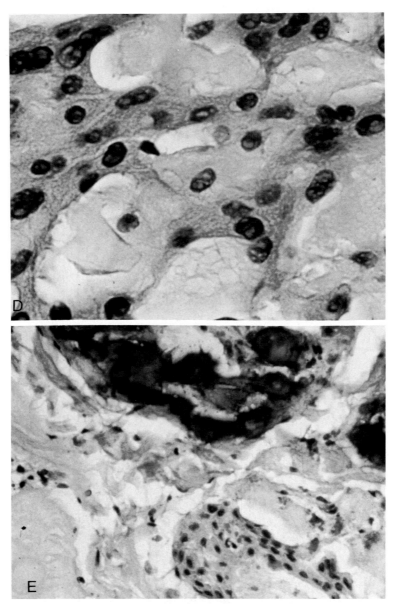

Figure 4–2 *Continued D,* The large nuclei and the cellular connections are apparent in this high-power view. *E,* Amorphic areas, which contain amyloid, and irregularly shaped calcifications are often seen. With maturation, the calcifications coalesce and produce radiographically visible radiopaque foci.

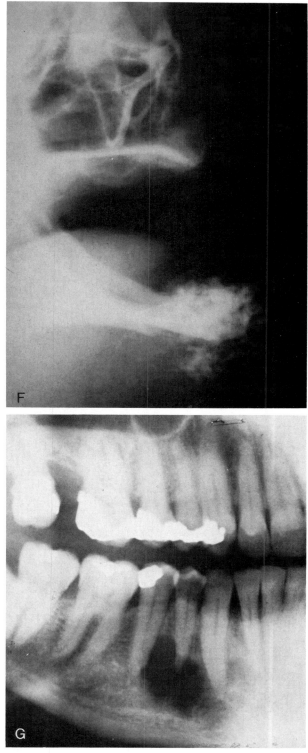

Figure 4–2 *Continued F,* This CEOT shows numerous radiopaque foci within a lesion in the anterior mandible of an elderly woman. This appearance has been described as "driven snow." (Courtesy of Dr. B. Harsanyi, Dalhousie University, Halifax, Nova Scotia.) *G,* The margins of this CEOT are well defined but not corticated. No evidence of internal radiopacities is present. The lesion is only slightly suggestive of a multilocular lesion. (Courtesy of Dr. C. Tomich, Indiana University School of Dentistry, Indianapolis, Indiana.)

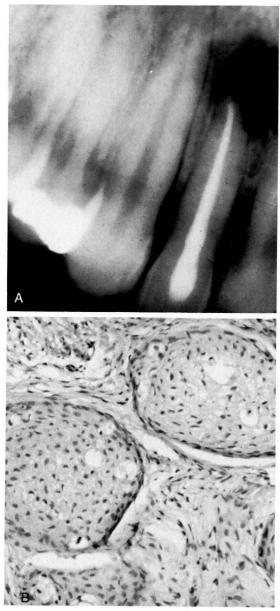

Figure 4–3. *A*, This squamous odontogenic tumor was radiographically very similar to a periapical granuloma or cyst. Other cases of squamous odontogenic tumor have mimicked periodontal disease. *B*, Numerous well-defined epithelial islands are present within a normal-appearing fibrous connective tissue stroma.

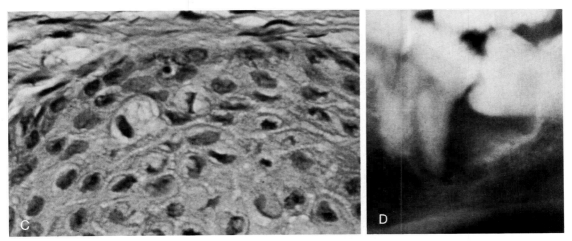

Figure 4–3 *Continued C*, The peripheral cells are flattened, and there is uniformity among the cells within the island. *D*, A squamous odontogenic tumor.

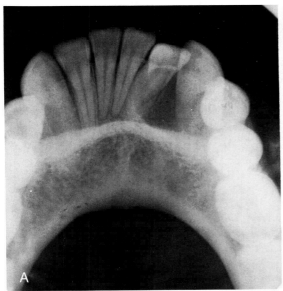

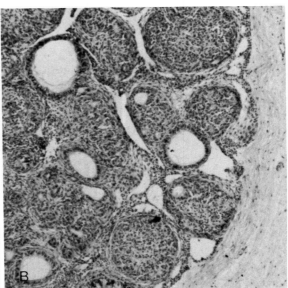

Figure 4–4. *A*, This adenomatoid odontogenic tumor was noted between the mandibular canine and the lateral incisor. Numerous small calcifications were present in this expansile lesion. (Courtesy of Dr. F. Woodlief, Richmond, Virginia.) *B*, A thick connective tissue capsule surrounds this lesion, which contains many well-defined solid nests as well as duct-like structures. Occasionally, foci of calcification and amyloid deposits are found. If the calcifications are present in adequate numbers, faint radiopacities will be seen on the radiograph.

Illustration continued on following page

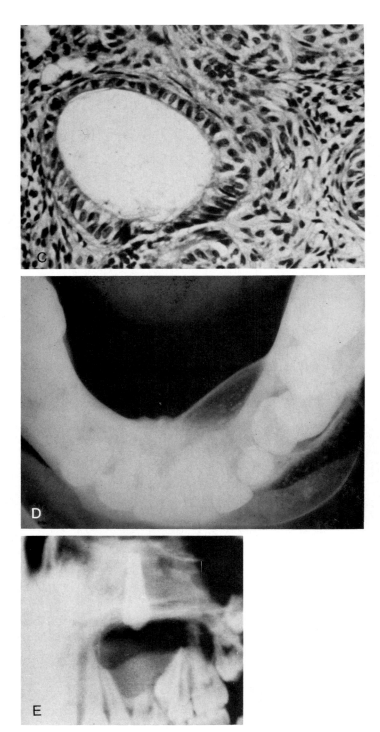

Figure 4–4 *Continued C,* The duct-like structures are lined by a layer of palisading cells, which is in contrast to the haphazard arrangement of the surrounding cells. *D,* A rare case of AOT in an anterior mandible shows gross expansion of both the lingual and the buccal cortical plates and multiple small, diffuse internal calcifications. Tooth displacement is also evident. (Courtesy of Dr. M. Murphy, Columbus, Ohio.) *E,* AOT in a left maxilla. Left maxillary canine has been extremely displaced. Root resorption is present on several teeth including retained primary canine and first molar. Lesion is well defined but contains no radiographically detectable calcifications.

Clinical Features

The mean age at time of diagnosis is 18 years, the majority of patients being in the second decade of life. Most patients (64%) are women, and 65% of the lesions are found in the maxilla. Of reported cases, 76% occurred between the canines (52% in the anterior maxilla, 24% in the anterior mandible), and very few were posterior to the second premolar. In at least 64% of cases, the patient presented with an intraoral swelling, which might be related to the fact that impacted teeth were associated with an AOT in 74% of the patients. An easy way to remember all this information is to remember the figure of 70%. Approximately 70% of patients are under the age of 20 and are women, and approximately 70% of tumors occur in the maxilla, between the canines, and are associated with an impacted tooth.

Radiographic Appearance

Almost all tumors (94%) are unilocular, frequently between the lateral incisor and the canine, and radiopaque foci are seen in 23 to 65% of the cases. The ability to visualize the radiopacities in any particular lesion is related to the amount of calcification present and the exposure factors utilized for exposing the radiograph. Separation of roots is relatively common (24.5%), but root resorption has been noted in only two cases.

The associated impacted teeth are unaffected, which suggests that the AOT forms after the completion of tooth formation.

Histopathologic Findings

The AOT is easily diagnosed in an adequate surgical specimen because of its thick connective tissue capsule, foci of calcification, and distinctive patterns of epithelial proliferation. Of the three epithelial patterns (solid nests, ducts, and cribriform) that are characteristic, the most common is the presence of solid nests. Scattered throughout the nests and islands of epithelial cells are small areas of basophilic calcification as well as an eosinophilic material that is thought to be produced by the basement membrane or to represent amyloid.

Treatment

Conservative excision is adequate because no recurrences have been reported, even after incomplete removal.

References

Abrams, A.M., Melrose, R.J., and Howell, F.V.: Adenoameloblastoma: A clinical pathologic study of ten new cases. Cancer, 22:175–185, 1968.

Courtney, R.M., and Kerr, D.A.: The odontogenic adenomatoid tumor: A comprehensive study of twenty new cases. Oral Surg. Oral Med. Oral Pathol., 39:424–435, 1975.

Giansanti, J.S., Someren, A., and Waldron, C.A.: Odontogenic adenomatoid tumor (adenoameloblastoma): Survey of 111 cases. Oral Surg. Oral Med. Oral Pathol., 30:69–86, 1970.

Shafer, W.G., Hine, M.K., and Levy, B.M.: A Textbook of Oral Pathology, 4th ed. Philadelphia: W. B. Saunders, 1983, pp. 289–291.

Swinson, T.W.: An extraosseous adenomatoid odontogenic tumor: A case report. Br. J. Oral Surg., 15:32–36, 1977.

CENTRAL ODONTOGENIC FIBROMA

This is an unusual neoplasm that is difficult to categorize because of subjective histologic criteria and the small number of reported cases (Fig. 4–5). To add to the confusion, there are two separate histologic types of central odontogenic fibroma (COF). One point of general agreement is that **this tumor is not related to the two soft tissue lesions with similar names**—peripheral odontogenic fibroma and peripheral ossifying fibroma.

Clinical Features

The range in age at time of diagnosis is 11 to 80 years. Eighty percent of the tumors were in the mandible and were characterized by a slow-growing expansion.

Radiographic Appearance

Although the tumor is traditionally described as multilocular, one review found only 20% of cases with this characteristic. It is reasonable to assume that with early diagnosis the percentage of unilocular lesions would be even higher. The COF usually has a well-defined sclerotic border. One of the subjective criteria for diagnosis of this lesion has been that it should be of sufficient size to be considered a neoplasm compared with the normal size of a dental follicle. This is a problem because there is no widely accepted definition for what constitutes a minimum pathologic size.

Histopathologic Findings

Gardner compared the two histologic types of COF: simple and the type defined by the World Health Organization (WHO). The simple type resembles the connective tissue of a dental follicle. Despite the tumor's name, islands of odontogenic epithelium do not have to be noted to render the diagnosis. If present, the islands do not contain stellate reticulum nor is there palisading of the peripheral cells. These features help separate it from an ameloblastoma. The WHO type of COF is similar except that it also contains calcifications that are considered to be dentin or cementum because of their proximity to odontogenic epithelium. Of the two types, the simple type is more common.

There has been discussion about a possible relationship between the COF and odontogenic myxoma. One theory is that a COF is the mature terminal stage of a myxoma, whereas another supposes that a myxoma simply represents myxomatous change within a COF. Too few cases of either lesion have been reported to decide whether there is an association.

Treatment

Surgical removal is adequate because the recurrence rate is only 13%. However, one tumor did recur 9 years after the initial surgery.

References

Dahl, E.C., Wolfson, S.H., and Haugen, J.C.: Central odontogenic fibroma: Review of literature and report of cases. J. Oral Surg., 39:120–124, 1981.

Doyle, J.L., Lamster, I.B., and Baden, E.: Odontogenic fibroma of the complex (WHO) type: Report of six cases. J. Oral Maxillofac. Surg., 43:666–674, 1985.

Dunlap, C.L., and Barker, B.F.: Central odontogenic fibroma of the WHO type. Oral Surg. Oral Med. Oral Pathol., 57:390–394, 1984.

Gardner, D.G.: The central odontogenic fibroma: An attempt at clarification. Oral Surg. Oral Med. Oral Pathol., 50:425–432, 1980.

Heimdal, A., Isacsson, G., and Nilsson, L.: Recurrent central odontogenic fibroma. Oral Surg. Oral Med. Oral Pathol., 50:140–145, 1980.

Slootweg, P.J., and Muller, H.: Central fibroma of the jaw, odontogenic or desmoplastic: A report of five cases with reference to differential diagnosis. Oral Surg. Oral Med. Oral Pathol., 56:61–70, 1983.

Svirsky, J.A., Abbey, L.M., and Kaugars, G.E.: A clinical review of central odontogenic fibroma: With the addition of three new cases. J. Oral Med., 41:51–54, 1986.

Wesley, R.K., Wysocki, G.P., and Mintz, S.M.: The central odontogenic fibroma: Clinical and morphologic studies. Oral Surg. Oral Med. Oral Pathol., 40:235–245, 1975.

ODONTOGENIC MYXOMA

The intraosseous myxoma is an enigma because of the difficulty in separating the myxoma histologically from other fibrous lesions. There is reason to believe that this lesion may be either a variant of the central odontogenic fibroma or prominent myxomatous degeneration in a central fibrous lesion. Some authors have attached the term odontogenic to this lesion because there is some evidence that it occurs only in the jaws. Even with electron microscopic examination, it has not been possible to identify the cell of origin of the myxoma. The cases reported in the condyle rule out a purely odontogenic source, but the peculiar affinity for the jaw is still unexplained (Fig. 4–6).

Clinical Features

The age at the time of diagnosis ranges from 5 months to 62 years. Most lesions occur in the posterior mandible, but two have been reported in the mandibular condyle. The most common presenting sign is painless clinical expansion of the jaw.

Radiographic Appearance

The classic appearance is a "soap bubble" or irregular radiolucency that is traversed by fine bony trabeculae. The majority are multilocular, but 37.5% are unilocular. In most cases, at least a portion of the lesion's border is indefinite. There is greater variability with maxillary lesions, especially those that involve the antrum.

Histopathologic Findings

As implied by the name, the overall appearance is predominantly myxomatous. Malignancy is occasionally suggested because hyperchromatic, binucleated cells demonstrating mitotic activity are common. Surprisingly, the presence of odontogenic epithelium is not required for the diagnosis, and, indeed, in only 17% of the cases are there nests of epithelium.

Text continued on page 79

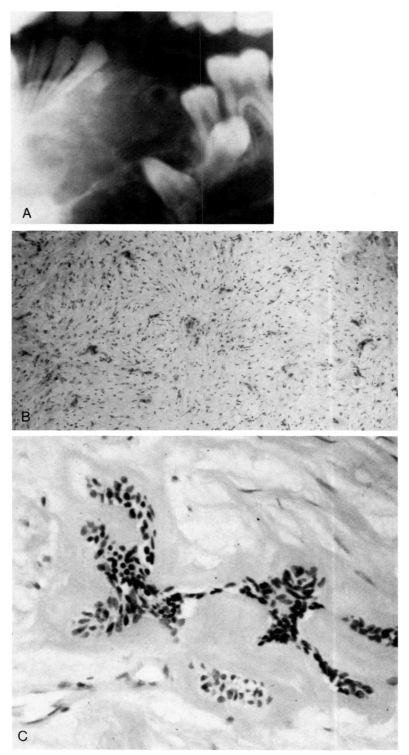

Figure 4–5. *A,* Large, multilocular, expansile lesion in a mandible that contains some opacities. The lesion has displaced erupted and unerupted teeth alike in this 9-year-old boy. (Courtesy of Dr. C. Tomich, Indiana University School of Dentistry, Indianapolis, Indiana.) *B,* Many islands of odontogenic epithelium are scattered throughout this specimen. *C,* This high-power view shows a dense eosinophilic material, which is interpreted as dentinoid, surrounding the islands.

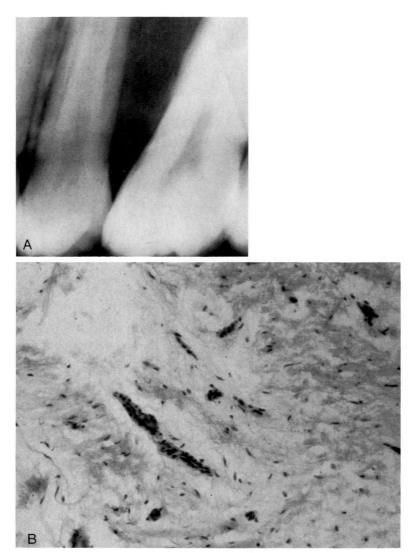

Figure 4–6. *A,* The radiolucency between the maxillary second premolar and the first molar in this 20-year-old woman was diagnosed as an odontogenic myxoma. The intraoral radiograph reveals only a portion of the lesion. *B,* Scattered islands of odontogenic epithelium are present in the hypocellular fibrous connective tissue. No evidence of a capsule is seen.

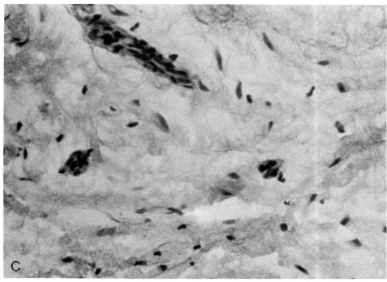

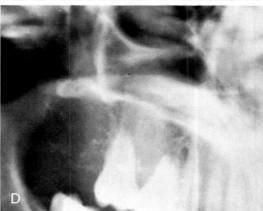

Figure 4–6 *Continued C,* The epithelial islands are unremarkable and may even be difficult to find in some cases. *D,* Odontogenic myxoma of the right maxilla including the tuberosity. Note also the cloudy maxillary sinus. The tumor makes the antrum appear radiopaque. Some mild displacement of the maxillary first molar and the maxillary second premolar is present. (Courtesy of Dr. C. Tomich, Indiana University School of Dentistry, Indianapolis, Indiana.)

Illustration continued on following page

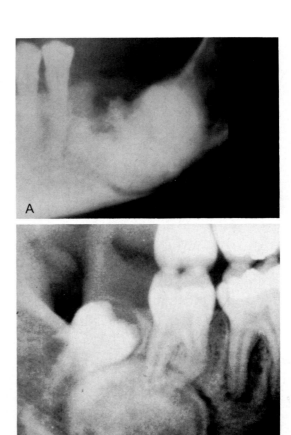

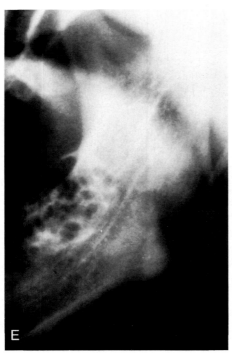

Figure 4–6 *Continued E*, Soap-bubble appearance of odontogenic myxoma in the posterior mandible.

Figure 4–7. *A*, The characteristic radiographic features of a benign cementoblastoma are present in this case: a well-defined radiopacity that had obscured the roots of a mandibular molar (now extracted) and that is surrounded by a radiolucent band. These features help to distinguish this abnormality from other lesions such as the central ossifying fibroma or odontoma that may appear radiographically similar. (Courtesy of Dr. C. Tomich, Indiana University School of Dentistry, Indianapolis, Indiana.) *B*, Cementoblastoma at apex of the second permanent molar. Note the radiolucent rim about the lesion. Note also that the root apices can be detected "within" the radiopacity. Compare this lesion with a second view taken 6 months later in *C*.

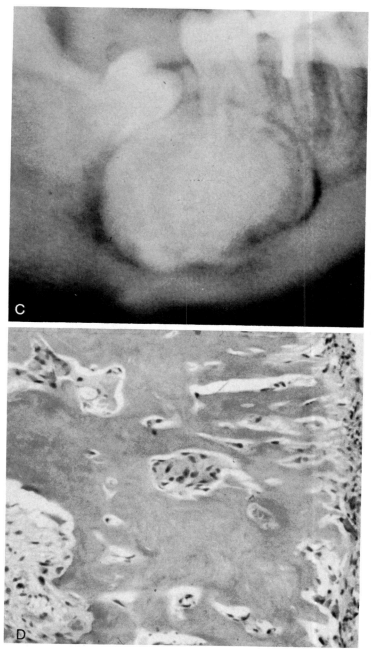

Figure 4–7 *Continued C,* The tumor has increased in size. Reactive bone is seen at the periphery of the lesion, but the radiolucent rim representing the fibrous connective tissue capsule or "tumor front" is still apparent. *D,* The peripheral portion of a benign cementoblastoma typically contains spicules of calcified material that are at a 90-degree angle to the edge of the lesion. The areas closer to the tooth consist of dense sheets of cementum-like material. If the tooth and lesion are removed intact, the continuity with the root of the tooth is readily apparent.

Illustration continued on following page

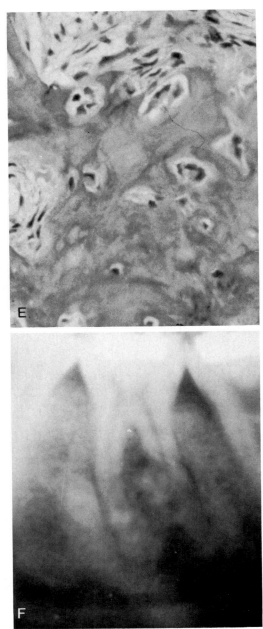

Figure 4–7 *Continued E,* Increased cellular activity is evident in this histologic section. This histologic feature is commonly seen and should not be mistaken for malignant change. *F,* An "early," possibly just developing, cementoblastoma showing less radiodensity. (Courtesy of Dr. G. Terezhalmy, Case Western Reserve University, Cleveland, Ohio.)

Treatment

Although recurrence rates as high as 33% have been quoted, analysis of several series reveals a recurrence rate of 12.5% in cases treated with curettage. Therefore, the reputation of the myxoma as a clinically aggressive lesion that is difficult to remove may not be entirely accurate.

References

Ghosh, B.C., Huvos, A.G., and Whiteley, H.W.: Myxoma of the jaw bones. Cancer, 31:237–240, 1973.

Goldblatt, L.I.: Ultrastructural study of an odontogenic myxoma. Oral Surg. Oral Med. Oral Pathol., 42:206–220, 1976.

Kangur, T.T., Dahlin, D.C., and Turlington, E.G.: Myxomatous tumors of the jaws. J. Oral Surg., 33:523–528, 1975.

Shafer, W.G., Hine, M.K., and Levy, B.M.: A Textbook of Oral Pathology, 4th ed. Philadelphia: W. B. Saunders, 1983, pp. 295–297.

Slootweg, P.J., and Wittkampf, A.R.M.: Myxoma of the jaws: An analysis of 15 cases. J. Oral Maxillofac. Surg., 14:46–52, 1986.

Stabholz, A., Heling, I., Friedman, S., and Azaz, B.: Odontogenic myxoma in the maxillary premolar region. J. Endodont., 13:182–185, 1987.

White, D.K., Chen, S., Mohnac, A.M., et al: Odontogenic myxoma: A clinical and ultrastructural study. Oral Surg. Oral Med. Oral Pathol., 39:901–917, 1975.

BENIGN CEMENTOBLASTOMA

This neoplasm is also known as a true cementoma because it arises from cementoblasts. Although the terms may sound similar, the benign cementoblastoma is not related to lesions known as cementoma (periapical cemental dysplasia), central cementifying fibroma, or gigantiform cementoma (Fig. 4–7).

Clinical Features

More than half the cases are diagnosed in patients less than 20 years of age. Most benign cementoblastomas are found in the posterior mandible, and almost half are associated with a mandibular permanent first molar. Only one case involving a deciduous tooth has been reported. Bony expansion has been present in 73% of patients.

Radiographic Appearance

The benign cementoblastoma, which is attached to a tooth, is characterized by a well-defined circular radiopacity surrounded by a thin radiolucent line. The root of the tooth is not radiographically visible because of the proliferation of cementum. There is no other odontogenic lesion that has these radiographic findings.

Histopathologic Findings

The central portion of the specimen is usually a solid sheet of cementum, but the periphery has trabeculae of cementum with prominent cementoclastic and cementoblastic activity. The large pleomorphic cementoblasts can lead to an erroneous diagnosis of benign osteoblastoma or osteosarcoma. Care is necessary when submitting a biopsy specimen because an accurate diagnosis may not be possible if only a portion of the periphery is examined.

Treatment

Excision of the lesion and extraction of the associated tooth have long been advocated, but one case report demonstrated that endodontic therapy prior to surgery could save the tooth. There have been no reported recurrences.

References

Corio, R.L., Crawford, B.E., and Schaberg, S.J.: Benign cementoblastoma. Oral Surg. Oral Med. Oral Pathol., 41:524–530, 1976.

Farman, A.G., Kohler, W.W., Nortjé, C.J., and Van Wyk, C.W.: Cementoblastoma: Report of a case. J. Oral Surg., 37:198–203, 1979.

Forsslund, H.G., Bodin, I., and Julin, P.: Undiagnosed benign cementoblastoma in a patient with a 6-year pain condition. Oral Surg. Oral Med. Oral Pathol., 66:243–248, 1988.

Goerig, A.C., Fay, J.T., and King, E.: Endodontic treatment of a cementoblastoma: Report of a case. Oral Surg. Oral Med. Oral Pathol., 58:133–136, 1984.

Shafer, W.G., Hine, M.K., and Levy, B.M.: A Textbook of Oral Pathology, 4th ed. Philadelphia: W.B. Saunders, 1983, pp. 301–303.

AMELOBLASTIC FIBROMA

The histologic appearance of this tumor displays many elements found in the development of a tooth (Fig. 4–8). The nests and strands of odontogenic epithelium resemble enamel organ, whereas the myxomatous connective tissue is similar to the embryonic dental papilla. **The term ameloblastic is misleading because these tumors are not a type of ameloblastoma.**

Clinical Features

The mean age at time of diagnosis is 15 years, and 71% of tumors are discovered in patients under the age of 20. A strong predilection (88%) for the mandible has been reported, and most tumors are in the posterior region. Slightly more than half of the patients have a clinically evident bony expansion.

Radiographic Appearance

The typical case shows a well-defined, **pericoronal** radiolucency—that is, a radiolucency occurring around the crown of an impacted mandibular molar. The majority of lesions (75%) are multilocular, and many (75%) are associated with an impacted tooth. There is a tendency for small lesions to be unilocular and to become multilocular with time.

Histopathologic Findings

Although the strands of odontogenic epithelium are at first glance the most prominent feature, the diagnosis is based on the presence of connective tissue that is embryonic in appearance. The epithelial islands can be quite numerous but rarely have a central area of stellate reticulum–like tissue as in an ameloblastoma.

Treatment

The appropriate therapy is hard to assess because the reported recurrence rates range from 18.8 to 43.5%. However, it is reasonable to assume that larger multilocular lesions are more likely to recur. **Treatment should probably be conservative because this lesion behaves more like a fibroma than an ameloblastoma.**

References

Tanaka, S.: Recurrent ameloblastic fibroma: Report of a case. Oral Surg. Oral Med. Oral Pathol., 33:944–950, 1972.

Trodahl, J.N.: Ameloblastic fibroma: A survey of cases from the Armed Forces Institute of Pathology. Oral Surg. Oral. Med. Oral Pathol., 33:547–558, 1972.

Zallen, R.D., Preskar, M.H., and McClary, S.A.: Ameloblastic fibroma. J. Oral Maxillofac. Surg., 40:513–517, 1982.

ODONTOMA

Although the odontoma is considered the most common odontogenic tumor in one large survey, other authors feel that it is better categorized as a hamartoma. The term odontoma was originated by Broca in 1868 and was initially applied to all odontogenic tumors. Gradually it evolved to its current usage indicating the presence of unorganized but recognizable enamel and dentin within a self-limiting hamartomatous process. Traditionally, compound odontomas were diagnosed by their radiographic similarity to teeth. Indeed, the lesion usually appears to contain multiple little tooth-like structures. Complex odontomas, on the other hand, are less organized. However, the distinction between compound and complex odontomas is vague, and there does not seem to be any clinical value in separating them (Fig. 4–9).

Clinical Features

More than half of these tumors (54%) are diagnosed in the second decade of life, and the median age at diagnosis is 16 years. Only 15% are discovered in patients 30 years or older. There is no sex predilection, but the incidence in blacks is double the expected rate. The lesions are evenly divided between the maxilla and the mandible, but 58% occur between the canines. Of all odontomas, 34% are in the anterior maxilla, and 24.5% are in the anterior mandible. Symptoms such as expansion are present in at least 15% of all patients.

Radiographic Appearance

As defined by WHO, a **complex odontoma** is a disorderly arrangement of dental tissues, and a **compound odontoma** has a more orderly pattern, in which tooth-like components are apparent. This subjectivity explains the range of values (38 to 68%) in the literature indicating the percentage of all odontomas that are compound. Classically, compound odontomas contain miniature tooth-like structures with foci of radiodense enamel and are surrounded by a thin radiolucent follicle. The complex odontoma is less structured but still has a follicle, and radiopacities with the density of enamel can occasionally be visualized. There does not seem to be sufficient **clinical** justification to separate the two types of odontoma.

Almost half (48%) of all cases are associated with an impacted tooth. Because not all odontomas occur adjacent to an unerupted tooth, this implies that either the odontoma develops after the tooth has begun to erupt or that a tooth can erupt around an odontoma.

Histopathologic Features

An odontoma contains all the parts of a normal tooth except that they are haphazardly arranged. Large, irregularly shaped pieces of dentin usually make up the bulk of the specimen. Eosinophilic sheets of enamel rods are often in close proximity to the dentin, but the enamel itself is lost during the decalcification of the specimen. Areas of pulp tissue surrounded by dentin are sometimes found. There are no histologic criteria that distinguish a compound odontoma from a complex one.

Treatment

Surgical removal is recommended because of the possibility of cystic or ameloblastic change within the follicle. Also, removal is important for the proper eruption of any impacted teeth. A surprisingly high percentage (28%) of odontomas are associated with a dentigerous cyst. This tendency for dentigerous cyst formation in an odontoma remains relatively constant for each decade of life.

References

Bodin, I., Julin, P., and Thomsson, M.: Odontomas and their pathological sequels. Dentomaxillofac. Radiol., 12:109–114, 1983.

Budnick, S.: Compound and complex odontomas. Oral Surg. Oral Med. Oral Pathol., 42:501–505, 1976.

Caton, R.B., Marble, H.B., and Topazian, R.G.: Complex odontoma in the maxillary sinus. Oral Surg. Oral Med. Oral Pathol., 36:658–662, 1973.

Kaugars, G.E., Miller, M.E., and Abbey, L.M.: Odontomas. Oral Surg. Oral Med. Oral Pathol., 67:172–176, 1989.

Regezi, J.A., Kerr, D.A., and Courtney, R.M.: Odontogenic tumors: Analysis of 706 cases. J. Oral Surg., 36:771–778, 1978.

Ruprecht, A., Batniji, S., and El-Neiveihi, E.: The incidence of odontomas in dental patients at King Saud University. Dentomaxillofac. Radiol., 13:77–79, 1984.

Slootweg, P.J.: An analysis of the interrelationship of the mixed odontogenic tumors—the ameloblastic fibroma, ameloblastic fibro-odontoma, and the odontomas. Oral Surg. Oral Med. Oral Pathol., 51:266–274, 1981.

Toretti, E.F., Miller, A.S., and Peezick, B.: Odontomas: An analysis of 167 cases. J. Pedodontics 8:282–284, 1984.

AMELOBLASTIC FIBRO-ODONTOMA

The ameloblastic fibro-odontoma (AFO) combines the histologic elements of an ameloblastic fibroma with those of an odontoma (Fig. 4–10). Despite the confusing name, most authorities feel that the AFO is an immature odontoma, because of the age of the patient at diagnosis and its most common anatomic location. However, with more reported cases it is possible that the AFO will emerge as a unique neoplasm.

Clinical Features

The mean age at time of diagnosis is 8 years, which is approximately 8 years younger than patients with an odontoma. A slight propensity (62%) has been shown for the mandible, and 72% of these tumors are located posterior to the canines. Patients usually present with a painless expansion of the jaw.

Radiographic Appearance

The AFO is a well-defined radiolucency that contains multiple radiopacities and is usually coronal to an impacted tooth (pericoronal).

Histopathologic Findings

The background connective tissue appears embryonic and contains strands of odontogenic epithelial cells similar to those found in an ameloblastic fibroma. The calcified portion has enamel matrix, dentin, and cementum in an irregularly shaped configuration. Overall, the histologic picture is that of an odontoma whose connective tissue contains foci of ameloblastic fibroma.

Treatment

Conservative excision is adequate because the recurrence rate is only 3%.

References

Hanna, R.J., Regezi, J.A., and Hayward, J.R.: Ameloblastic fibro-odontoma: Report of case with light and electron microscopic observations. J. Oral Surg., 34:820–825, 1976.

Hawkins, P.L., and Sadeghi, E.M.: Ameloblastic fibro-odontoma: Report of case. J. Oral Maxillofac. Surg., 44:1014–1019, 1986.

Miller, A.S., López, C.F., Pullon, P.A., et al: Ameloblastic fibro-odontoma: Report of seven cases. Oral Surg. Oral Med. Oral Pathol., 41:354–365, 1976.

Sanders, D.W., Kolodny, S.C., and Jacoby, J.K.: Ameloblastic fibro-odontoma: Report of case. J. Oral Surg., 32:281–285, 1974.

Shafer, W.G., Hine, M.K., and Levy, B.M.: A Textbook of Oral Pathology, 4th ed. Philadelphia: W.B. Saunders, 1983, pp. 307–308.

Slootweg, P.J.: An analysis of the interrelationship of the mixed odontogenic tumors—ameloblastic fibroma, ameloblastic fibro-odontoma, and the odontomas. Oral Surg. Oral Med. Oral Pathol., 51:266–276, 1981.

Warnock, G.R., Pankey, G., and Foss, R.: Well-circumscribed mixed-density lesion coronal to an unerupted permanent tooth. J. Am Dent. Assoc., 119:311–312, 1989.

AMELOBLASTIC ODONTOMA

This unique lesion may represent a mixed odontogenic tumor because it contains simultaneously epithelial islands of ameloblastoma and the mesodermal calcified elements of an odontoma (Fig. 4–11). Because of the small number of reported cases and the uncertainty concerning histogenesis, it is not known whether this is an ameloblastoma that matures to the point of producing calcified dental tissues, an odontoma that induces the formation of an ameloblastoma, or the fortuitous occurrence of two separate lesions. The clinical data are based on only 12 reported cases, so this information could change as more reports are published.

Clinical Features

The average age at diagnosis is 19 years, and the oldest patient was 50 years old at the time of diagnosis. The tumors were almost evenly divided between the maxilla and the mandible, and 67% were posterior to the canines. Almost all reported tumors have been expansile, and one-third of patients complained of pain.

Radiographic Appearance

This lesion produces a mixed radiographic appearance in which the radiopacity becomes more apparent with time. The lesion is usually well defined, but some tumors have demonstrated aggressive growth. Because of the size and density of the tumor, it is not always possible to visualize the enamel in the odontoma portion. An associated impacted tooth was noted in at least 5 of the 12 cases (42%).

Histopathologic Findings

There is a haphazard arrangement of a typical odontoma adjacent to islands of ameloblastoma. An important feature is that the connective tissue surrounding the ameloblastic islands appears mature in contrast to the embryonic tissue found in an ameloblastic fibroma or an ameloblastic fibro-odontoma.

Treatment

Of nine patients with follow-up, three experienced recurrences 6 to 49 months after the initial surgery. One patient had two documented recurrences. **In contrast to the ameloblastic fibroma, the ameloblastic odontoma should be treated like an ameloblastoma because of the demonstrated aggressive expansion and the 33% recurrence rate.**

References

Frissell, C.T., and Shafer, W.G.: Ameloblastic odontoma: Report of a case. Oral Surg. Oral Med. Oral Pathol., 6:1129–1133, 1953.

Kaugars, G.E., and Zussman, H.W.: Ameloblastic odontoma (odonto-ameloblastoma): Report of a case. Oral Surg. Oral Med. Oral Pathol. (in press, 1990).

CALCIFYING ODONTOGENIC CYST

There is confusion about whether this lesion is best classified as an odontogenic cyst or a tumor because it has features of both (Fig. 4–12). It is not known whether it is an odontogenic cyst that sometimes has the clinical and histologic features of a neoplasm or whether it is a neoplasm that often undergoes cystic degeneration. Regardless of their classification, calcifying odontogenic cysts are characterized by a unique histopathologic appearance that confirms their odontogenic origin.

Synonym: Gorlin cyst

Clinical Features

The calcifying odontogenic cyst can occur in either an intraosseous (75%) or an extraosseous (25%) location. Central lesions are usually diagnosed during the second decade of life, but a wide age range has been reported. Analysis of several studies shows variability in the most common location, which implies that it occurs throughout the jawbones. A relatively high number are associated with odontomas (47%) or dentigerous cysts (20%). Roughly half of the reported tumors caused clinical expansion.

Peripheral calcifying odontogenic cysts are diagnosed at a later age (mean, 45 years) and are evenly divided between the mandible and the maxilla. A majority occurred between the canines, and none was posterior to the first molar. Clinically, the lesions are usually less than 1 cm in diameter and present as a painless mass.

It is tempting to speculate that central and peripheral calcifying odontogenic cysts are two separate lesions or at least arise from two different sources of epithelium. No substantive proof exists for either theory.

Radiographic Appearance

Central lesions typically appear as well-defined radiolucencies that may contain small areas of opacification or, rarely, large foci that dominate the radiographic appearance. Multiloculation is more likely in larger lesions. The presence of an associated odontoma is a common finding, as is cystic degeneration. Saucerization of the cortical bone was seen in 17% of the peripheral lesions. These lesions may displace teeth. Twenty percent of reported cases are associated with impacted teeth (Langland et al, 1982).

Histopathologic Findings

Thickening of the stellate reticulum–type cystic epithelium, a distinctive hyperchromatic basal cell layer, eosinophilic ghost cells, and deposits of dystrophic calcification are the histologic hallmarks. Patients with tumors diagnosed as peripheral lesions should have a radiograph of the area taken to rule out the possibility of cortical perforation by a central lesion. The ghost cells and calcifications are not unique because they are found also with some frequency in odontomas.

Treatment

Because of the low recurrence rate, surgical enucleation is usually adequate for central lesions, and conservative excision is indicated for extraosseous cases.

References

Altini, M., and Farman, A.G.: The calcifying odontogenic cyst: Eight new cases and a review of the literature. Oral Surg. Oral Med. Oral Pathol., 40:751–759, 1975.

Freedman, P., Lumerman, H., and Gee, J.: Calcifying odontogenic cyst: A review and analysis of seventy cases. Oral Surg. Oral Med. Oral Pathol., 40:93–106, 1975.

Kaugars, C.C., Kaugars, G.E., and DeBiasi, G.F.: Extraosseous calcifying odontogenic cyst: Case report and a review of the literature. J. Am. Dent. Assoc., 119:715–718, 1989.

Langland, O.E., Langlais, R.P., Morris, C.R.: Principles and Practice of Panoramic Radiology. Philadelphia: W.B. Saunders, 1982, pp. 263–264.

Shamaskin, R.G., Svirsky, J.A., and Kaugars, G.E.: Intraosseous and extraosseous calcifying odontogenic cyst (Gorlin cyst). J. Oral Maxillofac. Surg., 47:562–565, 1989.

Praetorius, F., Hjorting-Hansen, E., Gorlin, R.J., et al: Calcifying odontogenic cyst: Range, variations and neoplastic potential. Acta Odontol. Scand., 39:227–240, 1981.

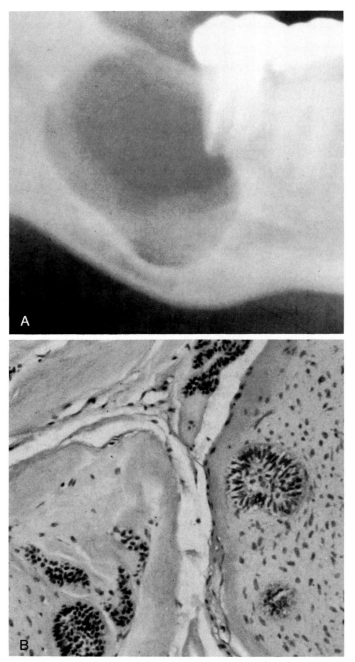

Figure 4–8. *A,* This recurrent ameloblastic fibroma shows the potential for aggressive growth in these tumors. (Courtesy of Dr. B. Malbon, Richmond, Virginia.) *B,* The diagnosis of ameloblastic fibroma is made primarily on the basis of the appearance of the connective tissue, not the presence of the odontogenic epithelial islands, which resemble those in ameloblastoma.

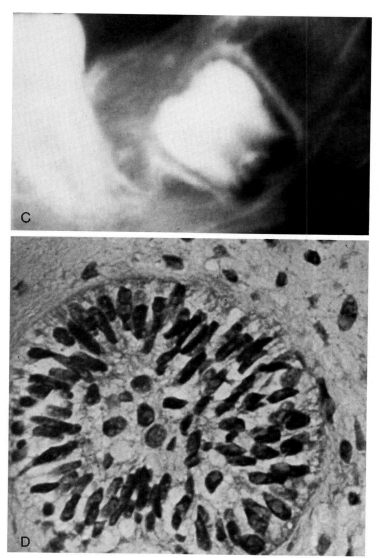

Figure 4–8 *Continued C,* This ameloblastic fibroma presented as a radiolucent area around an impacted mandibular second molar in a 10-year-old boy. The delayed eruption of one tooth in a child should prompt the clinician to obtain a radiograph to rule out the possibility of an odontogenic tumor. (Courtesy of Dr. J. Nelson, Richmond, Virginia.) *D,* Considerable similarity to ameloblastoma is evident in this section, but the embryonic appearance of the connective tissue is the diagnostic clue.

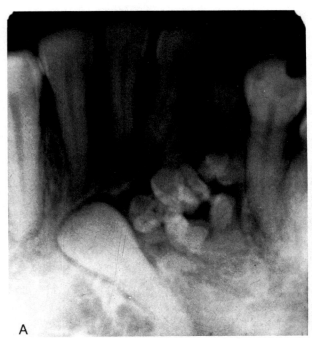

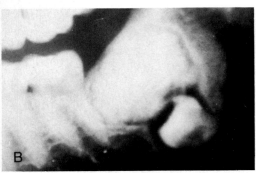

Figure 4–9. *A,* This lesion is unorganized, but the opacities resemble tooth-like structures. The diagnosis of odontoma is made because of the presence of foci of enamel radiodensities. *B,* A complex odontoma. No discernible separate tooth-like structures are present, simply a solid radiopaque mass with a radiolucent rim. (Part *F* shows another complex odontoma.)

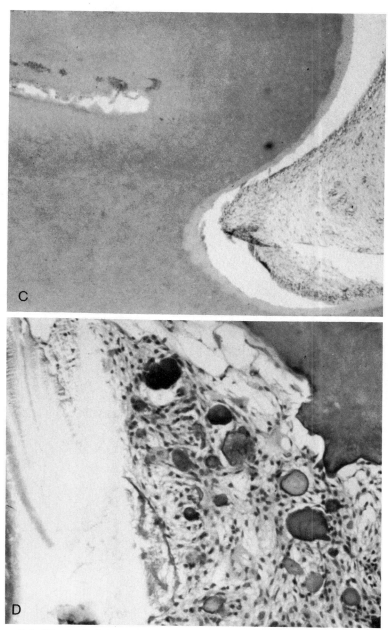

Figure 4–9 *Continued C,* Histologically, an odontoma can be best described as a tooth that was designed by a committee! Although all the components of a tooth are present, there is a haphazard arrangement. Some odontomas resemble recognizable teeth because they contain pulpal tissue within normal-appearing dentin. *D,* Other odontomas are less organized and have areas of enamel matrix, irregularly shaped pieces of dentin, and cementum-like droplets within the connective tissue. The probability of seeing enamel radiodensities on a radiograph decreases in the less organized odontomas.

Illustration continued on following page

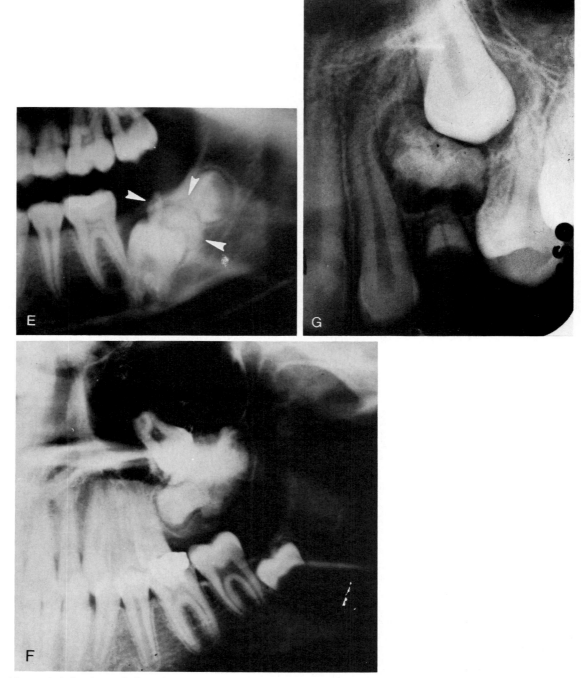

Figure 4–9 *Continued E,* Complex odontoma in mandibular molar region. Small opacity resembles a tooth (*arrow*). Eruption of the second permanent molar has been prevented. (Courtesy of Dr. C. Tomich, Indiana University School of Dentistry, Indianapolis, Indiana.) *F,* Large, well-defined radiopacity in the maxillary left quadrant. The lesion is surrounded by a cortical outline and a radiolucent rim, almost like a target lesion. Two molars are impacted because of this complex odontoma. *G,* Complex odontoma in the anterior maxilla preventing eruption of a permanent canine.

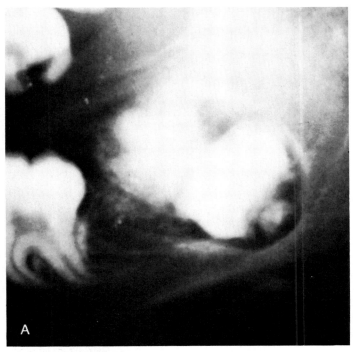

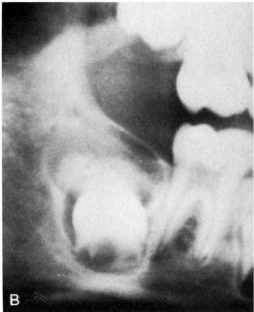

Figure 4–10. *A,* The ameloblastic fibro-odontoma is considered by some to be an immature odontoma. Its radiographic similarity to an odontoma is seen in this case, which shows an impacted tooth associated with a well-defined radiopacity surrounded by a radiolucent band. (Courtesy of Dr. J. Riviere, Richmond, Virginia.) *B,* Ameloblastic fibro-odontoma. A pericoronal radiolucency containing radiopacities. This patient was about 8 years old.
Illustration continued on following page

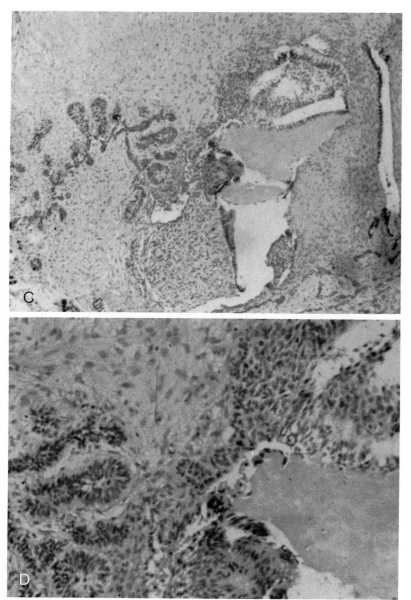

Figure 4–10 *Continued C,* This unique lesion contains the histologic features of both an ameloblastic fibroma and an odontoma. The former usually makes up the bulk of the specimen, but areas of typical odontoma are easily located. *D,* The amorphic areas in close proximity to the epithelial cells represent portions of the odontoma. In light of present thinking, the calcifications would be expected to increase with time because this lesion is generally thought to be an immature odontoma.

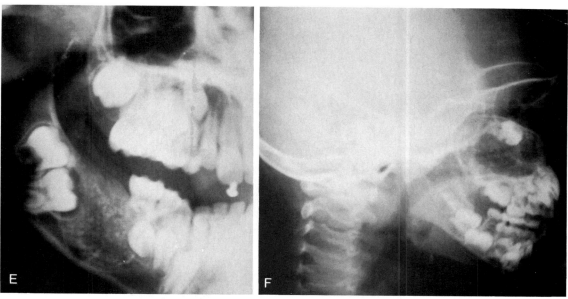

Figure 4–10 *Continued E,* A large, well-defined radiolucency with a cortical rim around much of its periphery. There are numerous radiopaque flecks within the lesion. Displacement of multiple teeth is seen. This is an ameloblastic fibro-odontoma in a young man. *F,* Ameloblastic fibro-odontoma filling the entire maxillary sinus. Developing first molar has been displaced up to the orbit in a 4-year-old. Note internal opacities.

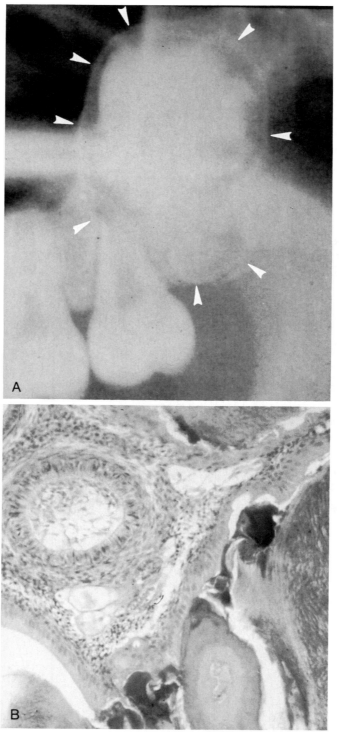

Figure 4–11. *A,* This is an example of a rare ameloblastic odontoma *(arrows)* found in the posterior maxilla of a 15-year-old boy. The patient had been aware of a slow-growing expansion during the previous 2 years before this lesion was removed. A resemblance to an odontoma is noted, but the large size is more suggestive of an ameloblastic odontoma. (Courtesy of Dr. H. Zussman, Fairfax, Virginia.) *B,* Ameloblastic islands placed randomly among elements of an odontoma describe this rare tumor. However, the ameloblastic islands do not appear to be actively producing any of the calcified structures.

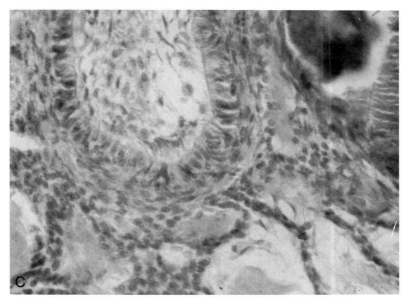

Figure 4–11 *Continued C,* The ameloblastic islands demonstrate prominent peripheral palisading and polarization with a central area that is similar to stellate reticulum.

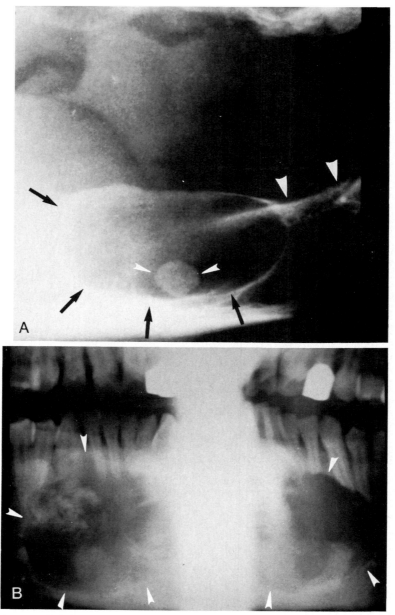

Figure 4–12. *A,* A large, well-defined, expansile, unilocular COC *(black arrows)* with a solitary radiopacity within the cyst *(small white arrowheads)*. Note the cortical outline. *Large white arrowheads* point to the external oblique ridge. This COC has not perforated or remodeled the external oblique ridge or the inferior cortical border of the mandible. *B,* Another COC. This large, expansile, mixed radiolucent-radiopaque lesion in the anterior mandible *(arrowheads)* has displaced teeth and resorbed roots—more like tumor behavior than cystic behavior. Note that there are several foci of calcifications internally. The opacity near the apices of the lower right premolars is a coexisting torus.

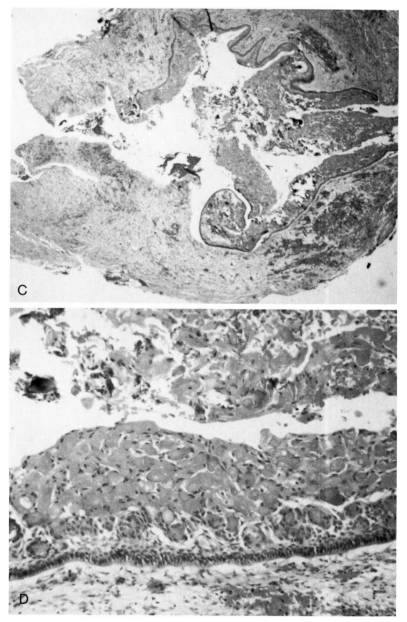

Figure 4–12 *Continued C,* Thickened cystic epithelium with a prominent basal cell layer and foci that resemble stellate reticulum are seen in this low-power view. *D,* A high-power view shows ghost cells (epithelial cells that have lost their nuclei) and deeply staining calcifications.

MALIGNANT NEOPLASMS

J. Lovas

PRIMARY NONODONTOGENIC MALIGNANT NEOPLASMS WITHIN JAWBONES
OSTEOSARCOMA (Osteogenic Sarcoma)
CHONDROSARCOMA
EWING'S SARCOMA
MYELOMA (Multiple Myeloma)
LYMPHOMA
  Hodgkin's Lymphoma
  Non-Hodgkin's Lymphoma (Burkitt's Lymphoma)

LEUKEMIA
Acute
Chronic

PRIMARY ODONTOGENIC MALIGNANT NEOPLASMS

PRIMARY MALIGNANCIES ADJACENT TO JAWS (SQUAMOUS CELL CARCINOMA, VERRUCOUS CARCINOMA, ADENOCARCINOMA)

METASTASES TO THE JAWS

The diagnosis of all lesions, but especially those involving bone, requires careful correlation of all pertinent information. Rarely is a single type of data, be it clinical, radiographic, or histologic, adequate for diagnosis of jaw lesions. Likewise, radiographic examination of an important lesion should never be limited to a single view.

The cause of malignant neoplasms is in general unknown. In most cases, even knowledge of risk factors or premalignant lesions is minimal. Iatrogenic or accidental exposure to ionizing radiation is the major exception. There is an increased risk of developing a variety of **radiation-induced sarcomas** years after exposure. Radiation therapy (e.g., for squamous cell carcinomas of the oral mucosa) does not destroy all the normal cells at the periphery of the radiation field but can transform these cells (e.g., osteocytes) into malignant cells after a latent period of, on average, 10 to 14 years. With increasing long-term survival following cancer treatment, the incidence of radiation-induced sarcomas is also likely to increase.

Malignant neoplasms of the jaws, like those affecting the rest of the skeleton, are described as primary or secondary and central or peripheral. **Primary** refers to de novo origin within normal bone, **secondary** to origin within a preexisting benign bony lesion. Unfortunately, the adjective secondary is often also used as a synonym for metastatic. **Central** refers to an intraosseous origin, whereas **peripheral** refers to an extraosseous (i.e., soft tissue) origin.

PRIMARY NONODONTOGENIC MALIGNANT NEOPLASMS WITHIN JAWBONES

OSTEOSARCOMA (Osteogenic Sarcoma)

Osteosarcoma is defined as a malignant neoplasm in which malignant connective tissue cells directly form osteoid (the organic matrix of bone). A histologic definition is necessary because other malignant, some benign neoplastic, and some reactive processes can closely resemble osteosarcoma clinically, radiographically, and even histologically. Chondrosarcomas and fibrosarcomas resemble chondroblastic and fibroblastic osteosarcomas, respectively. Osteoblastomas and healing fracture calluses can also be difficult to differentiate histologically from osteosarcoma.

After myeloma, osteosarcoma is the most common primary malignant neoplasm of bone. The distal femur and proximal tibia of young adults are most frequently involved. Only about 9% of osteosarcomas affect the craniofacial bones (Dahlin and Unni, 1986).

Although most osteosarcomas are idiopathic, patients with Paget's disease of bone or fibrous dysplasia and those who have had previous irradiation are at increased risk. **Radiation-induced osteosarcoma** is an iatrogenic form of osteosarcoma that usually occurs in a much older age group than ordinary (idiopathic) osteosarcoma. There are also numerous rare subtypes of osteosarcoma —peripheral, parosteal, periosteal, telangiectatic, and so on—that are beyond the scope of this text.

Clinical Features

A rapidly growing, painless or minimally painful mass is the most common presenting feature of osteosarcomas of the jaw. Oral mucosal ulceration, tooth mobility, displacement and loosening of teeth, paresthesia, and toothache have all been reported in varying frequencies (Garrington et al, 1967; Clark et al, 1983; Forteza et al, 1986). Regional lymph node metastasis is usually absent at the time of initial diagnosis. The average age of patients with craniofacial osteosarcoma is 34, a decade older than those with lesions of long bone (Lee et al, 1988).

Radiographic Appearance

An ill-defined osteolytic, osteoblastic, or mixed lesion with either an osteoid or a chondroid type of tumor matrix mineralization and soft tissue extension is strongly suggestive of osteosarcoma (Lee et al, 1988). Maxillary lesions frequently arise from the alveolar ridge. Mandibular lesions tend to arise from the body of the mandible. Periosteal reaction is infrequent in craniofacial osteosarcomas, especially in the maxilla. Even though the most common histologic form is chondroblastic, the most common radiographic type of tumor matrix mineralization is osteoid calcification (Lee et al, 1988).

The earliest and most subtle radiographic signs are a unilateral, symmetrically widened, periodontal ligament space about the root of a tooth (Garrington et al, 1967) and irregular widening of the mandibular canal with areas of narrowing and loss of the cortical margins (Yagan et al, 1985).

Osteomyelitis is the most common non-neoplastic disease simulating a malignant process in the mandible (Finkelstein, 1970). The most common form of osteomyelitis mimicking osteosarcoma is the chronic focal sclerosing type (see Chapter 2). Focal periapical osteopetrosis is another common condition that must be distinguished from osteosarcoma.

Computed tomography (CT) is excellent for detecting tumor calcification, cortical involvement, and soft tissue as well as intramedullary extension. Magnetic resonance imaging (MRI) is even better than CT for demonstrating intramedullary and extraosseous tumor components (Lee et al, 1988).

Histopathologic Findings

Neoplastic cells are oval or spindle-shaped with hyperchromatic nuclei. The periphery of the lesion tends to be richly cellular, whereas the central areas tend to exhibit a "lacy" pattern of ossification (osteoblastic pattern) (Figs. 5–1*B* and 5–2*C*). Cartilage may predominate (chondroblastic pattern) (Fig. 5–3*B*), or the lesion may be composed primarily of spindle cells (fibroblastic pattern) (Fig. 5–4*B*). Direct osteoid formation by malignant osteoblasts must be present for a diagnosis of osteosarcoma.

Treatment

Radical surgery appears to offer the best prognosis. Every attempt should be made to excise the neoplasm completely at the initial definitive surgery (Verner et al, 1984). The survival rates are 35% for 5 years, 30% for 10 years, and 15% for 15 years. Metastases tend to occur within 2 years of primary therapy and tend to involve the lungs and brain (Garrington et al, 1967; Batsakis et al, 1980).

References

Batsakis, J.G., Solomon, A.R., and Rice, D.H.: The pathology of head and neck tumors: Neoplasms of cartilage, bone and notochord. Head Neck Surg., 3:43–57, 1980.

Clark, J.L., Unni, K.K., Dahlin, D.C., and Devine, K.D.: Osteosarcoma of the jaw. Cancer, 51:2311–2316, 1983.

Dahlin, D.C., and Unni, K.K.: Bone Tumors. General Aspects and Data on 8,542 Cases, 4th ed. Springfield, Ill.: Charles C Thomas, 1986, p. 271.

Finkelstein, J.B.: Osteosarcoma of the jaw bones. Radiol. Clin. North Am., 8:425–443, 1970.

Forteza, G., Colmenero, B., and Lopez-Barea, F.: Osteogenic sarcoma of the maxilla and mandible. Oral Surg. Oral Med. Oral Pathol., 62:179–184, 1986.

Garrington, G.E., Scofield, H.H., Cornyn, J., and Hooker, S.P.: Osteosarcoma of the jaws: Analysis of 56 cases. Cancer, 20:377–391, 1967.

Lee, Y.Y., Van Tassel, P., Nauert, C., Raymond, A.K., and Edeiken, J.: Craniofacial osteosarcomas: Plain film, CT, and MR findings in 46 cases. Am. J. Radiol., 150:1397–1402, 1988.

Verner, J., Rice, D.H., and Newman, A.N.: Osteosarcoma and chondrosarcoma of the head and neck. Laryngoscope, 94:240–242, 1984.

Yagan, R., Radivoyevitch, M., and Bellon, E.M.: Involvement of the mandibular canal: Early sign of osteogenic sarcoma of the mandible. Oral Surg. Oral Med. Oral Pathol., 60:56–60, 1985.

CHONDROSARCOMA

Chondrosarcoma is defined histologically as a malignant neoplasm characterized by malignant connective tissue cells directly forming cartilage. Cartilage can ossify in normal cartilaginous tissue and in chondrosarcomas as well as in chondroblastic osteosarcomas. The critical distinction between osteosarcomas and chondrosarcomas is that only in osteosarcomas is there direct formation of osteoid or bone by malignant cells (Cotran et al, 1989).

Only about 10% of all primary malignant neoplasms of bone are chondrosarcomas, and only 1 to 10% of all these occur in the head and neck, mostly in the jaws. Osteosarcomas are about twice as common and Ewing's sarcomas half as common as chondrosarcomas. Cartilage, a normal finding in the incisive papillar area, is a possible site of origin for maxillary chondrosarcomas.

Mesenchymal chondrosarcoma is a rare, somewhat distinctive type of chondrosarcoma with a predilection for the facial bones (and ribs); it tends to occur in the second and third decades of life, is associated with a poor prognosis, and has a distinct histologic appearance (Christensen, 1982).

Chondrosarcomas are often difficult to diagnose clinically and radiographically as well as histologically. As with any jaw lesion, careful correlation of all pertinent data is essential.

Clinical Features

Preceding trauma, a benign bony or cartilaginous lesion, and a family history of sarcoma of bone appear to be risk factors. The most common initial complaint is the presence of a firm swelling or mass. A lobular periphery, typical of chondrosarcoma, may be clinically apparent. In fewer than half the cases, dull or sharp pain is present. Other symptoms can include loose, separated teeth, paresthesia, and nasal obstruction. The mean age is 33, and the age range is 16 to 67 (Garrington and Collett, 1988a and 1988b). The mandibular condyle is rarely involved (Nortjé et al, 1976).

Radiographic Appearance

Chondrosarcomas share the radiographic features of malignant neoplasms in general and osteosarcomas in particular. The majority are osteolytic with poorly defined margins. Scattered radiopaque foci represent calcification in neoplastic cartilage.

On one end of the spectrum of appearances are highly calcified lesions in which the central area is most densely radiopaque, with the opacity diminishing peripherally in a sunburst pattern. On the other end are purely radiolucent lesions in which the lobular pattern of growth mimics multilocular cysts. Characteristic of chondrosarcoma are discrete striae, ringlets, and pinpoint areas of radiopacity within an area of radiolucency (Nortjé et al, 1976). Chondrosarcomas, like certain other lesions with an infiltrative growth pattern, can occasionally escape radiographic detection by permeating marrow spaces without destroying normal bone trabeculae. Subtle extension of malignant neoplasms into adjacent bone is the principal reason why clinically and radiographically normal-appearing bony margins must be routinely excised or included in the field of therapeutic radiation.

An early radiographic sign of chondrosarcoma (like osteosarcoma) is unilateral, symmetric widening of the periodontal ligament space about the root of a tooth (Garrington and Collett, 1988a and 1988b).

Computed tomography is very useful in determining the margins of the lesion, especially extension into adjacent structures such as sinuses and soft tissues.

Histopathologic Findings

Cartilage containing cytologically atypical chondrocytes is the main histologic feature. Plump chondrocyte nuclei, binucleate chondrocytes, and occasional giant chondrocytes are seen (Figs. 5–5B and 5–6). The peripheral portions of the tumor lobules are the most cellular and least differentiated and thus should undergo biopsy to facilitate accurate histopathologic diagnosis. Calcification, sometimes extensive, and ossification are common. Histologic grading is useful for estimating prognosis—the less differentiated, the poorer the prognosis (Garrington and Collett, 1988a and 1988b).

Treatment

Early radical surgery appears to offer the best prognosis. Recurrence following incomplete excision is usually prompt but has occurred after 13 years. Death usually results from uncontrolled local disease with direct extension into the brain. Because regional lymph node involvement is uncommon, neck dissection does not appear to be beneficial. Metastases are usually to the lungs. The survival rates are 32% for 5 years, 15% for 10 years, and 0% for 15 years—somewhat worse than for osteosarcoma (Garrington and Collett, 1988a and 1988b).

References

Christensen, R.E.: Mesenchymal chondrosarcoma of the jaws. Oral Surg. Oral Med. Oral Pathol., 54:197–206, 1982.

Cotran, R.S., Kumar, V., and Robbins, S.L.: Robbins Pathologic Basis of Disease, 4th ed. Philadelphia: W.B. Saunders, 1989, pp. 1340–1342.

Garrington, G.E., and Collett, W.K.: Chondrosarcoma. I. A selected literature review. J. Oral Pathol., 17:1–11, 1988a.

Garrington, G.E., and Collett, W.K.: Chondrosarcoma. II. Chondrosarcoma of the jaws: Analysis of 37 cases. J. Oral Pathol., 17:12–20, 1988b.

Nortjé, C.J., Farman, A.G., Grotepass, F.W., and Van Zyl, J.A.: Chondrosarcoma of the mandibular condyle. Report of a case with special reference to radiographic features. Br. J. Oral Surg., 14:101–111, 1976.

EWING'S SARCOMA

Ewing's sarcoma is a rare, aggressive, primary malignant neoplasm of bone, most frequently affecting the long bones of children between 10 and 15 years of age. Only 4 to 6% of primary malignant bone neoplasms are Ewing's sarcomas, and only 1 to 4% of these involve the head and neck. Location of the primary site is the most important predictor of clinical behavior; pelvic bone involvement is associated with the worst prognosis, long bone involvement with intermediate prognosis, and jaw bone involvement with the best prognosis. The combination of prompt diagnosis and multimodal therapy including surgery, chemotherapy, and radiotherapy is resulting in markedly improved outcomes (Cotran et al, 1989).

Clinical Features

The average age at diagnosis of Ewing's sarcoma of the head and neck is 11 years, and the age range is 3 to 23. There is a slight male predominance. In the United States the majority of patients are white.

The most frequent presenting feature is a painful bony-hard swelling or soft tissue mass. Elevation of the periosteum, caused by the neoplasm breaking through the cortex, gives rise to pain. Teeth can be displaced without root resorption. Invasion of the orbital floor can give rise to rotation of the eye. With head and neck lesions, fever, weight loss, and changes in alkaline phosphatase, blood urea nitrogen (BUN) and aspartate aminotransferase (AST) are uncommon. In the head and neck, the most common primary sites (in decreasing order) are the skull, mandible, maxilla, and ethmoid sinuses (Siegal et al, 1987).

Asymptomatic metastases, primarily to the lungs and other bones, can occur up to 6 months after diagnosis.

Radiographic Appearance

The radiographic features are not pathognomonic, only suggestive of a malignancy or infectious process. On plain films a poorly defined, permeative lesion with a lamellated (onion-skin) or spiculated (sun-ray) periosteal reaction and an associated soft tissue mass is typically described in long bones. However, periosteal reaction, cortical thickening, and sclerotic change (the latter representing necrotic bone) were infrequently observed in a series of 32 cases involving the head and neck (Siegal et al, 1987). Lamellated periosteal reactions are less frequently seen in the jaws, possibly because of the complex anatomy (de Santos and Jing, 1978). Purely lytic change, honeycombing, bone expansion, and cortical violation are more common than in long bones because the cortices of the thinner bones of the head and neck are more easily violated (Siegal et al, 1987). Displacement of teeth and developing tooth buds, without resorption, has been reported (de Santos and Jing, 1978). In the head and neck, because of differences in presentation on plain films and because of the difficulty in demonstrating soft tissue extension, computed tomography has been strongly recommended for staging prior to therapy.

Histopathologic Findings

Ewing's sarcoma appears to be of neuroectodermal origin (Cotran et al, 1989). Lesions are highly cellular, often with prominent areas of necrosis and hemorrhage. Viable round cells with relatively large nuclei often cluster around blood vessels. This is one of the few malignant neoplasms that does not have prominent nuclear pleomorphism, prominent nucleoli, or many mitoses. Cells are poorly cohesive and exhibit little intercellular stroma (Figs. 5–7*E* and 5–8*B*). Intracytoplasmic glycogen, a frequent (but not constant) finding, is useful in differentiating this neoplasm from primary lymphoma of bone.

Treatment

Like Ewing's sarcoma of long bones, jaw lesions are treated by multimodal therapy including radiotherapy and multicourse chemotherapy with or without surgery. If there is no relapse or metastasis 3 years after treatment of the primary tumor, cure is highly probable. As in any irradiated site, there is a low but long-term risk of developing radiation-induced sarcoma.

References

Cotran, R.S., Kumar, V., and Robbins, S.L.: Robbins Pathologic Basis of Disease, 4th ed. Philadelphia: W.B. Saunders, 1989, pp. 1342–1343.
de Santos, L.A., and Jing B.S.: Radiographic findings of Ewing's sarcoma of the jaws. Br. J. Radiol., 51:682–687, 1978.
Siegal, G.P., Oliver, W.R., Reinus, W.R., Gilula, L.A., Foulkes, M.A., Kissane, J.M., and Askin, F.B.: Primary Ewing's sarcoma involving the bones of the head and neck. Cancer 60:2829–2840, 1987.

MYELOMA (Multiple Myeloma)

Myeloma is the most common primary malignant neoplasm of bone in adults. It usually arises in marrow spaces and later disseminates throughout the body. As in other malignancies, the proliferating cells are **monoclonal** (all derived from a single cell) and therefore produce the same cell product—in this case, the same immunoglobulin. Elevated levels of complete or incomplete monoclonal immunoglobulins can be detected in the plasma or urine. **Bence Jones proteins** are monoclonal light-chain components of immunoglobulin found in the urine of patients with myeloma (Cotran et al, 1989).

The key steps in diagnosing myeloma include a positive history of bone pain, radiographic documentation of multiple punched-out radiolucencies in bones, serum electrophoretic identification of myeloma proteins in the blood or urine, and histologic identification of monoclonal plasma cell infiltrates (Cotran et al, 1989).

In decreasing order of frequency, the vertebrae, ribs, skull, pelvis, femur, clavicles, and scapula are affected. Patients are usually around age 55. Bone pain, pathologic fractures, and hypercalcemia result from infiltration and destruction of medullary and then cortical bone. Infections and renal failure, due to suppression of normal B cells by the neoplasm, and renal toxicity resulting from Bence Jones proteins are the chief causes of death. Despite chemotherapy, the average survival time is around 3 years (Cotran et al, 1989).

Myeloma is closely related to three relatively rare forms of plasma cell dyscrasia: **plasma cell myelomatosis, solitary plasmacytoma of bone (solitary myeloma),** and **extramedullary plas-**

macytoma. A variable proportion of these are transformed to myeloma within 20 years (Cataldo and Meyer, 1966; Batsakis, 1979; Corwin and Lindberg, 1979). The remainder of the discussion is about myeloma.

Clinical Features

The mandible is involved in 5 to 30% of cases of myeloma (maxillary lesions are rare) (Cataldo and Meyer, 1966; Lambertenghi-Deliliers et al, 1988). The angle, molar, and premolar regions are most frequently affected. Patients are usually asymptomatic. Complaints of local pain, swelling, and paresthesia are associated with large lytic lesions (Lambertenghi-Deliliers et al, 1988).

Radiographic Appearance

Diffuse, often marked osteoporosis, frequently combined with multiple small punched-out radiolucencies, is characteristic (Fig. 5–9). There is usually no osteosclerotic bone reaction to the well-delineated, circular radiolucencies (Cataldo and Meyer, 1966). Mandibular lesions may be the initial manifestation of myeloma but more often are found after diagnosis, usually along with skull lesions (Lambertenghi-Deliliers et al, 1988).

Histopathologic Findings

The histologic picture is dominated by sheets of atypical plasma cells that replace the normal bony trabeculae (Figs. 5–8*B* and 5–10*A*). Although the cells can exhibit varying degrees of differentiation, they may closely resemble reactive plasma cells. Only myelomas with surface ulceration contain a mixture of inflammatory cells among the plasma cells, thus mimicking a purely inflammatory process. Immunoperoxidase staining is very useful for distinguishing reactive (inflammatory, polyclonal) plasma cell infiltrates in patients with chronic periodontitis from neoplastic (monoclonal) ones (Wright et al, 1981).

Treatment

No treatment regimen for myeloma is curative. Remission is achieved with combination chemotherapy, sometimes combined with autologous bone marrow transplants and total body irradiation (Durie, 1989). Mean survival is around 3 years. The presence of mandibular lesions suggests an advanced clinical stage (Lambertenghi-Deliliers et al, 1988).

References

Batsakis, J.G.: Tumors of the Head and Neck. Clinical and Pathological Considerations, 2nd ed. Baltimore: Williams & Wilkins, 1979, pp. 383–387.

Cataldo, E., and Meyer, I.: Solitary and multiple plasma-cell tumors of the jaws and oral cavity. Oral Surg. Oral Med. Oral Pathol., 22:628–639, 1966.

Corwin, J., and Lindberg, R.D.: Solitary plasmacytoma of bone vs. extramedullary plasmacytoma and their relationship to multiple myeloma. Cancer 43:1007–1013, 1979.

Cotran, R.S., Kumar, V., and Robbins, S.L.: Robbins Pathologic Basis of Disease, 4th ed. Philadelphia: W.B. Saunders, 1989, p. 743.

Durie, B.G.M.: Approach to the management of plasma cell disorders. *In* Kelley, W.N. (ed.): Textbook of Internal Medicine, Vol. 1. Philadelphia: J.B. Lippincott, 1989, pp. 1324–1331.

Lambertenghi-Deliliers, G., Bruno, E., Cortelezzi, A., Fumagalli, L., and Morosini, A.: Incidence of jaw lesions in 193 patients with multiple myeloma. Oral Surg. Oral Med. Oral Pathol., 65:533–537, 1988.

Wright, B.A., Wysocki, G.P., and Bannerjee, D.: Diagnostic use of immunoperoxidase techniques for plasma cell lesions of the jaws. Oral Surg. Oral Med. Oral Pathol., 52:615–622, 1981.

LYMPHOMA

Lymphomas are malignant neoplasms characterized by monoclonal proliferation of cells native to lymphoid tissue, i.e., most often lymphocytes but sometimes histiocytes or their precursors. All forms of lymphoma have the potential to disseminate from the lymphatics to the spleen, liver, and bone marrow and eventually into the blood stream. Clinical staging (Ann Arbor classification) for lymphomas is based on the number and distribution of nodal and extranodal sites involved as well as the presence or absence of fever, night sweats, and weight loss. Lymphomas are classified as Hodgkin's or non-Hodgkin's types (Cotran et al, 1989).

Hodgkin's Lymphoma

Hodgkin's lymphoma is a relatively uncommon malignancy. This form of lymphoma tends to remain restricted to the lymphoid tissues. Involvement of Waldeyer's ring or other extranodal sites such as the jaws is uncommon. The disease is characterized histologically by the presence of neoplastic giant cells called the **Reed-Sternberg cells,** usually accompanied by a reactive inflammatory cell infiltrate. The average age at diagnosis is 32. This disease is now curable in most cases (Cotran et al, 1989).

Non-Hodgkin's Lymphoma
(Burkitt's Lymphoma)

Non-Hodgkin's lymphoma (NHL), although most often presenting as a generalized or localized lymphadenopathy, arises extranodally in a third of cases—e.g., in Waldeyer's ring, bone marrow. The currently accepted classification of NHL is called the Working Formulation for Clinical Usage. It has three major prognostic groupings, each with a different probability for 5-year survival: low grade, 50 to 70%; intermediate, 35 to 45%; and high grade, 23 to 32% (Cotran et al, 1989). **Burkitt's lymphoma** is an uncommon form of NHL that is endemic in Africa but uncommon in North America. Unlike African Burkitt's, the American form involves the jaws relatively infrequently.

Clinical Features. Although extranodal presentation of NHL is common, oral lesions are uncommon. When oral lesions do occur, they are more likely to be part of a more generalized regional involvement than a primary. Oral soft tissues are more often involved than the jawbones. Fourteen of the 31 oral cases (45%) reviewed by Eisenbud et al (1984) arose in the jaws—i.e., were **primary lymphomas of bone** (formerly known as primary reticulum cell sarcomas). The posterior maxilla and mandible were the most common sites. Presenting symptoms and signs include painful or painless, ulcerated or nonulcerated, soft or firm swellings, paresthesia, and tooth mobility. Primary Hodgkin's lymphoma of the jawbones is rare, but secondary involvement occurs in 5 to 15% of cases (Cohen et al, 1984). Extranodal lymphomas in general and primary lymphomas of the jawbones in particular are more difficult to diagnose and classify than lymphomas arising in nodal tissue (Robbins et al, 1986).

Radiographic Appearance. Initially, radiographic changes consist of subtle osteoporosis. The neoplasm can be present in the medullary bone and inferior alveolar canal, causing nerve compression and paresthesia before radiographically detectable change develops (Wang and Fleishil, 1968). Later, large, ill-defined radiolucent lesions are characteristic. The intramedullary mass can expand, erode, or perforate the cortex, giving rise to a soft tissue mass.

Histopathologic Findings. Sheets of monoclonal lymphocytes replacing the normal bony trabeculae are characteristic (Figs. 5–11C and D). The complex and everchanging histologic classification of lymphomas is beyond the scope of this book. Burkitt's lymphomas have been shown to devitalize teeth by completely replacing the pulp with neoplastic cells.

Treatment. Hodgkin's lymphoma is treated with radiotherapy alone, chemotherapy alone, or a combination of both. NHL is treated with combination chemotherapy (Longo and Urba, 1989). The prognosis for lymphomas of the jaws appears to be similar to that of lymphomas of extragnathic sites with a corresponding clinical stage and histologic type and frequency of mitoses (Eisenbud et al, 1983; Robbins et al, 1986; Fukuda et al, 1987).

References

Cohen, M.A., Bender, S., and Struthers, P.J.: Hodgkin's diseases of the jaws. Review of the literature and report of a case. Oral Surg. Oral Med. Oral Pathol., 57:413–417, 1984.

Cotran, R.S., Kumar, V., and Robbins, S.L.: Robbins Pathologic Basis of Disease, 4th ed. Philadelphia: W.B. Saunders, 1989, pp. 708–722.

Eisenbud, L., Sciubba, J., Mir, R., and Sachs, S.A.: Oral presentations in non-Hodgkin's lymphoma: A review of thirty-one cases. Part I. Data analysis. Oral Surg. Oral Med. Oral Pathol., 56:151–156, 1983.

Eisenbud, L., Sciubba, J., Mir, R., and Sachs, S.A.: Oral presentations in non-Hodgkin's lymphoma: A review of thirty-one cases. Part II. Fourteen cases arising in bone. Oral Surg. Oral Med. Oral Pathol., 57:272–280, 1984.

Fukuda, Y., Ishida, T., Fujimoto, M., Ueda, T., and Aozasa. K.: Malignant lymphoma of the oral cavity: Clinicopathologic analysis of 20 cases. J. Oral Pathol., 16:8–12, 1987.

Longo, D.L., and Urba, W.J.: Differential diagnosis of lymphadenopathy and approach to the management of lymphomas. In Kelley, W.N. (ed.): Textbook of Internal Medicine, Vol. 1. Philadelphia: J.B. Lippincott, 1989, pp. 1311–1323.

Robbins, K.T., Fuller, L.M., Manning, J., Goepfert, H., Velasquez, W.S., Sullivan, M.P., and Finkelstein, J.B.: Primary lymphoma of the mandible. Head Neck Surg., 8:192–199, 1986.

Wang, C.C., and Fleishil, D.J.: Primary reticulum cell sarcoma of bone. Cancer 28:994–998, 1968.

LEUKEMIA

Leukemias are malignant neoplasms of hematopoietic stem cells characterized by replacement of the bone marrow by neoplasm (Fig. 5–12B). The most dramatic manifestation of leukemia is the presence of excessive numbers of neoplastic cells in the peripheral blood. Any organ can become involved, but the most

Text continued on page 117

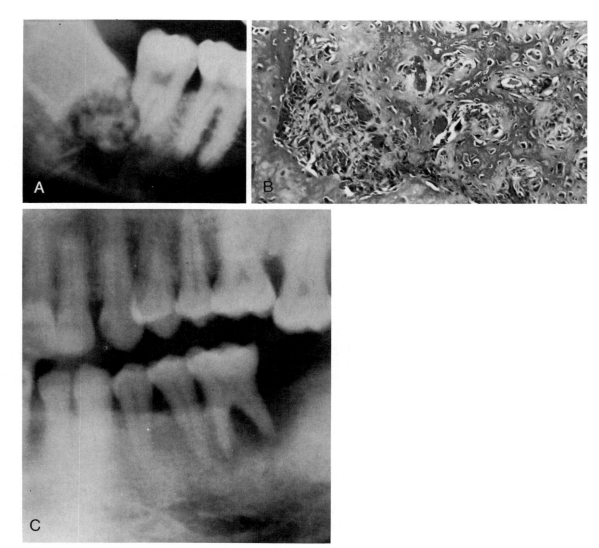

Figure 5–1. *A,* This ill-defined, mixed radiolucent-radiopaque lesion associated with the apex of the second permanent molar shows some radiating trabeculae from the inferior aspect of the lesion. This is consistent with an osteosarcoma. *B,* Osteosarcoma, osteoblastic type. Medium-power view shows "lacy" malignant osteoid formation in a well-differentiated osteoblastic osteosarcoma. *C,* This malignant tumor, which proved to be an osteosarcoma, began as a symmetric widening about the distal root of the lower left first molar.

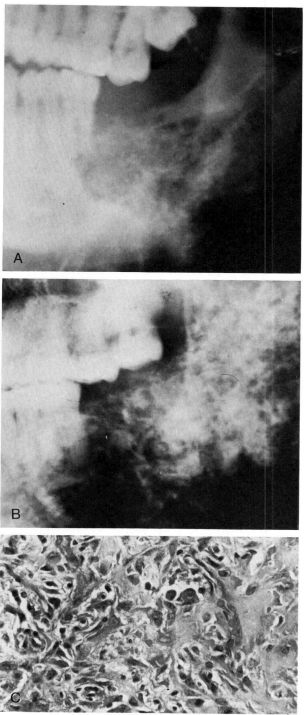

Figure 5–2. *A,* This large, expansile, moth-eaten, and ill-defined radiolucency shows evidence of the "sun-ray" appearance in the inferior portion. This was a malignant osteosarcoma. *B,* A rather large, mixed, ill-defined, radiolucent-radiopaque lesion also proved to be an osteosar-coma. *C,* Osteosarcoma, osteoblastic type. Higher power view of the same case shows malignant osteocytes, with pleomorphic hyperchromatic nuclei forming osteoid directly.

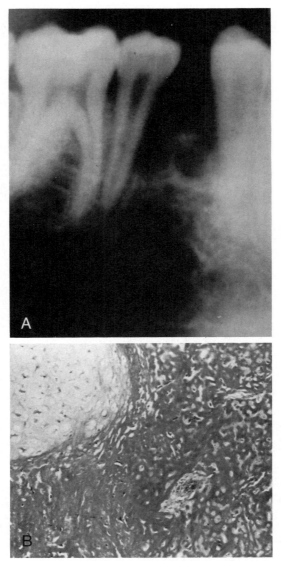

Figure 5–3. *A,* This moth-eaten radiolucency appeared between the two permanent premolars. The borders are ragged, and there is evidence of a sequestrum or bone production within the central portion of the lesion. The radiolucency below the apices of the teeth in this quad- rant is artifactual. The lesion turned out to be an osteo- sarcoma, chrondroblastic type. *B,* Osteosarcoma, osteo- blastic and chondroblastic type. Medium-power view shows a chondroblastic area *(top left)* in an otherwise osteoblastic osteosarcoma.

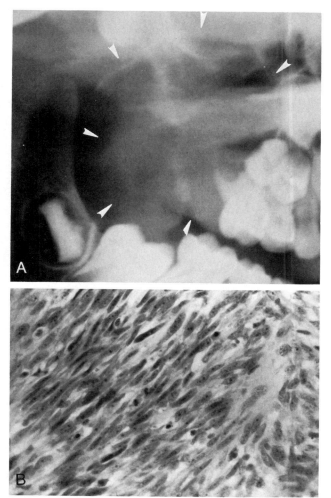

Figure 5–4. *A,* Most of the posterior portion of the right maxilla has been destroyed by an ill-defined radiolucent lesion (*arrows*). This tumor also displaced a developing permanent tooth. *B,* Osteosarcoma, fibroblastic type. High-power view of an osteosarcoma composed primarily of spindle cells and resembling a fibrosarcoma except for small areas (not shown) of direct osteoid formation by the malignant cells.

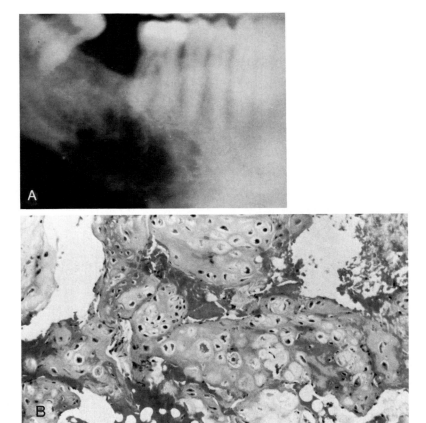

Figure 5–5. *A,* This chondrosarcoma appeared as a moth-eaten, ill-defined radiolucent lesion at the inferior border of the mandible. *B,* Chondrosarcoma. Medium-power view showing markedly enlarged pleomorphic, malignant chondrocytes.

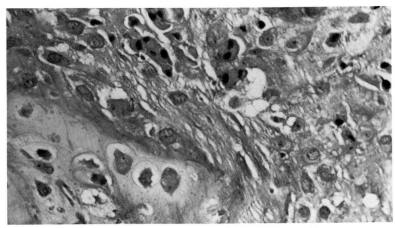

Figure 5–6. Chondrosarcoma. Higher power view showing enlarged pleomorphic, malignant, often binucleate chondrocytes.

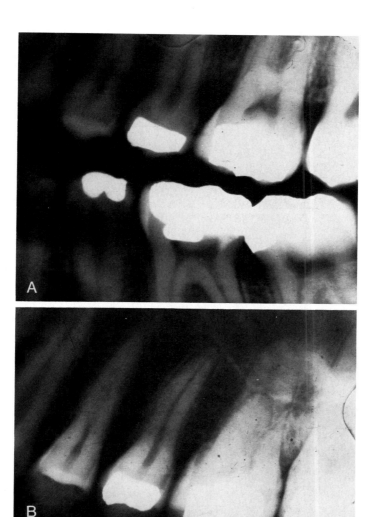

Figure 5–7. *A* and *B,* These figures should be compared with *C* and *D*. Bone is still present between the premolar and the first molar in the maxilla in *A.* In *C,* bone destruction is apparent in this same region. On the periapical film *(B),* we can still see the lamina dura and periodontal ligament space about the premolar. The bone pattern, although obscured, is somewhat normal. In *D,* the bone pattern about these premolars and molars is rather moth-eaten. The lamina dura is absent from both these teeth, and large areas of horizontal bone destruction are noted. The interval of time between these two sets of films was 2 years for development of this Ewing's sarcoma.

Illustration continued on following page

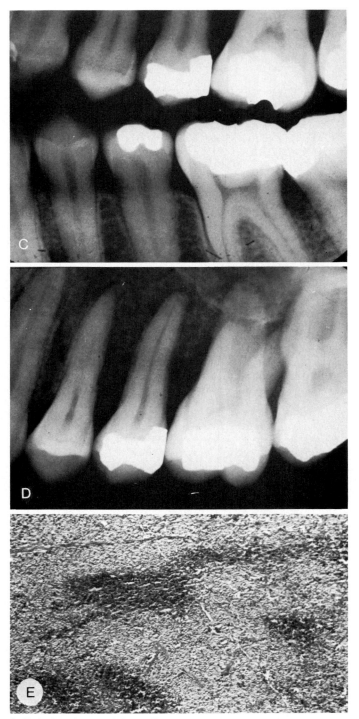

Figure 5–7 *Continued C,* Ewing's sarcoma, left maxilla. *D,* Ewing's sarcoma, left maxilla. *E,* Ewing's sarcoma. Low-power view showing small islands of viable tumor centered around blood vessels among large areas of necrotic tumor.

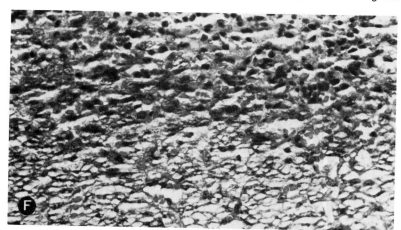

Figure 5–7 *Continued F* Ewing's sarcoma. High-power view showing small, uniform tumor cells with basophilic nuclei and inconspicuous cytoplasm *(top half)* and necrotic tumor cells *(bottom half)*.

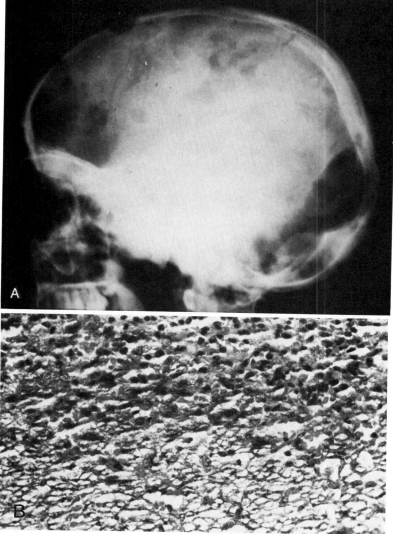

Figure 5–8. *A,* Lateral skull radiograph of patient with multiple punched-out radiolucencies of multiple myeloma. *B,* Myeloma. Low-power view showing massive infiltration of the marrow space by malignant plasma cells.

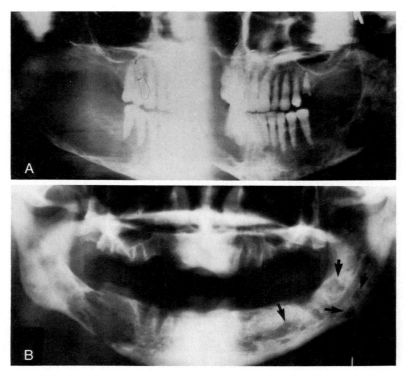

Figure 5–9. *A*, Multiple bilateral radiolucent areas in the mandible are consistent with multiple myeloma. *B*, Recurrence of persistence of multiple myeloma. Note multiple "punched-out" radiolucencies (*arrows*). Lesion in right mandible is so large it has caused a pathologic fracture.

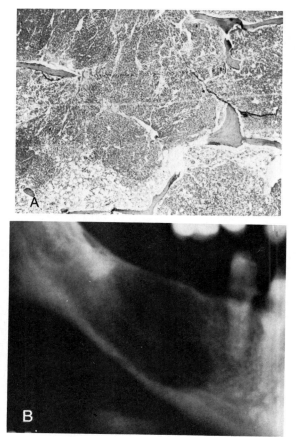

Figure 5–10. *A*, Myeloma. Higher power view showing an infiltrate composed entirely of malignant plasma cells. *B*, A case of multiple myeloma primarily in the mandible appearing as punched-out radiolucency.

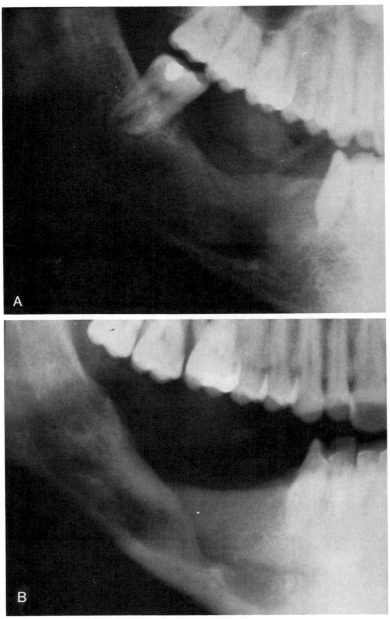

Figure 5–11. *A*, Hodgkin's lymphoma in a 25-year-old woman. (Courtesy of Dr. C. Tomich, Indiana University School of Dentistry, Indianapolis, Indiana.) *B*, Follow-up radiograph some 3 years after radiation therapy.

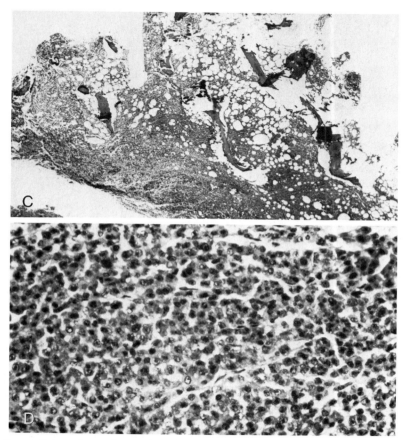

Figure 5–11 *Continued C*, Lymphoma. Low-power view shows massive infiltration of the marrow space by malignant lymphocytes. *D*, Lymphoma. Higher power view showing an infiltrate composed entirely of malignant lymphocytes.

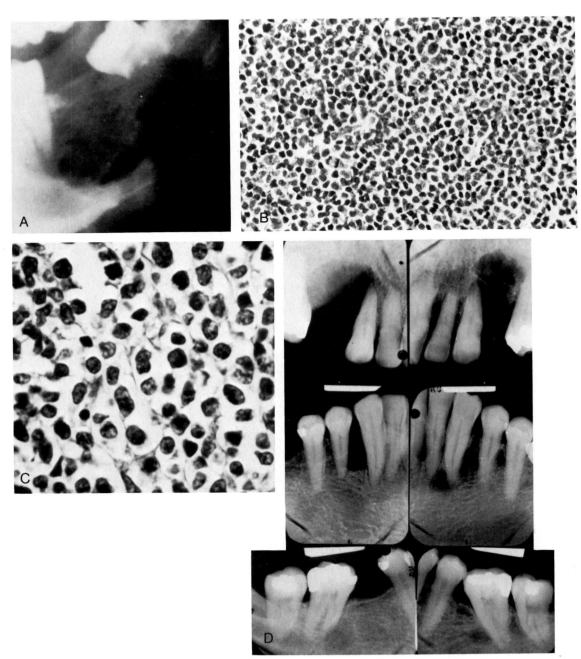

Figure 5–12. *A,* Some of the features of leukemic involvement of bone can be seen in this case: loss of crestal bone, root resorption, loss of periodontal ligament space, and bone destruction. *B,* Leukemia, acute myelomonocytic. *C,* High-power view shows an infiltrate composed entirely of malignant leukocytes. *D,* Leukemic changes in the maxilla and mandible.

striking changes occur in the bone marrow, spleen, lymph nodes, and liver. Many leukemias exhibit chromosomal (karyotypic) abnormalities, usually translocations, in the leukemic cells. Proto-oncogenes in new locations appear to derange growth regulation, producing a cell line that is autonomous. It is not known what actually initiates the mutation (translocation), but ionizing radiation, chemicals, and viruses are possibilities.

It is difficult to classify this group of related neoplasms in a manner that is scientifically accurate and at the same time clinically useful. Clinically, leukemias are usually classified as either acute or chronic.

Acute

Acute leukemia is characterized by an accumulation of undifferentiated white blood cell precursors ("leukemic blasts"). It is subdivided into acute lymphoblastic leukemia (ALL), which primarily affects children, and acute myeloblastic leukemia (AML), which primarily affects young adults. Because neoplastic leukemic cells fill the bone marrow, red blood cell, granulocyte, and platelet formation is severely impaired, and the clinical picture is dominated by anemia, infections, and hemorrhage. Untreated, it is rapidly fatal.

Chronic

Chronic leukemia is characterized by well-differentiated leukocytes and slow progression. It is subdivided into chronic myeloid leukemia (CML), primarily affecting adults, and chronic lymphocytic leukemia (CLL), which primarily affects the elderly (Cotran et al, 1989).

Clinical Features. Early oral symptoms and signs of undiagnosed disease are common in acute but uncommon in chronic leukemia. The most common oral problems leading to professional consultation and diagnosis are oral manifestations of thrombocytopenia (gingival oozing, petechiae, hematomas, or ecchymoses), cervical lymphadenopathy, sore throat, pharyngitis, nonspecific ulceration, mucosal pallor, and pain (Lynch and Ship, 1967; White, 1970; Stafford et al, 1980). Except in the monocytic form, diffuse gingival enlargement and markedly increased gingivitis are uncommon in acute leukemia (White, 1970). Dental pain and loss of pulp vitality can occur owing to replacement of the pulp by leukemic infiltrate. Endodontic therapy may eliminate the symptoms, possibly delaying diagnosis, unless the pulp contents are submitted for histopathologic examination (Sela and Pisanti, 1977).

Radiographic Appearance. Lytic lesions of any part of the skeleton can occur during the course of acute leukemia. Loss of trabeculation about the apices of mandibular molars, destruction of bony crypts of developing teeth, thinning or disappearance of the lamina dura of erupted teeth, asymmetric widening of periodontal ligament spaces, and loss of alveolar crestal bone are characteristic but not constant features (Stern and Cole, 1973).

Histopathologic Findings. Diagnosis is usually based on peripheral blood smears and bone marrow biopsies. Oral biopsies are contraindicated when there is a risk of prolonged bleeding or increased susceptibility to infection. Oral biopsies do reveal a dense infiltrate of atypical leukocytes, but the frequent presence of inflammatory cells makes definitive diagnosis difficult. Leukemic infiltrates can devitalize teeth by completely replacing the pulp (Sela and Pisanti, 1977).

Treatment. Leukemia is treated with combination chemotherapy. Prognosis continues to improve with new combinations of chemotherapeutic agents.

References

Cotran, R.S., Kumar, V., and Robbins, S.L.: Robbins Pathologic Basis of Disease, 4th ed. Philadelphia: W.B. Saunders, 1989, pp. 722–734.

Lynch, M.A., and Ship, I.I.: Oral manifestations of leukemia: A postdiagnostic study. J. Am. Dent. Assoc., 75:1139–1144, 1967.

Sela, M.N., and Pisanti, S.: Early diagnosis and treatment of patients with leukemia, a dental problem. J. Oral Med., 32:46–50, 1977.

Stafford, R., Sonis, S., Lockhart, P., and Sonis, A.: Oral pathoses as diagnostic indicators in leukemia. Oral Surg. Oral Med. Oral Pathol., 50:134–139, 1980.

Stern, M.H., and Cole, W.L.: Radiographic changes in the mandible associated with leukemic infiltration in a case of acute myelogenous leukemia. Oral Surg. Oral Med. Oral Pathol., 36:343–348, 1973.

White, G.E.: Oral manifestations of leukemia in children. Oral Surg. Oral Med. Oral Pathol., 29:420–427, 1970.

PRIMARY ODONTOGENIC MALIGNANT NEOPLASMS

These lesions are extremely rare (Regezi et al, 1978; Weir et al, 1987). Therefore, the much more common primary squamous cell carcinomas of the oral mucosa, which involve the jaws by direct extension, and metastatic neoplasms to the jaws must first be ruled out. The 1971 WHO classification of malignant odontogenic neoplasms (Pindborg and Kramer, 1971) is as follows:

ODONTOGENIC CARCINOMAS

Malignant ameloblastoma
Primary intraosseous carcinoma
Other carcinomas arising from odontogenic epithelium (including those arising from odontogenic cysts)

ODONTOGENIC SARCOMAS

Ameloblastic fibrosarcoma (ameloblastic sarcoma)
Ameloblastic odontosarcoma

The reader is referred to the following references for further details: Browne and Gough, 1972; Eversole et al, 1975; Larsson and Almeren, 1978; Elzay, 1982; Slootweg and Muller, 1984; Gingell et al, 1984; and Dorner et al, 1988. Figure 5–13 is a case of a squamous cell carcinoma arising in the lining of a dentigerous cyst.

References

Browne, R.M., and Gough, N.G.: Malignant change in the epithelium lining odontogenic cysts. Cancer 29:1199–1207, 1972.

Dorner, L., Sear, A.J., and Smith, G.T.: A case of ameloblastic carcinoma with pulmonary metastases. Br. J. Oral Maxillofac. Surg., 26:503–510, 1988.

Elzay, R.P.: Primary intraosseous carcinoma of the jaws. Oral Surg. Oral Med. Oral Pathol., 54:299–303, 1982.

Eversole, L.R., Sabes, W.R., and Rovin, S.: Aggressive growth and neoplastic potential of odontogenic cysts. With special reference to central epidermoid and mucoepidermoid carcinomas. Cancer 35:270–282, 1975.

Gingell, J.C., Beckerman, T., Levy, B.A., and Snider, L.A.: Central mucoepidermoid carcinoma. Review of the literature and report of a case with an apical periodontal cyst. Oral Surg. Oral Med. Oral Pathol., 57:436–440, 1984.

Larsson, A., and Almeren, H.: Ameloblastoma of the jaws. An analysis of a consecutive series of cases reported to the Swedish cancer registry during 1958–1971. Acta Pathol. Microbiol. Scand. [A] 86:337–349, 1978.

Pindborg, J.J., and Kramer, I.R.H.: Histological Typing of Odontogenic Tumors, Jaw Cysts, and Allied Lesions. Geneva: World Health Organization, 1971.

Regezi, J.A., Kerr. D.A., and Courtney, R.M.: Odontogenic tumors: Analysis of 706 cases. J. Oral Surg., 36:771–778, 1978.

Slootweg, P.J., and Muller, H.: Malignant ameloblastoma or ameloblastic carcinoma. Oral Surg. Oral Med. Oral Pathol., 57:168–176, 1984.

Weir, J.C., Davenport, W.D., and Skinner, R.L.: A diagnostic and epidemiologic survey of 15,783 oral lesions. J. Am. Dent. Assoc., 115:439–442, 1987.

PRIMARY MALIGNANCIES ADJACENT TO JAWS (Squamous Cell Carcinoma, Verrucous Carcinoma, Adenocarcinoma)

Any malignant neoplasm of the mucosa, skin, or soft tissues can involve adjacent bone by direct extension, causing cortical erosion and penetration of medullary bone. **Squamous cell carcinoma** of the oral mucosa, by far the most common form of oral malignancy, often involves the jawbones. Up to 50% of gingival squamous cell carcinomas involve alveolar bone, but this is sometimes difficult to appreciate, even on intraoral radiographs (Whitehouse, 1976). **Verrucous carcinoma,** unlike most other malignancies, tends to erode bone with little medullary infiltration. This well-differentiated form of squamous cell carcinoma metastasizes late, often only after radiotherapy or after repeated surgical attempts at removal. **Adenocarcinoma** of the major or minor salivary glands or mucous glands of the antra is a far less common cause of cortical erosion of the jawbones.

In cases of soft tissue lesions immediately adjacent to bone it is obviously prudent to rule out radiographically primary bone involvement (lesions arising in bone) or secondary involvement (lesions affecting bone but arising in soft tissue). Bone scans, magnetic resonance imaging (MRI), computed tomography (CT), intraoral radiographs, and panoramic radiographs are, in roughly descending order of sensitivity, important for presurgical assessment of secondary bone involvement by oral carcinoma (Baker et al, 1982; Belkin et al, 1988). It is essential to interpret the results of facial bone scintigraphy in the light of a thorough oral examination because areas of inflammation/infection (e.g., periodontitis or apical periodontitis) within the jaws also take up radioactive phosphate.

Clinical Features

Carcinoma of the gingiva, unlike most other malignancies, tends to be painful early in its development. Because of the pain and localized radiographic changes, it is often misdiagnosed as periodontitis or apical periodontitis, and tooth extraction is performed (Saxby and Soutar, 1989).

Carcinoma as well as inflammatory/infectious processes initially stimulates the periosteum to undergo a fibrous tissue reaction and to lay down periosteal new bone. As a result, the periosteum becomes more difficult to elevate off the bone, and the cortex exhibits an exophytic, roughened surface. Occasionally, the neoplasm invades between the periosteal new bone and the original cortex, suggesting that surgeons should include portions of the jaw exhibiting periosteal new bone in their excision (McGregor and MacDonald, 1988b).

Radiographic Appearance

The initial radiographic lesion is a reasonably well defined, radiolucent "cupping out" of the cortex, often surrounded by a "ground glass" or finely trabeculated zone of radiopacity (Fig. 5–14). Later, the underlying medullary bone exhibits a somewhat less well defined radiolucency, which is continuous with the cortical defect. The radiopaque ground glass border persists. Such radiolucencies with finely trabeculated radiopaque peripheries, especially when associated with teeth, can closely mimic focal sclerosing osteomyelitis (Schwartz and Shklar, 1967).

Histopathologic Findings

Carcinomas penetrate the marrow spaces of bone as thin projections, cords, or islands of cells (Fig. 5–13B) rather than as large sheets. Adjacent marrow spaces are replaced by fibrous connective tissue and chronic inflammatory cells (the latter probably an immunologic reaction to the neoplasm). Immediately adjacent to the neoplasm, the osseous margins (**zone of invasion**) exhibit active osteoclastic resorption, necrotic bone spicules, and little evidence of osteoblastic activity. Peripheral to the zone of invasion is the **peripheral zone,** which shows active osteogenesis. Much new bone with a prominent osteoblast layer and osteoid seams is present. The stimulus for this reactive new bone formation can be attributed to either pressure from the neoplasm or release of chemical mediators by the neoplasm or by the inflammatory cells (Schwartz and Shklar, 1967).

As expected, jaws that have been previously irradiated fail to mount an osteoblastic reaction to invading carcinoma (McGregor and MacDonald, 1988b).

Treatment

Bone involvement has an unfavorable effect on prognosis and complicates surgical as well as radiation therapy. Invasion of the medullary cavity of **nonirradiated, edentulous mandibles** by squamous cell carcinoma occurs primarily through the residual alveolar ridge. Only in about 9% of cases has entry through the foramina (e.g., mental foramen) been documented. Based on these observations, in patients with minimal bony invasion, excision of only the superficial aspect (preserving the inferior border) of the edentulous mandible is recommended. When there is gross jaw involvement by carcinoma, segmental resection becomes mandatory (McGregor and MacDonald, 1988a).

Invasion of the medullary cavity of **irradiated, edentulous mandibles** by squamous cell carcinoma also occurs primarily through the residual alveolar ridge, but multifocal sites of infiltration through buccal and lingual cortical plates is frequently observed also. Radiation appears to destroy the barrier to cortical infiltration by damaging osteoblasts and soft tissues. Osteoblasts can no longer mount a reactive endosteal osteoblastic response to the carcinoma (Schwartz and Shklar, 1967; McGregor and MacDonald, 1988b). The integrity of tissue planes between muscle, loose connective tissue, periosteum, and bone is lost. Therefore, when carcinoma is in close proximity to the irradiated edentulous mandible, segmental resection appears to be appropriate (McGregor and MacDonald, 1988a).

References

Baker, H.L., Woodbury, D.H., Krause, C.J., Saxon, K.G., and Stewart, R.C.: Evaluation of bone scan by scintigraphy to detect subclinical invasion of the mandible by squamous cell carcinoma of the oral cavity. Otolaryngol. Head Neck Surg., 90:327–336, 1982.

Belkin, B.A., Papageorge, M.B., Fakitsas, J., and Bankoff, M.S.: A comparative study of magnetic resonance imaging versus computed tomography for the evaluation of maxillary and mandibular tumors. J. Oral Maxillofac. Surg., 46:1039–1047, 1988.

McGregor, A.D., and MacDonald, D.G.: Routes of entry of squamous cell carcinoma to the mandible. Head Neck Surg., 10:294–301, 1988a.

McGregor, A.D., and MacDonald, D.G.: Reactive changes in the mandible in the presence of squamous cell carcinoma. Head Neck Surg., 10:378–386, 1988b.

Saxby, P.J., and Soutar, D.S.: Intra-oral tumours presenting after dental extraction. Br. Dent. J., 166:337–338, 1989.

Schwartz, S., and Shklar, G.: Reaction of alveolar bone to invasion of oral carcinoma. Oral Surg. Oral Med. Oral Pathol., 24:33–37, 1967.

Whitehouse, G.H.: Radiological bone changes produced by intraoral squamous carcinomata involving the alveolus. Clin. Otolaryngol., 1:45–47, 1976.

METASTASES TO THE JAWS

About 1% of all oral malignancies are metastases (Meyer and Shklar, 1965). The majority of lesions are carcinomas (84%). Neuroblastomas (9%), sarcomas (6%), and melanomas (1%) are relatively rare (Oikarinen et al, 1975). The most common sites of origin (64%) of oral metastases are the breast, lung, and kidney (Oikarinen et al, 1975). Primary neoplasms from the breast, bronchus, thyroid, prostate, and ovaries commonly metastasize to bone. Adenocarcinomas, especially from breast primaries, are the most common metastatic neoplasms to the jaws (Meyer and Shklar, 1965). The jaws are far more often involved than the oral soft tissues. The ratio of mandibular to maxillary involvement is 5:1 (Oikarinen et al, 1975). Metastases are the most common malignant neoplasms of both the jaws and the extragnathic skeleton. Premolar and molar areas of the body and angle of the mandible are most commonly affected (Oikarinen et al, 1975). Condylar involvement is rare (Giles and McDonald, 1982).

Because establishment of a metastatic lesion in bone is partially dependent on the presence of hematopoietic marrow, the incidence of jaw metastases is relatively low, and these lesions primarily affect the more highly vascularized, posterior regions of the mandible (Spott, 1985; Zachariades, 1989). Factors that determine the localization of metastases are not well understood. There is experimental and some clinical evidence to suggest that sites of injury or inflammation are predisposed (Cohen and Laszlo, 1972; MacGregor and Lewis, 1972). Metastases reach bones hematogenously; therefore metastatic disease in the jaws suggests that widespread dissemination has already occurred. Nevertheless, if bone scans reveal only one or a few operable metastases, treatment of these as well as the primary is warranted. Jaw metastases are usually solitary.

In general, the longer the disease-free state has existed, the lower the probability of recurrence or metastasis. Even 10 years after successful treatment of a primary, silent metastatic deposits can be activated to rapid growth by local injury or inflammation (Cohen and Laszlo, 1972). Because about 30% (Oikarinen et al, 1975) of jaw metastases originate from occult (hidden or subclinical) primary lesions, a negative history of previous or current malignancy should not deter the clinician from suspecting metastatic disease.

Clinical Features

Typically, a patient with a past history of malignancy complains of pain in the posterior mandible. Most oral metastases appear 1 to 5 years after diagnosis of the primary (Oikarinen et al, 1975). The mandible is involved far more often than the maxilla. The molar or premolar areas are most commonly involved. Patients are in the fourth to seventh decade of life. About a third of oral metastatic tumors are the initial manifestation of malignancy. Common clinical features are swelling, pain, and altered sensation (paresthesia, hyperesthesia, numbness, and anesthesia dolorosa) (Oikarinen et al, 1975). Tooth mobility, tooth displacement, and pathologic fracture are rare (Oikarinen et al, 1975; Zachariades, 1989). Apical periodontitis may be very closely simulated by these tumors (Spott, 1985). Metastases may preferentially localize to a preexistent area of apical periodontitis (Cohen and Laszlo, 1972).

Radiographic Appearance

Most often the lesion is radiolucent, but it can have some radiopaque components. The margins are always ill defined (ragged, "moth-eaten"). Occasionally, cortical expansion is seen (Yagan and Bellon, 1984). Primaries from the prostate, breast, and urinary tract are notable for giving rise to osteoblastic metastases.

At least initially, radiographic change is subtle or nonexistent despite localized pain and inexplicable loss of vitality (Spott, 1985). In the early stages, the metastatic tumor infiltrates marrow spaces without destroying the intervening bony trabeculae, but the neurovascular supply of teeth is vulnerable.

Histopathologic Findings

Although metastases may be less differentiated, their histologic appearance is usually similar to that of the primary. This is an important feature, especially when the primary is occult and must be found (Fig. 5–15*B*). Histochemistry, electron microscopy, and immunohistochemistry are particularly useful in helping to determine the tissue of origin of poorly differentiated metastatic (as well as primary) neoplasms because these have a "primitive" or unspecialized histomorphology and produce very little cell product. For example, a poorly differentiated carcinoma may be composed of small round cells, histologically mimicking lymphoma. Immunohistochemistry of such a lesion would show an absence of antigenic determinants characteristic of lymphocytes but the presence of those characteristic of epithelial cells (i.e., keratin).

Treatment

Unless widespread metastases have already been documented, a biopsy is required for definitive diagnosis, prognosis, and treatment planning. Prognosis depends on the number and distribution of the metastases and on whether the primary has been or can be treated. In general, an osseous metastasis represents one of many hematogenously disseminated metastases, and thus the prognosis is usually grave. Survival following diagnosis of a jaw metastasis is usually less than 1 year (Oikarinen et al, 1975).

References

Cohen, H.J., and Laszlo, J.: Influence of trauma on the unusual distribution of metastases from carcinoma of the larynx. Cancer 29:466–471, 1972.

Giles, D.L., and McDonald, P.J.: Pathologic fracture of mandibular condyle due to carcinoma of the rectum. Oral Surg. Oral Med. Oral Pathol., 53:247–249, 1982.

MacGregor, A.J., and Lewis, D.A.: Metastasis of carcinoma of the lung by implantation in tooth sockets. Br. J. Oral Surg., 9:195–199, 1972.

Meyer, I., and Shklar, G.: Malignant tumors metastatic to the mouth and jaws. Oral Surg. Oral Med. Oral Pathol., 20:350–362, 1965.

Oikarinen, V.J., Calonius, P.E.B., and Sainio, P.: Metastatic tumors to the oral region. I. An analysis of cases in the literature. Proc. Finn. Dent. Soc., 71:58–65, 1975.

Spott, R.J.: Metastatic breast carcinoma disguised as periapical disease in the maxilla. Oral Surg. Oral Med. Oral Pathol., 60:327–328, 1985.

Yagan, R., and Bellon, E.M.: Breast carcinoma metastatic to the mandible mimicking ameloblastoma. Oral Surg. Oral Med. Oral Pathol., 57:189–194, 1984.

Zachariades, N.: Neoplasms metastatic to the mouth, jaws and surrounding tissues. J. Craniomaxillofac. Surg., 17:283–290, 1989.

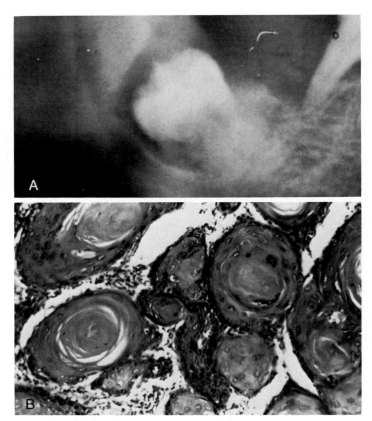

Figure 5–13. *A,* This radiograph illustrates a squamous cell carcinoma arising in the lining of a dentigerous cyst. (Courtesy of Dr. C. Tomich, Indiana University School of Dentistry, Indianapolis, Indiana.) *B,* Squamous cell carcinoma, well differentiated. Medium-power view of neoplastic islands of epithelium that are attempting to differentiate (forming "keratin pearls") in the center.

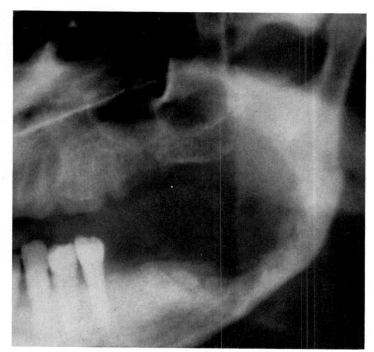

Figure 5–14. Squamous cell carcinoma in the floor of the mouth with secondary invasion into the mandibular alveolar bone. This cupped-out, ill-defined radiolucency is characteristic of secondary invasion of squamous cell carcinoma into bone.

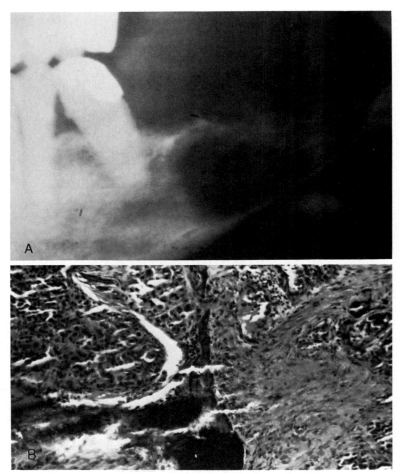

Figure 5–15. *A,* Ill-defined, multilocular destructive radiolucency in the posterior mandible. This was an adenocarcinoma that had metastasized from the lung. *B,* Poorly differentiated adenocarcinoma that has metastasized to the mandible from an occult primary. Medium-power view of the neoplastic cells surrounding residual trabeculae of normal bone *(center).*

BENIGN FIBRO-OSSEOUS LESIONS

G. Kaugars

CENTRAL OSSIFYING FIBROMA

CONDENSING OSTEITIS

OSTEOSCLEROSIS

PERIAPICAL CEMENTAL DYSPLASIA

FLORID OSSEOUS DYSPLASIA

FIBROUS DYSPLASIA

PAGET'S DISEASE

The term benign fibro-osseous lesion (BFOL) is used in a generic fashion for a diverse group of bone conditions that share a similar histologic appearance. Therefore, BFOL is not a specific diagnosis but rather a broad category. Nomenclature has always presented a problem with BFOLs because of the many terms that have been utilized. As an example, the term fibrous dysplasia was previously used for several of the entities that are now called BFOLs. This has made it difficult to compare studies because the diagnostic criteria have changed, and in some cases, a widely accepted definition is still not available. A number of classifications have been proposed for BFOLs, some based on whether or not the lesions are of periodontal ligament origin and others on the type of calcification present within the lesion. Although these classifications are of some academic interest, they have limited clinical usefulness because the treatment is generally determined by the clinical and radiographic features in a particular case. Table 6–1 contains a summary of characteristics of BFOLs.

Some general observations will make it easier to understand the nuances of BFOLs.

1. The diagnosis of a BFOL is based primarily on its clinical and radiographic findings; if necessary, the diagnosis is confirmed by biopsy.

2. There is a strong correlation between the radiographic appearance and the histopathologic features. The degree of radiopacity is reflected by the amount of bone, cementum, and other calcified material within a lesion. Some BFOLs begin as a radiolucency that evolves into a radiopacity as the percentage of calcification increases.

Table 6–1. BENIGN FIBRO-OSSEOUS LESIONS

Lesion	Age (yr)	Sex	Race	Solitary or Multiple	Maxilla or Mandible	Anterior or Posterior	Radiolucent or Radiopaque	Well-defined or Diffuse	Expansion
Central ossifying fibroma	Average = 30	80% F	50% blacks	Solitary	75% mandible	Posterior	RL→RO	Well-defined	Yes
Condensing osteitis	10–30	—	—	Either	Mandible	Posterior	RO	Either	No
Osteosclerosis	10–30	—	—	Either	Mandible	Posterior	RO	Either	No
Periapical cemental dysplasia	30–45	93% F	71% blacks	Multiple	Mandible	Anterior	RL→RO	Well-defined	No
Florid osseous dysplasia	Average = 50	90% F	90% blacks	Multiple	Mandible	Posterior	RL→RO	Either, but usually well-defined	Yes or no
Monostotic fibrous dysplasia	10–30	M = F	—	Solitary	Maxilla	Posterior	RO	Diffuse	Yes
Polyostotic fibrous dysplasia	<10	F	—	Multiple	Maxilla	Posterior	RO	Diffuse	Yes
Paget's disease	>40	65% M	Caucasian	90% multiple	Maxilla	Either	RL→RO	Diffuse	Yes

3. A variety of calcifications may be found within any one particular lesion.

4. The treatment is usually predicated on determining the correct diagnosis from the clinical findings and the radiographic appearance. The importance of this concept cannot be overstated because the range of treatment for BFOLs ranges from benign neglect to radical surgery.

5. Nomenclature is a problem because some of the diagnostic terms are similar. There is even a geographic variation in the popularity of some of the terms. The most widely used synonyms are included in the description of each lesion to help the reader.

CENTRAL OSSIFYING FIBROMA

The term central ossifying fibroma (COF) was first used in 1927, but not until recently was this lesion separated from other BFOLs. Of all the BFOLs, the COF is the only one considered to be a true neoplasm. Difficulty in distinguishing bone from cementum as well as the presence of a variety of calcifications within the same specimen has led most pathologists to recognize the central cementifying fibroma and the central cemento-ossifying fibroma as histologic variants of the COF. One theory is that the COF is of periodontal ligament origin because it has the capability of producing bone or cementum.

Synonyms: *Central cementifying fibroma, central cemento-ossifying fibroma.*

Clinical Features

The reported average age at time of diagnosis has consistently been between 26 and 36 years of age. The predilection of this lesion for this age group is confirmed by the fact that 56% of the cases are diagnosed in either the third or the fourth decade of life. A higher incidence in females (61 to 100%) and non-Caucasians (42 to 53%) has also been reported. The mandible is the most common site (62 to 89%), a majority of tumors (77%) being found in the premolar-molar region. The COF is asymptomatic in the early stages, but slow, gradual growth eventually produces a noticeable localized swelling.

Radiographic Appearance

This solitary, well-defined lesion becomes more radiopaque with time because of the increased amount of calcification. The COF usually maintains its circular configuration during expansion, but rarely erosion of cortical bone is noted. The initial radiolucent phase can easily be mistaken for periapical pathosis or an odontogenic cyst. With time, the radiopaque foci become more apparent in the gradually expanding lesion. Divergence of roots (17%) as well as root resorption (11%) is occasionally noted.

Although the COF is usually found in the tooth-bearing regions of the jaws, there has been at least one case in which the lesion had no apparent connection to dental structures.

Histopathologic Findings

The typical COF contains irregularly shaped pieces of bone or cementum surrounded by hypercellular fibrous connective tissue. These calcifications correspond to the radiopaque foci seen on radiographs. The lesions usually have a mixture of various types of calcification, but immature woven bone is the most common. Mature lesions are characterized by dense lamellar bone with little connective tissue, which is responsible for the uniformly dense radiopacity seen on radiographs.

Treatment

Surgical removal is indicated because of the potential continued expansion of the COF. There is usually a thin connective capsule surrounding the lesion, so that at the time of surgery the COF easily "shells out." Despite this characteristic, patients with multiple recurrences have been reported, and one series demonstrated an initial recurrence rate of 28% among patients available for follow-up.

The well-defined radiographic appearance and the ability to shell out the COF separate it from fibrous dysplasia, which is diffuse and difficult to remove.

References

Eversole, L.R., Leider, A.S., and Nelson, K.: Ossifying fibroma: A clinicopathologic study of sixty-four cases. Oral Surg. Oral Med. Oral Pathol., 60:505–511, 1985.

Eversole, L.R., Merrell, P.W., and Strub, D.: Radiographic characteristics of central ossifying fibroma. Oral Surg. Oral Med. Oral Pathol., 59:522–527, 1985.

Eversole, L.R., Sabes, W.R., and Rovin, S.: Fibrous dysplasia: A nosologic problem in the diagnosis of fibro-osseous lesions of the jaws. J. Oral Pathol., 1:189–220, 1972.

Gay, I., Sela, J., Tcherdakoff, P., et al: Ossifying fibroma: Report of a case. J. Oral Surg., 33:368–371, 1975.

Langdon, J.D., Rapidis, A.D., and Patel, M.F.: Ossifying fibroma—one disease or six? An analysis of 39 fibro-osseous lesions of the jaws. Br. J. Oral Surg., 14:1–11, 1976.

Mayo, K., and Scott, R.F.: Persistent cemento-ossifying fibroma of the mandible: Report of a case and review of the literature. J. Oral Maxillofac. Surg., 46:58–63, 1988.

Shafer, W.G., Hine, M.K., and Levy, B.M.: A Textbook of Oral Pathology, 4th ed. Philadelphia: W.B. Saunders, 1983, pp. 142–144.

Waldron, C.A.: Fibro-osseous lesions of the jaws. J. Oral Maxillofac. Surg., 43:249–262, 1985.

CONDENSING OSTEITIS

Condensing osteitis is the term widely used to describe a periapical radiopacity associated with a tooth that has a large carious lesion or that has had extensive restorative procedures. It is difficult to find a term for this lesion that is concise, clinically descriptive, and histologically accurate. This difficulty is reflected in the number of synonyms that have been applied. In general, condensing osteitis is considered an innocuous entity that is a proliferative bony response to a low-grade bacterial infection. A surprisingly small amount of published information is available concerning condensing osteitis despite its reported incidence of 4 to 8% in the adult population.

Synonyms: *Chronic focal sclerosing osteomyelitis, focal periapical osteopetrosis, sclerosing osteitis.*

Clinical Features

Condensing osteitis is most commonly diagnosed in the second and third decades of life but is rarely seen before the age of 10 years. The radiopacity is likely to persist for many years or even for the lifetime of the patient once it has been established. Almost all cases reported have been located in the mandible, the largest number occurring in the mandibular first molar. Condensing osteitis itself is asymptomatic, but the associated tooth may have signs or symptoms related to caries or previous dental restorations.

Radiographic Appearance

Typically, the lesion is a radiopacity in close proximity to the apex of a tooth that does not obscure the root outline. The radiopacity may be well defined or may diffuse into the surrounding bone. The density of the radiopacity is fairly uniform, and there is no radiolucent phase that precedes its characteristic appearance. Condensing osteitis is also occasionally seen adjacent to an area of periapical pathosis in an apparent response to the inflammation.

Histopathologic Features

Irregular trabeculae of bone associated with a small amount of fibrous connective tissue that usually contains a few chronic inflammatory cells are noted. However, some lesions demonstrate a mass of dense viable bone and an absence of inflammatory cells. The presence of ossification in the histologic specimens explains the radiopaque appearance of this lesion. Neither condensing osteitis nor chronic focal sclerosing osteomyelitis is a completely accurate term because occasional cases lack inflammatory cells.

Treatment

Whatever dental care is required for the associated tooth should be rendered, but the condensing osteitis itself does not require any treatment. It is not unusual to see residual areas of condensing osteitis persist for many years after the extraction of the tooth. However, one study showed that after nonsurgical endodontic treatment, 85% of the lesions regressed.

References

Eliasson, S., Halvarsson, C., and Ljungheimer, C.: Periapical condensing osteitis and endodontic treatment. Oral Surg. Oral Med. Oral Pathol., 57:195–199, 1984.

Eversole, L.R., Stone, C.E., and Strub, D.: Focal sclerosing osteomyelitis/focal periapical osteopetrosis: Radiographic patterns. Oral Surg. Oral Med. Oral Pathol., 58:456–460, 1984.

Farman, A.G., de V Joubert, J., and Nortjé, C.J.: Focal osteosclerosis and apical periodontal pathoses in "European" and Cape coloured dental outpatients. Int. J. Oral Surg., 7:549–557, 1978.

Hedin, M., and Polhage, L.: Follow-up study of periradicular bone condensations. Scand. J. Dent. Res., 79:436–440, 1971.

OSTEOSCLEROSIS

There is considerable similarity between osteosclerosis and condensing osteitis; indeed, they may be the same entity but with different causes. Although osteosclerosis is relatively common, there have been very few published reports. Trauma and the retention of primary teeth have been implicated as initiating factors in osteosclerosis, whereas bacterial infection is the initial cause in condensing osteitis. Despite the occasional difficulty in distinguishing between these lesions, it should be kept in mind that the appropriate clinical management for both is the same because they represent incidental radiographic findings and do not require treatment.

Synonym: *Enostosis, dense bone island.*

Clinical Features

Almost all lesions are first noticed incidentally on routine radiographs in young people and persist into adulthood. The lesions are asymptomatic and do not cause expansion. Many are found in the mandible but do not have the same predilection for the first molar as noted with condensing osteitis. Osteosclerotic lesions are diagnosed with some frequency in the mandibular canine area, a fact that may be related to bruxism, and between the mandibular premolars, a situation that may be associated with retained deciduous root tips. In addition, osteosclerosis occurs in the body of the mandible and adjacent to third molar extraction sites. Patients rarely can remember a specific traumatic incident that caused the lesion, which supports the hypothesis that even minor trauma may stimulate the occurrence of one of these lesions. The teeth are vital.

Radiographic Appearance

The radiographic findings are similar to those typical of condensing osteitis because the lesions can be either well defined or diffuse and do not have a radiolucent phase. The principal difference is that osteosclerosis is less likely to be located at the apex of a tooth.

A similar lesion, called a bone island, occurs in the orthopedic radiology literature. It resembles osteosclerosis in that it is asymptomatic, the incidence increases with age, it has an unknown etiology, it appears radiographically as a discrete homogeneous radiopacity, and normal bone is present in a biopsy specimen. The only significance of a bone island is that it needs to be differentiated from osteoblastic metastases in a patient with a primary tumor (see discussion in Chapter 5).

Histopathologic Findings

A biopsy is generally not indicated, but a mixture of irregular trabeculae of bone and fibrous connective tissue has been found in the lesions that have been examined. Inflammatory cells are usually not present.

Treatment

None is indicated other than diagnosis by recognition. The lesions are likely to persist for years, and their removal is not justified.

References

Goaz, P.W., and White, S.C.: Oral Radiology: Principles and Interpretation, 2nd ed. St. Louis: C.V. Mosby, 1987, pp. 470–471.
Resnick, D., and Niwayama, G.: Diagnosis of Bone and Joint Disorders. Philadelphia: W.B. Saunders, 1981, pp. 2963–2970.

PERIAPICAL CEMENTAL DYSPLASIA

This lesion presents the perplexing problem of an entity that is found in 0.3% of the adult population and has well-known clinical parameters, yet its etiology remains a mystery. The term cementoma is widely used, but its usage is discouraged because of the confusion in terminology with benign cementoblastoma (true cementoma), central cementifying fibroma, and gigantiform cementoma.

Synonym: *Cementoma.*

Clinical Features

The typical case of periapical cemental dysplasia (PCD) is diagnosed in an asymptomatic black woman over the age of 30 years. The predilection for blacks (71%) and woman (93%) is unexplained but closely matches that of florid osseous dysplasia. A majority of cases (52%) are diagnosed in patients between 31 and 45 years of age; only rarely are they less than 20 years old. Almost all lesions are located between the mandibular canines, and multiple lesions usually must be present before the diagnosis of PCD can be rendered with any confidence. If a solitary lesion is present, an alternative diagnosis should be considered. The associated teeth are vital and asymptomatic unless coincidentally involved by other dental disease.

Radiographic Appearance

Multiple well-defined lesions are commonly found at the apices of the mandibular anterior teeth. The sequential radiographic stages and their frequency at the time of diagnosis are as follows: radiolucent (28.7%), mixed (53.6%), and radiopaque (17.7%). There is considerable radiographic similarity between an early radiolucent lesion of PCD and periapical pathosis. It is not unusual to see several lesions at various stages of development in the same patient, which may mean that the lesions do not begin at the same time or progress at the same rate. The amount of calcification within a lesion increases with time, so an older lesion appears as a homogeneous radiopacity. A radiolucent rim usually persists about the periphery of the lesion and may be interposed between the tooth apex and the bulk of the lesion.

Histopathologic Findings

The histologic appearance is related to the radiographic stage of development, but in general, there is a mixture of "cementoid" and "osteoid" calcifications as well as trabeculae of woven bone. As with some of the other BFOLs, the terms PCD and cementoma are not accurate because the lesions also contain bone and osteoid. The hypercellular fibrous connective tissue usually contains some chronic inflammatory cells.

Treatment

None is indicated in the cases that have a classic clinical and radiographic presentation. Testing the vitality of the teeth is useful in evaluating the possibility of periapical pathosis if radiolucent lesions are noted.

References

Chaudhry, A.P., Spink, J.H., and Gorlin, R.J.: Periapical fibrous dysplasia. J. Oral Surg., 16:483–488, 1958.
Shafer, W.G., Hine, M.K., and Levy, B.M.: A Textbook of Oral Pathology, 4th ed. Philadelphia: W.B. Saunders, 1983, pp. 297–298.
Zegarelli, E.V., Napoli, N., and Hoffman, P.: The cementoma: A study of 230 patients with 435 cementomas. Oral Surg. Oral Med. Oral Pathol., 17:219–224, 1974.

FLORID OSSEOUS DYSPLASIA

Florid osseous dysplasia (FOD) is characterized by multiple radiolucent/radiopaque areas in the jawbones of middle-aged black women. This is an interesting process that has given rise to numerous terms in an attempt to explain all the associated features. Because of the uncertainty about pathogenesis and the wide range of clinical and radiographic appearances, it is doubtful that one term can ever adequately describe this condition. The choice of FOD over the other terms was made because it is currently the most popular one, not because it is a more accurate description. Despite the plethora of synonyms, it appears that various authors are describing the same process. Many words have been devoted to discussing the etiology, but it can be summarized by only one—unknown. The theory that this is a proliferative bony response to a chronic low-grade infection such as periodontal disease is attractive but does not explain all the cases. It is possible that several different etiologic factors could produce the same features. There have been isolated reports of hereditary transmission of FOD, but this is quite rare.

Synonyms: *Chronic diffuse sclerosing osteomyelitis, gigantiform cementoma, multiple enostosis, sclerotic cemental masses.*

Clinical Features

The average age at the time of diagnosis is approximately 50 years. Most (77 to 100%) of the patients are women, and one series reported that more than 85% are black. The age, sex, and race data closely approximate those typical of periapical cemental dysplasia. When considering the radiographic and histologic features, it is reasonable to conclude that

Text continued on page 145

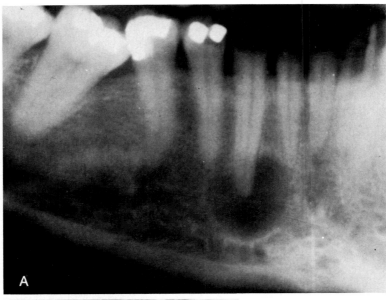

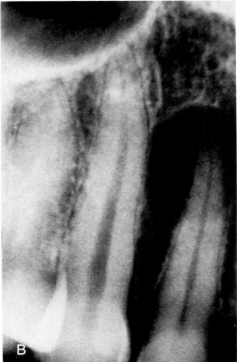

Figure 6–1. *A,* A well-defined solitary radiolucency resembling a periapical cyst. This was a central ossifying fibroma without evidence of internal calcifications. *B,* This well-defined radiolucency at the apex of the lateral incisor is an unusual presentation of a COF because it occurred in the anterior maxilla, and there is no apparent calcification radiographically. The amount of calcification in a COF increases with time until the lesion develops a solid radiopaque appearance.

Illustration continued on following page

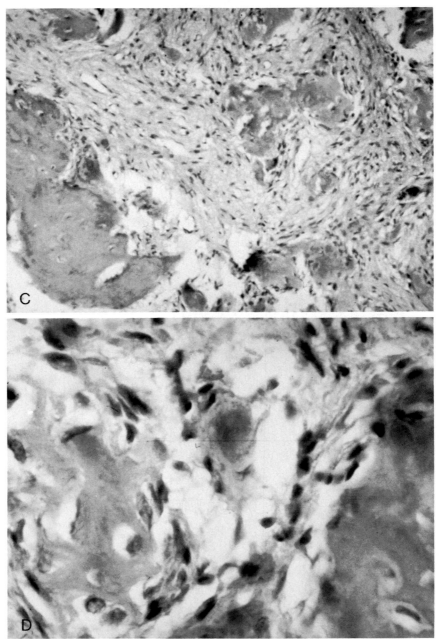

Figure 6–1 *Continued C,* The hypercellular fibrous connective tissue is apparent in this low-power view, and there is a range in maturity among the calcifications within the specimen. The presence of trabeculae of woven bone or lamellar bone increases the likelihood of seeing radiopacities on the radiograph. It is not unusual to find cementum-like deposits in these lesions, in which case the diagnosis of "central cemento-ossifying fibroma" is appropriate. *D,* This high-power view shows prominent osteoblastic activity in association with foci of immature osteoid.

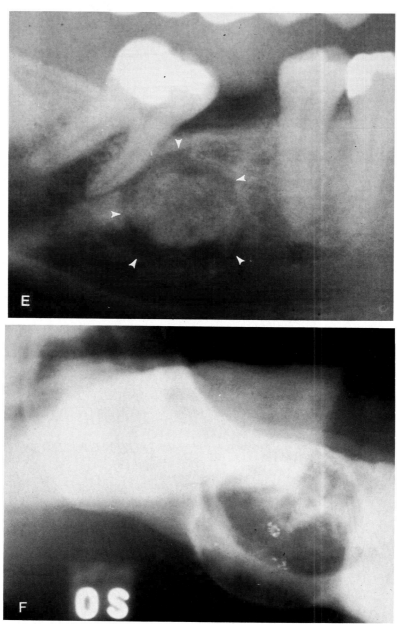

Figure 6–1 *Continued E,* This well-defined radiopacity *(arrows)* was noted on the right mandible of a 37-year-old woman. A COF is characterized by an increase in radiographic density with time but is usually surrounded by a radiolucent rim. *F,* A large cemento-ossifying fibroma that has a somewhat multilocular appearance. (Courtesy of Dr. C. Tomich, Indiana University School of Dentistry, Indianapolis, Indiana.)

Illustration continued on following page

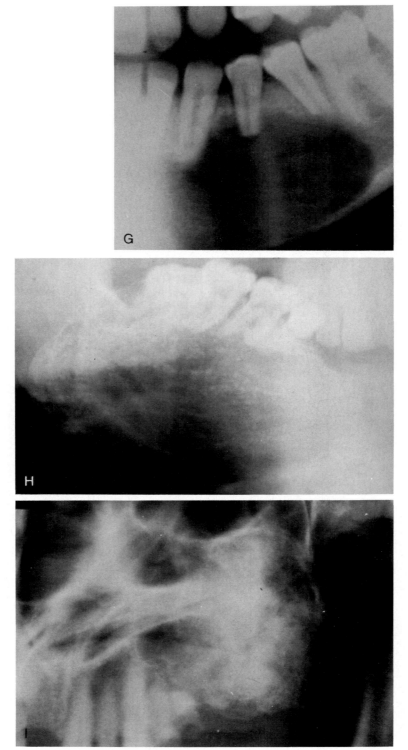

Figure 6–1 *Continued G,* A large, well-defined, expansile, unilocular radiolucency in the left mandible has resorbed roots, displaced teeth, and remodeled the inferior cortical border. This was termed a juvenile aggressive ossifying fibroma and may represent a specific type of COF. This lesion occurred in a 14-year-old boy. *H,* Another very large COF showing internal calcifications. Note the tremendous expansion of the mandible and the gross displacement of teeth. *I,* A large, diffuse radiopaque lesion in the posterior maxilla that proved to be a COF.

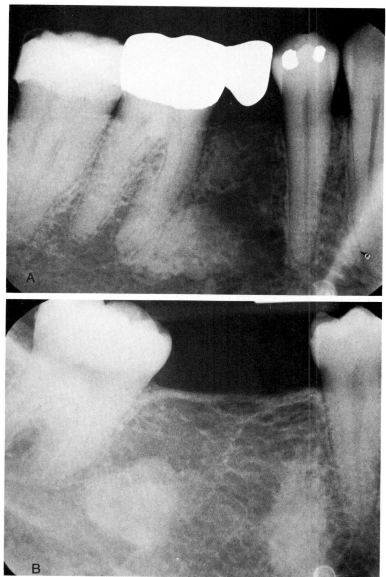

Figure 6–2. *A,* Condensing osteitis is associated with teeth with large carious lesions or teeth that have had extensive restorative work. This case shows a poorly defined radiopacity adjacent to the root of a mandibular molar restored with a crown. The radiographic density and border definition can vary widely in cases of con-densing osteitis. *B,* The term residual condensing osteitis implies that the area of condensing osteitis persisted after the associated tooth had been extracted. In this example there are two areas still visible many years after the molar was extracted. These lesions require no treatment.

Illustration continued on following page

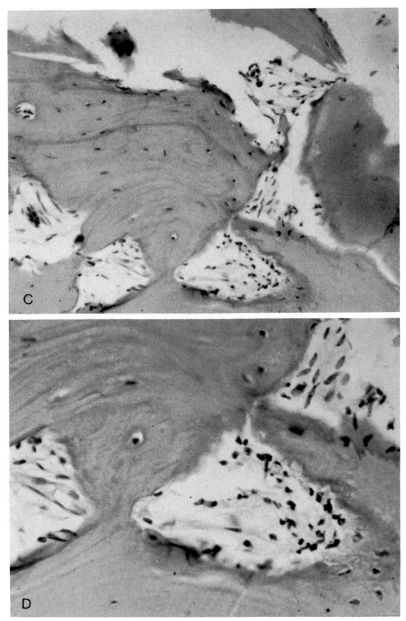

Figure 6–2 *Continued C,* This example of condensing osteitis contained primarily trabeculae of dense viable bone that corresponded to a well-defined radiopacity on the radiograph. In general, it is not necessary to perform a biopsy of these lesions unless this is justified by unusual circumstances. *D,* The small dark cells in this histologic section are lymphocytes that are interspersed among the trabeculae of bone. In spite of the term osteitis, inflammatory cells are not found in every specimen and need not be present in order to render the diagnosis. There are no substantive histologic differences between condensing osteitis and osteosclerosis.

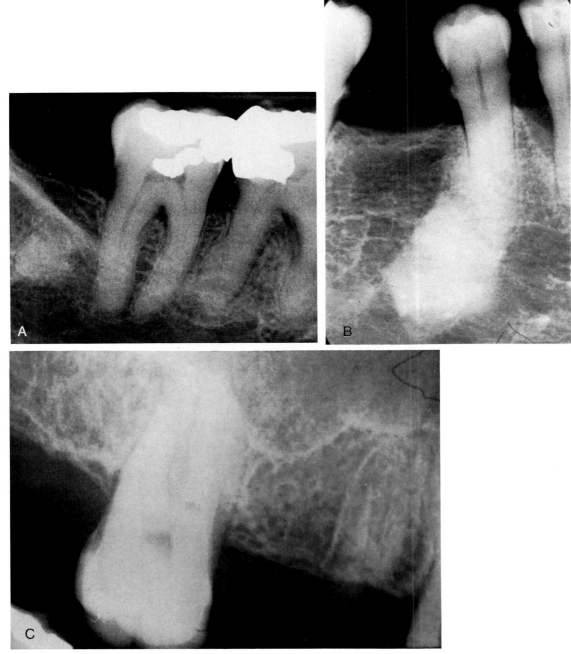

Figure 6–3. *A,* Although the well-defined radiopacity distal to the second molar resembles condensing osteitis, it is termed osteosclerosis because it occurred secondary to extraction of the third molar. Like condensing osteitis, this "lesion" requires no treatment. *B,* Traumatic occlusion from the opposing maxillary molar perhaps precipitated this well-defined radiopacity that is consistent with idiopathic osteosclerosis. *C,* One variation of osteosclerosis has been termed socket sclerosis. This anomaly of postextraction socket healing often gives the radiographic impression of a retained root tip. Some authors believe that this appearance might be a radiographic sign of either malabsorption (gastrointestinal) or renal problems.

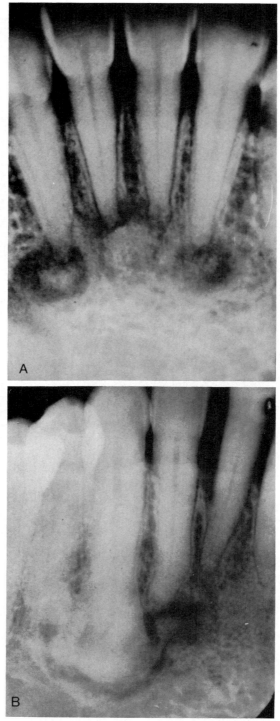

Figure 6–4. *A,* The classic radiographic features of periapical cemental dysplasia (PCD) are multiple radiolucent-radiopaque lesions at the apices of the lower central incisors. Typically, the lesions are at various stages of maturation, so that some are totally radiolucent, some are mixed radiolucent-radiopaque, and some are totally radiopaque. *B,* This illustration shows a mixed lesion in the anterior mandible.

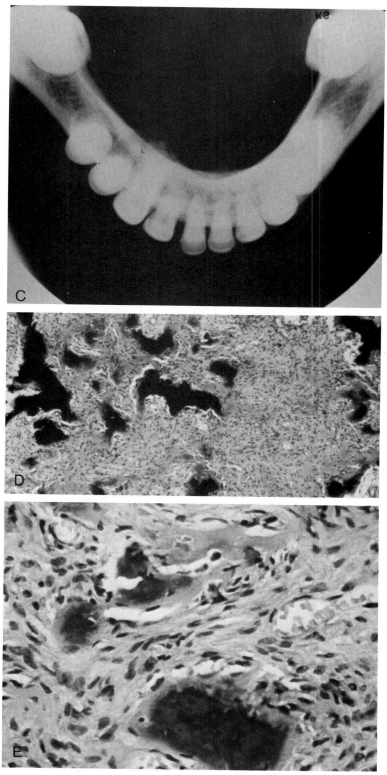

Figure 6–4 *Continued C,* Although PCD is said never to produce expansion, the occlusal view shows lingual cortical expansion. Expansion of the lingual aspect of the mandible by a lesion of PCD. *D,* Multiple, irregularly shaped calcifications are found within a hypercellular connective tissue stroma. A lesion may contain areas of osteoid or cementoid calcification in various degrees of maturation. *E,* The osteoid in this section appears dark because it was not decalcified prior to staining. A small number of inflammatory cells are present.

Illustration continued on following page

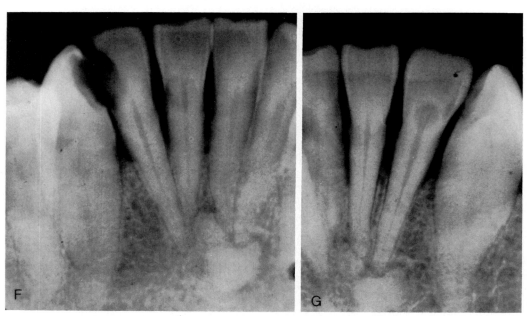

Figure 6–4 *Continued F*, This radiograph and that in G show two views of a mature lesion of PCD. Note that the lesion still has a radiolucent rim, which distinguishes it from lesions such as condensing osteitis and idiopathic osteosclerosis. *G*, Periapical cemental dysplasia, mature form.

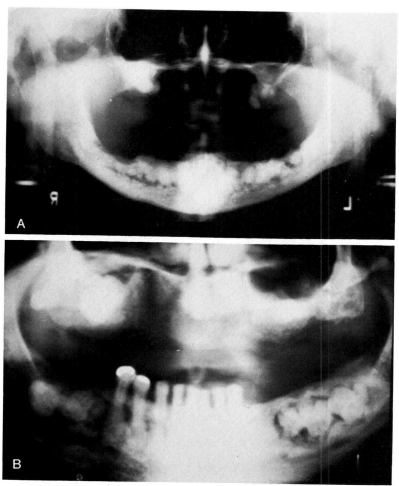

Figure 6–5. *A,* This panoramic radiograph demonstrates the typical multiple quadrant involvement seen in florid osseous dysplasia (FOD). These lesions are usually asymptomatic and do not show clinical expansion. *B.* Another case of FOD. Note that the large radiopaque mass in the lower left quadrant still has some areas of radiolucent rimming.

Illustration continued on following page

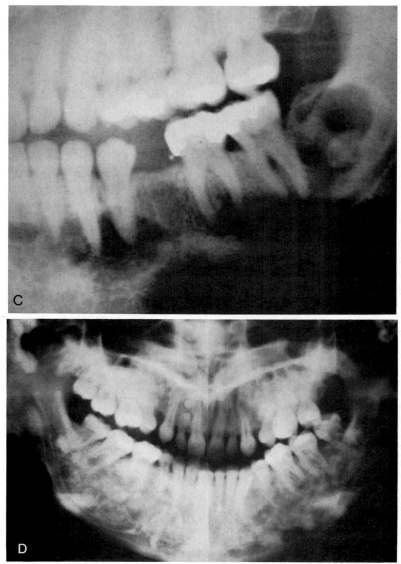

Figure 6–5 *Continued C,* The occasional simultaneous occurrence of FOD and traumatic bone cyst is seen in the left mandible of this 33-year-old woman. On surgical exploration, the area distal to the lower left second molar was found to contain only a hollow cavity consistent with the findings of a traumatic bone cyst. (Courtesy Dr. R. O'Neill, Petersburg, Virginia.) *D,* A case of FOD. This lesion looks as if it has expanded the mandible; however, the **apparent** expansion was due to a positioning error in which the patient's head was tipped too low, distorting the size of the mandible radiographically.

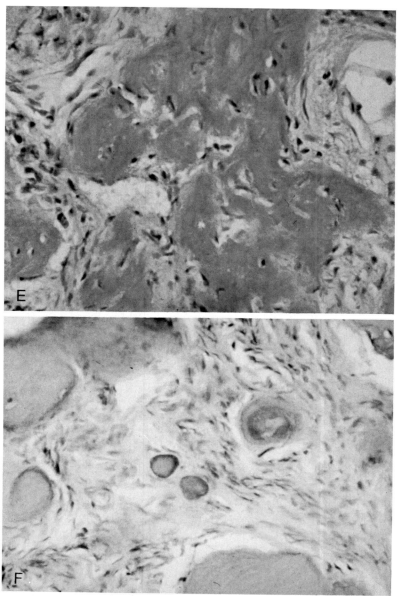

Figure 6–5 *Continued E,* The histologic features of FOD are very similar to those of periapical cemental dysplasia. Multiple lesions within any one patient can demonstrate large variations in the type of calcifications and their maturation. This area showed osteoid associated with prominent osteoblastic activity. *F,* Another area from the same specimen contained cementum-like droplets within the connective tissue.

Illustration continued on following page

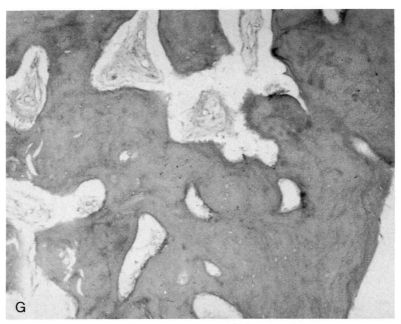

Figure 6–5 *Continued G*, Trabeculae of dense viable bone were prominently featured in another portion of the same specimen. The degree of inflammation is variable, and its presence is not required to make the diagnosis.

FOD represents a variant of periapical cemental dysplasia that affects multiple quadrants. In FOD there is a high propensity (87%) for occurrence in the mandible, and all four quadrants are affected in a majority (59%) of patients. It is difficult to assess the percentage of cases that are symptomatic because such cases are more likely to be seen by a practitioner and subsequently reported in the literature. Of the reported cases, almost half the patients have demonstrated a painful expansion, and about 25% have had a mucosal ulceration. It is our experience that most lesions are asymptomatic and are discovered on a routine radiographic examination.

Radiographic Appearance

Multiple, diffuse, radiolucent/radiopaque lesions are noted throughout the jawbones, especially the mandible; the lesions resemble periapical cemental dysplasia except for their propensity to reach a larger size. Increased calcification with time ultimately results in a pagetoid (cotton-wool) appearance. The development of radiolucent foci in a radiopaque lesion should prompt the clinician to evaluate the possibility of an osteomyelitis. A history of radiation therapy might suggest a diagnosis of osteoradionecrosis if the lesions are confined to the mandible.

Histopathologic Findings

There is great diversity of opinion concerning the percentage of bone or cementum in FOD because of the difficulty of distinguishing histologically between the two. However, this distinction does not have any clinical significance. As also seen in periapical cemental dysplasia, the amount of calcified tissue in any one particular lesion increases with time as the fibrous connective tissue concomitantly decreases. The osseous component can mature to such an extent that it resembles the mosaic bone pattern of Paget's disease. Inflammatory cells within the fibrous connective tissue have been reported in about half of all cases.

Treatment

No treatment is indicated in asymptomatic cases other than periodic assessment of the presence of an associated traumatic bone cyst, which occurs in about one-third of all cases. Avoidance of trauma such as extractions or osseous surgery is prudent in asymptomatic patients because of the bone's compromised healing ability due to its decreased vascularity. If osseous intervention is required in an asymptomatic patient, postoperative antibiotic coverage should be given.

For symptomatic patients with acute problems, short-term antibiotics are indicated even though the pathogenic organisms are difficult to isolate. Chronic problems should be treated with long-term antibiotic therapy of at least 3 months. Unfortunately, relapses are common after discontinuation of antibiotics. Dramatic improvement has been noted in some cases with an initial dose of 20 mg of prednisone followed by a maintenance dose of 10 mg every other day. In severe cases, both long-term intravenous antibiotics and sequestrectomy may be necessary.

References

Bhaskar, S.N., and Cutright, D.E.: Multiple enostosis: Report of 16 cases. J. Oral Surg., 26:321–325, 1968.

Jacobsson, S., and Hollender, L.: Treatment and prognosis of diffuse sclerosing osteomyelitis (DSO) of the mandible. Oral Surg. Oral Med. Oral Pathol., 49:7–14, 1980.

Melrose, R.J., Abrams, A.M., and Mills, B.G.: Florid osseous dysplasia. Oral Surg. Oral Med. Oral Pathol., 41:62–82, 1976.

Rabe, W.C., Angelillo, J.C., and Leipert, D.W.: Chronic sclerosing osteomyelitis: Treatment considerations in an atypical case. Oral Surg. Oral Med. Oral Pathol., 49:117–121, 1980.

Shafer, W.B., Hine, M.K., and Levy, B.M.: A Textbook of Oral Pathology, 4th ed. Philadelphia: W.B. Saunders, 1983, pp. 303, 503–506.

Van Merkesteyn, J.P.R., Groot, R.H., Bras, J., and Bakker, D.J.: Diffuse sclerosing osteomyelitis of the mandible: Clinical, radiographic and histologic findings in twenty-seven patients. J. Oral Maxillofac. Surg., 46:825–829, 1988.

Waldron, C.A., Giansanti, J.S., and Browand, B.C.: Sclerotic cemental masses of the jaws (so-called chronic sclerosing osteomyelitis, sclerosing osteitis, multiple enostosis, and gigantiform cementoma). Oral Surg. Oral Med. Oral Pathol., 39:590–604, 1975.

FIBROUS DYSPLASIA

Fibrous dysplasia has two distinct forms of involvement—monostotic (one bone) and polyostotic (multiple bones). The diagnosis is based principally on its unique clinical and radiographic features rather than on the histologic appearance. Either the monostotic or the polyostotic type can affect the jaws, but the former is more common. Some authorities feel that the two types of fibrous dysplasia may be separate entities because of the clinical differences and the fact that the monostotic type has never been reported to progress to the polyostotic type.

Clinical Features

The skull is involved in 10 to 25% of cases of monostotic fibrous dysplasia (MFD) and in approximately 50% of cases of polyostotic fibrous dysplasia (PFD). Most cases of MFD are diagnosed in patients between the ages of 10 and 30 years. Because of the greater severity of PFD, two-thirds of those patients are diagnosed before 10 years of age. There does not seem to be a predilection for either sex in MFD, but in PFD there are more women. A slight majority of jaw lesions (60%) occur in the maxilla, with most involving the area around the first molar. Mandibular lesions are usually found between the mental foramen and the mandibular angle. MFD usually presents as a slow-growing expansion that is asymptomatic. MFD involving the jaws has a propensity to expand in a buccal direction. Patients with PFD involving the jaws are more likely to be symptomatic because of the increased rate of growth and higher degree of involvement. Curiously, the cases of PFD that have been reported have a tendency to be unilateral.

A cutaneous marker for PFD is the presence of irregularly shaped light brown areas known as "café-au-lait" spots. The McCune-Albright syndrome is a combination of PFD, café-au-lait spots, and an endocrine disorder such as sexual precocity.

Radiographic Appearance

The typical lesion of fibrous dysplasia begins as a radiolucency that evolves into a poorly defined radiopacity that appears to blend into the surrounding bone. Lesions in the jaws are more likely to be radiopaque than are those in other bones. The most common (73%) presentation in the jaws shows numerous small unorganized trabeculae of bone that have been described as ground glass, salt and pepper, or orange peel. This appearance corresponds to the histologic finding of many delicate, unorganized pieces of osteoid that are undergoing calcification. However, lesions of fibrous dysplasia can also be multilocular and have a mottled appearance in which the multilocularity is obscured by increased trabeculation that renders the lesion more opaque. Partial loss of lamina dura may also be present as in Paget's disease and hyperparathyroidism.

Histopathologic Findings

Irregular trabeculae of bone (C-shaped or Chinese character) are scattered throughout the fibrous connective tissue of the specimen. With maturation, a greater percentage of lesions will contain lamellar instead of woven bone. Jaw lesions usually have more bone than lesions in other locations, which explains their greater likelihood to be radiopaque. Osteoblastic rimming of the bony trabeculae is now accepted as being compatible with the diagnosis of fibrous dysplasia. There is no apparent histologic difference between MFD and PFD.

Treatment

The possibility of polyostotic involvement and endocrine disorders should be considered in any patient with the diagnosis of fibrous dysplasia. A bone scan is useful for finding other lesions because of the increased vascularity and altered bone metabolism. If possible, surgery should be postponed until after puberty because these lesions have a tendency to stop growing at that time. Unfortunately, 20% of the lesions continue their growth after conservative surgery. Surgery on younger patients may be complicated by excessive bleeding. Older patients are more likely to develop postoperative infections. Radiation therapy is contraindicated because of the possibility of radiation-induced sarcoma.

Malignant transformation occurs in fewer than 0.5% of cases, is more common in PFD, and has a latent period of approximately 13.5 years after the initial diagnosis. Osteosarcoma is the most commonly associated malignancy; in one study, 35% of the transformations occurred in craniofacial lesions.

References

El Deeb, M., Waite, D.E., and Jaspers, M.T.: Fibrous dysplasia of the jaws. Oral Surg. Oral Med. Oral Pathol., 47:312–318, 1979.

Greenfield, G.B.: Radiology of Bone Diseases, 4th ed. Philadelphia: J.B. Lippincott, 1986, pp. 127–141.

Nance, F.L., Fonseca, R.J., and Burkes, E.J.: Technetium bone imaging as an adjunct in the management of fibrous dysplasia. Oral Surg. Oral Med. Oral Pathol., 50:199–206, 1980.

Resnick, D., and Niwayama, G.: Diagnosis of Bone and Joint Disorders. Philadelphia: W.B. Saunders, 1981, pp. 2949–2961.

Schwartz, D.T., and Alpert, M.: The malignant transformation of fibrous dysplasia. Am. J. Med. Sci., 247:1–20, 1964.

Waldron, C.A., and Giansanti, J.S.: Benign fibro-osseous lesions of the jaws: A clinical-radiologic-histologic review of 65 cases. Oral Surg. Oral Med. Oral Pathol., 35:190–201, 1973.

Zimmerman, D.C., Dahlin, D.C., and Stafne, E.C.: Fibrous dysplasia of the maxilla and mandible. Oral Surg. Oral Med. Oral Pathol., 11:55–68, 1958.

PAGET'S DISEASE

Paget's disease is a bone condition characterized by relatively common occurrence (2 to 4% of people over the age of 50), slow growth, and markedly elevated serum alkaline phosphatase. Although considerable effort has been expended in trying to determine the cause of Paget's disease, the etiology remains uncertain. A "slow" virus has been strongly suggested. As is the case with fibrous dysplasia, Paget's disease can occur in either a monostotic (one-bone) or a polyostotic (multiple-bone) form, but the latter is far more common. One difference between the two diseases is that polyostotic involvement in fibrous dysplasia is usually unilateral, but in Paget's disease it is bilateral.

The designation Paget's disease of bone is necessary to separate it from Paget's disease of the breast and extramammary Paget's disease, both of which are cutaneous malignancies.

Synonym: *Osteitis deformans.*

Clinical Features

Paget's disease is rare before the age of 40 years but is increasingly more common with each decade until about 10% of people over the age of 80 years have some manifestation. The diagnosis may be difficult because many cases are asymptomatic, and approximately 10% are monostotic. A slight predilection for men (65%) has been reported. An interesting geographic distribution is noted because Paget's disease is more common in the northern United States than in the south. There is also an increased incidence in northern Europe. The percentage of patients with Paget's disease who have clinical or radiographic involvement of the jaws is difficult to determine but is probably quite low. However, the skull is involved in 65% of all patients. The symptoms in Paget's disease are related to the slow, progressive bone enlargement that can occur anywhere in the body. Involvement of the cranial foramina causes a myriad of neuralgia-type pains in the head and neck. Patients may also complain that a denture no longer fits because of the increased size of the jaw and flattening of the alveolar ridges. Increased vascularity of a pagetic bone explains the warmth that one can sometimes sense when palpating an involved bone. Patients with Paget's disease of bone are more susceptible to osteomyelitis and osteosarcoma in involved bones. As can be surmised from this discussion, the signs and symptoms of Paget's disease are protean and can easily be overlooked or misdiagnosed in the early stages. The use of laboratory tests is useful in confirming the diagnosis. Increased urinary hydroxyproline indicates osteolysis and is often accompanied by a marked increase in serum alkaline phosphatase during the osteoblastic phase.

Radiographic Appearance

The radiographic stages of Paget's disease correlate with the histologic changes. An initial deossification phase is followed by reossification, which evolves into mature ossification. The classic cotton-wool appearance is evident during the later stages of this transition. Thickening of the inner and outer tables of the skull results in a prominent intervening diploë and is termed **osteoporosis circumscripta.** Hypercementosis, loss of lamina dura, and pulp stones have been reported in patients with jaw lesions, but the significance of these signs is unknown. Pathologic fracture of the jaw and other bones has been reported.

Histopathologic Findings

Osteoclasts are prominent during the early stages because of the bone resorption. Basophilic reversal lines begin to appear when partial resorption is quickly followed by bone deposition. This process produces the classic "mosaic" bone pattern. In advanced lesions the osteoblastic/osteoclastic activity is minimal, and the lesion involves primarily mature lamellar bone.

Treatment

Dental surgery in the early phases of Paget's disease can lead to complications because of increased bleeding, and a susceptibility to developing infections is associated with in mature lesions. Postoperative antibiotics are recommended for these patients. In addition, patients with Paget's disease have a higher associated incidence of cardiovascular disease.

In general, asymptomatic patients are not treated unless they are young. Calcitonin is popular in the treatment of symptomatic Paget's disease, especially in the osteolytic phase, because it inhibits bone resorption by inactivating osteoclasts. However, calcitonin has the drawbacks of being expensive and having to be administered by subcutaneous injection. Once a patient is in remission, calcitonin can be discontinued until symptoms or abnormal laboratory values are detected. A diphosphonate, disodium etidronate, is useful in the treatment of Paget's disease because it can inhibit bone resorption and the growth of hydroxyapatite crystals. Although less expensive and easier to administer than calcitonin, disodium etidronate does not appear to be as effective in bone healing.

Prior to extensive bone surgery, consideration should be given to the preoperative administration of calcitonin for 3 months to decrease the vascularity of the bone and enhance healing.

The two main complications of Paget's disease are pathologic fracture (10%) and sarcomatous degeneration, which occurs in about 1% of patients. Fortunately, both pathologic fractures and malignant change are even rarer in a jawbone affected by Paget's disease.

References

Freeman, D.A.: Paget's disease of bone. Am. J. Med. Sci., 295:144–158, 1988.

Greenfield, G.B.: Radiology of Bone Diseases, 4th ed. Philadelphia: J.B. Lippincott, 1986, pp. 110–127.

Marks, J.M., and Dunkelberger, F.B.: Paget's disease. J. Am. Dent. Assoc., 101:49–52, 1980.

Resnick, D., and Niwayama, G.: Diagnosis of Bone and Joint Disorders. Philadelphia: W.B. Saunders, 1981, pp. 1721–1752.

Shafer, W.G., Hine, M.K., and Levy, B.M.: A Textbook of Oral Pathology, 4th ed. Philadelphia: W.B. Saunders, 1983, pp. 688–693.

Smith, B.J., and Eveson, J.W.: Paget's disease of bone with particular reference to dentistry. J. Oral Pathol., 10:233–247, 1981.

Sofaer, J.A.: Dental extractions in Paget's disease of bone. Int. J. Oral Surg., 13:79–84, 1984.

Stafne, E.C., and Austin, L.T.: A study of dental roentgenograms in cases of Paget's disease (osteitis deformans), osteitis fibrosa cystica and osteoma. J. Am. Dent. Assoc., 25:1201–1214, 1938.

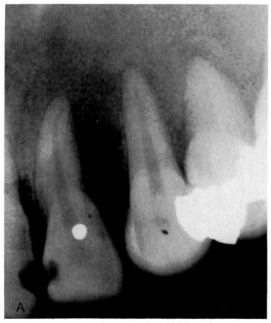
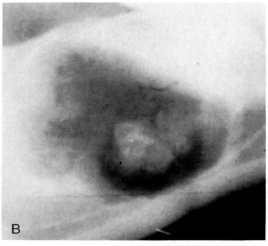

Figure 6–6. *A,* This periapical radiograph shows the typical "ground glass" appearance of fibrous dysplasia in the maxilla of an adolescent. Note also the loss of lamina dura. *B,* This "fibro-osseous" lesion reveals a well-defined, mixed radiolucent-radiopaque lesion in the mandible. The surrounding borders are quite hyperostotic. The diagnosis was fibrous dysplasia.

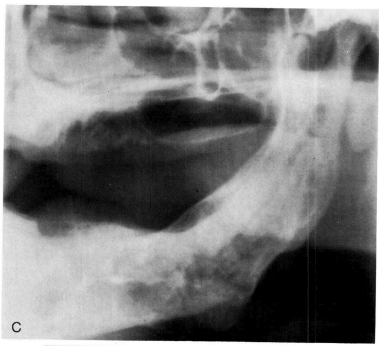

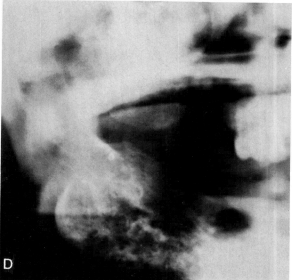

Figure 6–6 *Continued C,* A case of fibrous dysplasia that has remodeled a substantial portion of the posterior mandible. It appears as a rather diffuse, mixed radiolucent-radiopaque lesion. The changes extend from the canine region right up to the coronoid notch area. *D,* Another common appearance of fibrous dysplasia is multilocular. Such a lesion is seen in the right posterior mandible of this patient. Note the expansile appearance of this lesion.

Illustration continued on following page

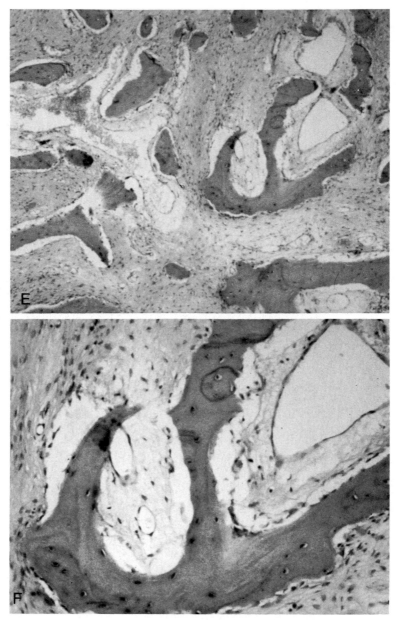

Figure 6–6 *Continued E*, This histologic section demonstrates the classic "Chinese character" orientation of the bony trabeculae. The bone can be of either the woven or the lamellar type. *F*, A high-power view shows the presence of several vascular spaces and a low level of osteoblastic activity along the periphery of the trabeculae.

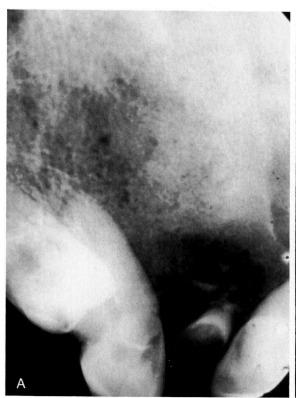 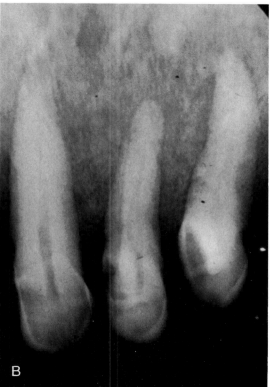

Figure 6–7. *A*, This illustration as well as those shown in *B* and *C* depicts the prominent trabecular changes seen in cases of Paget's disease of bone. *B*, Left anterior maxilla.

Illustration continued on following page

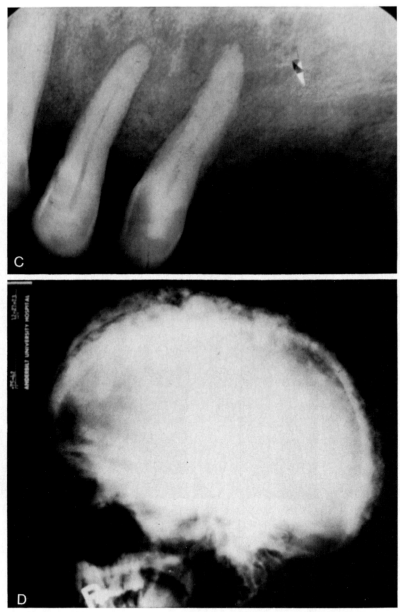

Figure 6–7 *Continued C,* Left posterior maxilla. *D,* Osteoporosis circumscripta of skull. Note cotton-wool appearance also.

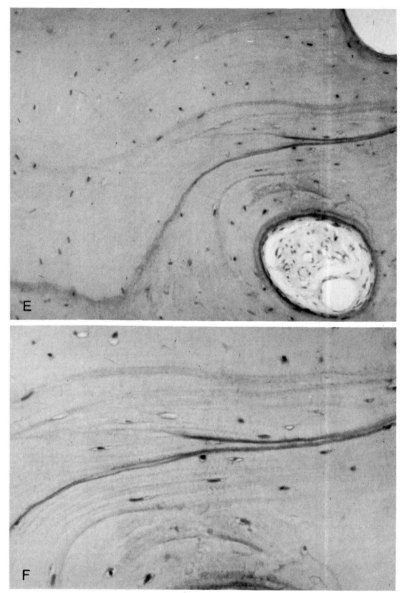

Figure 6–7 *Continued E*, This is an example of a mature lesion. Note the lack of osteoclastic or osteoblastic activity as well as the wavy reversal lines. Early lesions show increased osteoclastic activity (deossification), which is gradually replaced by increased osteoblastic activity (reossification). *F*, The reversal lines correspond to areas of bone that have been partially resorbed and subsequently reossified. The presence of these lines leads to the classic "mosaic" appearance of bone in the later stages of Paget's disease.

VASCULAR AND REACTIVE LESIONS

D. MILES

TRAUMATIC BONE CYST	**CENTRAL HEMANGIOMA**
ANEURYSMAL BONE CYST	**ARTERIOVENOUS MALFORMATION**
CENTRAL GIANT CELL GRANULOMA	

True vascular lesions are rare in the maxilla and mandible (Lund and Dahlin, 1964). Of the lesions to be discussed in this chapter, only the central hemangioma of bone is a bona fide neoplasm. A hemangioma is a tumor of childhood characterized by endothelial proliferation and a clinical course of rapid postnatal growth (Boyd et al, 1984). On the other hand, a vascular malformation such as the arteriovenous (A-V) malformation is a developmental anomaly with a normal endothelial cell cycle that, although present at birth, grows along with the child and can be modified by trauma, endocrine changes, and hemodynamic flow. The remainder of these lesions—the traumatic bone cyst, aneurysmal bone cyst, and central giant cell granuloma—are considered reactive lesions with varying degrees of vascularity. They too can be modified by vascular flow, trauma, endocrine changes, and giant cell involvement.

Radiographically, although appearances are variable, this group of lesions is commonly considered in the category of **multilocular lesions** when the clinician is developing the differential diagnosis. The traumatic bone cyst is one lesion that can be considered a great mimicker; that is, it can resemble many other lesions radiographically.

TRAUMATIC BONE CYST

The etiology of this lesion remains obscure. Despite the name traumatic bone cyst, there is rarely a history of trauma. Furthermore, this lesion is not really a true cyst at all. It has no identifiable epithelial lining histopathologically and thus fails to meet the main criterion for any cyst. Consequently, many additional names have been proposed for this lesion, among others, simple bone cyst, solitary bone cyst, hemorrhagic bone cyst, extravasation cyst, solitary bone cavity, unicameral cyst, idiopathic bone cavity, and progressive bone cavity (Kaugars and Cale, 1987). Nevertheless, the name that predominates in the literature is traumatic bone cyst (TBC). Rushton in 1946 described certain diagnostic criteria that define the TBC. These included the following:

1. The lesion should be single.
2. It should have no epithelial lining.
3. It should have no inflammation.
4. It should contain fluid or air and little or no soft tissue.
5. The margins of the cavity should be bony.
6. Histologic and chemical findings should not exclude the diagnosis of TBC.

More recently, these criteria have been modified to accept signs of inflammation and multiple lesions. Several authors have reported this lesion in association with florid osseous dysplasia (see Chapter 6), especially in black women over 30 years of age (Melrose et al, 1976; Kaugars and Cale, 1987), and other fibro-osseous lesions (Horner and Forman, 1988). Twenty-five percent of TBCs associated with florid osseous dysplasia are located in the anterior mandible. Theories of the origin of the TBC include a healing giant cell tumor (Monckeberg, 1904; Rushton, 1946; Hillerup and Hjørting-Hansen, 1978), intramedullary hemorrhage (Hansen et al, 1974), and a developmental anomaly (Jaffe, 1958).

Clinical Features

Most reports of TBC have noted a peak age incidence in the second decade of life. Ten of 12 reported cases by Poyton and Morgan in 1965 were in individuals under 20 years of age. There appears to be no sex predilection except in cases associated with florid osseous dysplasia. The posterior mandible is most commonly involved (Hansen et al, 1974). Most patients are asymptomatic; however, pain and swelling or expansion have been reported (Heubner and Turlington, 1971). In most instances, teeth in the region should be vital unless they are involved pulpally or periodontally. Several maxillary lesions have been reported (Poyton and Morgan, 1965; Hansen et al, 1974), and there has been a report of an unusual lesion of the mandibular condyle (Persson, 1985).

Radiographic Appearance

The classic appearance of a TBC is described as a solitary radiolucency of variable size with well-defined margins (which may or may not be sclerotic or corticated) that "scallop" between the roots of the teeth (Fig. 7–1A). However, many authors admit that the size, shape, and margins can be quite variable. Jacobs (1955) called these lesions "great imitators." Morris and coworkers (1970) described "a multiplicity of disguises." The lesion can be expansile but does not perforate the cortices of the mandible, only thins them (Fig. 7–1C and D) (Poyton and Morgan, 1965). The TBC does not displace teeth or resorb roots. The fact that the lesion has no epithelial boundary or tissue front to stimulate a bony response to "wall-off" the TBC might be a partial reason for the lack of a hyperostotic or sclerotic margin that delineates the cavity radiographically. Some authors describe this appearance as ill defined, when in fact the lesion is well defined but lacks the cortical rim seen at the periphery of other odontogenic lesions. Reports of lesions in the maxilla have not been very descriptive of the radiographic features. Most reports of lesions in this location cite the anterior maxilla as the site of predilection when the upper jaw is involved. Marlin and associates (1984) described a maxillary lesion with a scalloped outline surrounding the incisors and premolars that had a "corticated border in some areas."

Histopathologic Findings

The histopathologic findings in TBCs are less definitive than those seen with most lesions. Gross specimens consist of scant amounts of material. When tissue is present there are elements of fibrous connective tissue, hematopoietic or fatty marrow, and osteoid or new bone formation with osteoblasts. Inflammation is present in some specimens (contrary to Rushton's earlier postulates).

Treatment

Until very recently, treatment has consisted of surgical exploration or intervention at the time of biopsy. The cavity is curetted to obtain what little tissue is available; this procedure induces bleeding into the bony cavity that eventually organizes into a clot. Fibroblastic activity followed by osseous repair ensues. In patients with unicameral or simple bone cysts of other bones such as the femur, some clinicians have injected corticosteroids, usually methylprednisolone, and have achieved similar healing (Campana et al, 1984; Shindell et al 1987; Campanacci et al, 1986). Such trials have not been done in TBC lesions of the jaws. Autogenous blood has been injected into TBC to attempt repair with some success.

References

Boyd, J.B., Mulliken, J.B., Kaban, L.B., Upton, III, J., and Murray, J.E.: Skeletal changes associated with vascular malformations. Plast. Reconstr. Surg., 74:789, 1984.

Campana, R., Albisinni, U., Caroli, G.C., and Campanacci, M.: Contrast examination as a prognostic factor in the treatment of solitary bone cyst by cortisone injection. Skel. Radiol., 12:97, 1984.

Campanacci, M., Campana, R., and Picci, P.: Unicameral and aneurysmal bone cysts. Clin. Orthop. Rel. Res., 204:25–36, 1986.

Hansen, L.S., Sapone, J., and Sproat, R.C.: Traumatic bone cysts of jaws. Oral Surg., 37:899, 1974.

Heubner, R.B., and Turlington, E.G.: So-called traumatic bone cyst of the jaws. Oral Surg., 31:354, 1971.

Hillerup, S., and Hjørting-Hansen, E.: Aneurysmal bone cyst—simple bone cyst: Two aspects of the same pathologic entity. Int. J. Oral Surg., 7:16, 1978.

Horner, K., and Forman, G.M.: Atypical simple bone cysts of the jaws II: A possible association with benign fibro-osseous (cemental) lesions of the jaws. Clin. Radiol., 39:59–63, 1988.

Jacobs, M.H.: The traumatic bone cyst. Oral Surg., 8:940, 1955.

Jaffe, H.L.: Tumors and Tumorous Conditions of the Bones and Joints. Philadelphia: Lea & Febiger, 1958.

Kaugars, G.E., and Cale, A.E.: Traumatic bone cyst. Oral Surg., 63:318, 1987.

Lund, B.A., and Dahlin, D.C.: Hemangiomas of the mandible and maxilla. J. Oral Surg. Anesth. Hosp. Dent. Serv., 22:42/235, 1964.

Marlin, D.C., Barr, E.B., Zitterbart, P.A., and Sexauer, J.: Maxillary traumatic bone cyst: A case report. J. Ind. Dent. Assoc., 63:25, 1984.

Melrose, R.J., Abrams, A.M., and Mills, B.G.: Florid osseous dysplasia: A clinical-pathologic study of thirty-four cases. Oral Surg., 41:62, 1976.

Monckeberg, G.: Ueber Cystenbildung bei Ostitis Fibrosa. Verh. Deutsch. Gessellsch. Pathol., 7:232, 1904.

Morris, C.R., Steed, D.L., and Jacoby, J.J.: Traumatic bone cysts. J. Oral Surg. 28:188, 1970.

Persson, G.: An atypical solitary bone cyst. J. Oral Maxillofac. Surg., 43:905, 1985.

Poyton, H.G., and Morgan, G.A.: The simple bone cyst. Oral Surg., 20:188, 1965.

Rushton, M.A.: Solitary bone cysts in the mandible. Br. Dent. J., 81:37, 1946.

Shindell, R., Connolly, J.F., and Lippiello, L.: Prostaglandin levels in a unicameral bone cyst treated by corticosteroid injection. J. Pediatr. Orthop., 7:210, 1987.

ANEURYSMAL BONE CYST

Numerous theories have been proposed for the origin of the aneurysmal bone cyst (ABC). This lesion was first described in 1942 by Jaffe and Lichtenstein. Only 21 cases of aneurysmal bone cyst of the jaws had been described until 1980, and 48 by 1984 (Gingell et al, 1984). By 1986 the number of reported cases had reached 61 (Neuman, 1987). Many cases of aneurysmal bone cysts have been associated with other primary bone lesions such as fibrous dysplasia (Cornyn and Morris, 1978), central giant cell granuloma (Bernier and Bhaskar, 1958), ossifying fibroma (Buraczewski and Dabska, 1971), cementifying fibroma (Ellis and Walters, 1972), and osteosarcoma (Grushkin and Dahlin, 1968), as well as with other lesions.

Theories proposed to explain these findings include: (1) the presence of a localized circulatory disturbance leading to a dilated vascular bed with increased venous pressure, which in turn leads to bone remodeling; (2) an exaggerated response by connective tissue to repair a hematoma of bone; and (3) a secondary change in or response to a primary lesion (such as those described previously). Struthers and Shear (1984) published a comprehensive list of lesions that have been associated with the aneurysmal bone cyst (Table 7–1). You should note from the table that all the lesions in bold print are described in this chapter as vascular and reactive lesions.

The ABC has been described much more frequently in the long bones, especially the humerus and proximal femur (Campanacci et al, 1986). In these locations it has also been associated with benign conditions such as giant cell tumor, chondroblastoma, chondromyxoid

Table 7–1. LESIONS REPORTED IN ASSOCIATION WITH THE ANEURYSMAL BONE CYST

Cementifying fibroma	Giant cell tumor of bone
Nonossifying fibroma	**Solitary bone cyst (TBC)**
Ossifying fibroma	Hemangioendothelioma
Osteoblastoma	**Hemangioma**
Chondroblastoma	Fibrous dysplasia
Chondromyxoid fibroma	Osteosarcoma
Myxofibroma	Sarcoma
Central giant cell granuloma	

Modified from Struthers, P.J., and Shear, M.: Aneurysmal bone cyst of the jaws. I. Clinicopathologic features. Int. J. Oral Surg., 13:92–100, 1984. © 1984 Munksgaard International Publishers Ltd., Copenhagen, Denmark.

fibroma, and fibrous dysplasia and with malignant tumors including osteosarcoma, chondrosarcoma, and malignant endothelial tumors (Dahlin and McLeod, 1982).

In 1978 Hillerup and Hjorting-Hansen speculated that the aneurysmal bone cyst, the simple bone cyst, and the central giant cell granuloma were "different expressions of the same disease or failing healing process of bone lesions."

Clinical Features

The aneurysmal bone cyst in the head and neck region is primarily a lesion of younger age groups. Most lesions have been seen in patients under 20 years old. However, several cases in older individuals exist in the literature. Most reports also cite a predilection of the ABC for the mandible, especially in the body and ramus region (Bhaskar et al, 1959; Struthers and Shear, 1984; Dahlin and McLeod, 1982). Toljanic and colleagues (1987), in their review of the lesion, claimed that the common clinical presentation was a swelling of the soft tissues overlying the bony lesion. The mass could be painless or not and often had a firm or bone-hard consistency when palpated. Often the onset of the lesion, and thus the swelling, was rapid. There does not appear to be a sex predilection. Cases reported seem to be relatively equally distributed between men and women.

Radiographic Appearance

A case by Eisenbud et al (1987) illustrates and perhaps supports the concept of an altered circulatory disturbance in an area of compromised bone with remodeling resulting from hemodynamic forces. The initial radiographic presentation of a 48-year-old man with a right-side facial swelling was a diffuse, ill-defined osteolytic lesion that appeared to have eroded the inferior cortical border. Nine months after the initial visit the appearance had changed dramatically. The ABC was now a large expansile, somewhat multilocular radiolucent lesion that had a distinct margin. The second appearance was classic in the medical literature for an ABC, which is often described in the long bones as a "blow-out" lesion. Another presentation is a unilocular appearance. Expansion and cortical thinning are common (Fig. 7–2A and B). However, there is no characteristic or pathognomonic radiographic presentation for the ABC.

Hudson et al (1985) demonstrated fluid levels in multilocular ABCs of the skeleton with the use of magnetic resonance imaging (MRI) and computed tomography (CT). These imaging modalities allow the radiologist to look selectively for soft tissues in and around pathologic lesions. This has not yet been done with ABCs of the jaws. These imaging modalities, if performed on multilocular lesions, might help to separate vascular lesions such as the ABC, hemangioma, A-V malformation, and central giant cell granuloma (CGCG) from other multilocular odontogenic lesions without the need for more invasive procedures such as angiography. These imaging techniques and resultant views must, however, be coupled with the clinical and historic information of the patient. "Radiology comes to its greatest fruition in the hands of those who are best informed clinically" (Worth, 1963).

Histopathologic Findings

Microscopic examination of the ABC reveals multiple blood-filled sinusoidal spaces. A fibrous connective tissue stroma surrounds these spaces and contains numerous giant cells and scattered inflammatory cells. New bone trabeculae and osteoid are usually seen. These microscopic features are similar if not identical to those of the TBC and CGCG. On gross examination these lesions are not that similar.

Treatment

Treatment of the ABC of the jaws is conservative surgical curettage. However, many reports of recurrence exist, and some authors propose surgical resection. Struthers and Shear (1984) suggest that recurrence is most likely the result of technical management rather than the biologic behavior of the lesion. Radiotherapy has also been used in an attempt to fibrose vessels but probably should be avoided owing to potential induction of malignant transformation. Unlike the TBC, in which steroid injection has produced favorable results, surgery is the treatment of choice for the ABC.

References

Bernier, J.L., and Bhaskar, S.N.: Aneurysmal bone cysts of the mandible. Oral Surg., 11:1018–1028, 1958.

Bhaskar, S.N. Bernier, J.L., and Godby, F.: Aneurysmal bone cyst and other giant cell lesions of the jaws: Report of 104 cases. J. Oral Surg., 17:30–41, 1959.

Buraczewski, J., and Dabska, P.: Pathogenesis of aneurysmal bone cyst: Relationship between aneurysmal bone cyst and fibrous dysplasia of bone. Cancer 28:597–603, 1971.

Campanacci, M., Campanna, R., and Picci, P.: Unicameral and aneurysmal bone cyst. Clin. Orthop. Rel. Res., 20:425–436, 1986.

Cornyn, J., and Morris, C.R.: Different and unusual perspectives in diagnosis. Fifth Annual Continuing Education Program. American Academy of Dental Radiology (Case 8), 1978.

Dahlin, D.C., and McLeod, R.A.: Aneurysmal bone cyst and other non-neoplastic conditions. Skel. Radiol., 8:243–250, 1980.

Eisenbud, L., Attie, J., Garlick, J., and Platt, N.: Aneurysmal bone cyst of the mandible. Oral Surg., 64:202–206, 1987.

Ellis, D.J., and Walters, P.J.: Aneurysmal bone cyst of the maxilla. Oral Surg., 34:26–32, 1972.

Gingell, J.C., Leva, B.A., Beckerman, T., and Tilghman, D.M.: Aneurysmal bone cyst. J. Oral Maxillofac. Surg., 42:527–534, 1984.

Grushkin, S.E., and Dahlin, D.C.: Aneurysmal bone cysts of the jaws. J. Oral Surg., 26:523–528, 1968.

Hillerup, S., and Hjorting-Hansen, E.: Aneurysmal bone cyst, two aspects of the same pathologic entity? Int. J. Oral Surg., 7:16–22, 1978.

Hudson, T.M., Hamlin, D.J., and Fitzsimmon, J.R.: Magnetic resonance imaging of fluid levels in an aneurysmal bone cyst and in anticoagulated human blood. Skel. Radiol., 13:267–270, 1985.

Jaffe, H.L., and Lichtenstein, L.: Solitary unicameral bone cyst. Arch. Surg., 46:1004–1025, 1942.

Newman, L.: Aneurysmal bone cyst—A lesion in the mandibular ramus. Br. J. Oral Maxillofac. Surg., 25:74–78, 1987.

Struthers, P.J., and Shear, M.: Aneurysmal bone cyst of the jaws (I). Clinicopathologic features. Int. J. Oral Surg., 13:85–91, 1984.

Struthers, P.J., and Shear, M.: Aneurysmal bone cyst of the jaws (II). Pathogenesis. Int. J. Oral Surg., 13:92–100, 1984.

Toljanic, J.A., Lechewski, E., Huvos, A.G., Strong, E.W., and Schwiger, J.W.: Aneurysmal bone cysts of the jaws: A case study and review of the literature. Oral Surg., 64:72–77, 1987.

Worth, H.M.: Principles and Practice of Oral Radiologic Interpretation. Chicago: Year Book Medical Publishers, 1963, p. 275.

CENTRAL GIANT CELL GRANULOMA

In 1953, Jaffe wrote about the "giant-cell reparative granuloma." Comparing it with the giant cell tumor of bone, he said, "Actually, the jaw lesion in question only mimics the bona fide giant-cell tumor of bone, and it would probably be best to get away altogether from referring to it as a giant-cell tumor . . . the lesion is not a neoplasm in the true sense, but represents instead a local reparative reaction." He went on to say that "giant cell reparative granuloma of jawbones is not a common lesion." Thirty-five years later, Eisenbud and associates (1988) reported their experience with 37 cases and stated, "The central giant cell granuloma is one of the most commonly encountered expansile lesions of the jaws, second in frequency only to various odontogenic cysts." At least two things have changed in those 35 years. First and most obvious is the increase in reports of cases of CGCG. The second change, albeit less obvious initially, is the dropping of the term reparative from the histopathologic name of the lesion. The lesion when encountered is not in the process of repairing itself but, like the traumatic and aneurysmal bone cysts with their common and overlapping histopathology, probably represents a faulty response of healing altered by the presence of giant cells and disturbed circulation. Like Jaffe, Abrams and Shear (1974) and Batsakis (1979) believe that the CGCG and the giant cell tumor of bone are separate and distinct lesions, the latter being a true neoplasm. Most authors now believe the current hypothesis that the CGCG is one lesion in a spectrum of altered vascular and reactive responses in bone that include the ABC, the TBC, and the CGCG. As will be noted in the final section of this chapter, this spectrum of vascular lesions may also include the A-V malformation.

Very recently, Chuong and coworkers (1986) presented evidence that there is a difference in biologic behavior among CGCGs. They classified CGCGs into two groups—a "nonaggressive group" and an "aggressive group"—based on several histopathologic parameters including fractional surface area and relative size of the giant cells, stromal characteristics, mitotic index, presence of inflammatory cells, and amount of hemosiderin. They believe that the *aggressive* lesions have a higher relative size and that *recurrent* lesions are both larger and have a larger fractional surface area. Their findings may explain some of the difficulties that led earlier authors to confuse CGCGs and giant cell tumors of bone. Cases of CGCG have been reported outside the jaws (Merkow et al, 1985; Lorenzo and Dorfman, 1980; Picci et al, 1986), and the giant cell tumor of bone has been reported in the jaws (Sturrock et al, 1984; Abrams and Shear, 1974).

However, there are few reports of malignant giant cell lesions of any type of the jaws. Indeed, the first purportedly well-documented case of primary malignant giant cell tumor of the jawbones was reported by Mintz and colleagues in 1981. Obviously, it is very important to report any lesion of the mandible or maxilla that carries the diagnosis of CGCG or other giant cell lesion of the jaws.

Clinical Features

As early as 1965, Waldron and Shafer recognized and reported that the CGCG was primarily a lesion of children or young adults, with few cases occurring in adults over 50 years of age. Other authors have since confirmed this finding (Ficarra et al, 1987; Eisenbud et al, 1988). Table 7–2 illustrates the age range graphically in 37 cases. Eighty-nine percent of these lesions occurred in people under 50 years of age. Furthermore, there appears to be a predilection for women. In their paper, Waldron and Shafer reported that 26 of 38 patients were women (68%). Eisenbud and associates reported a 62% female predilection.

The CGCG is also one of the few lesions to cross the midline (Langland et al, 1982). Another clinical characteristic often reported of this lesion is its tendency to occur anterior to the first molars in both the maxilla and the mandible (Worth, 1963; Waldron and Shafer, 1966). However, the most recently reported series describes an equal distribution in the mandible (12 lesions in the anterior mandible and 13 in the posterior body and ramus) and a 2:1 occurrence in the posterior region of the maxilla (Eisenbud et al, 1988). Still, the mandible appears to be affected more than the maxilla. Various clinical appearances and behavior have been reported, ranging from a slow-growing painless swelling to a rapidly

Table 7–2. AGE RANGE OF CASES OF CENTRAL GIANT CELL GRANULOMA

Age Range	Number of Cases
1–9	3
10–19	16
20–29	6
30–39	6
40–49	2
50–59	0
60–69	2
70–79	1
80–89	1
Total	37

Modified from Eisenbud, L., Stern, M., Rotherberg, M., and Sachs, S.A.: Central giant cell granuloma of the jaws: Experiences in the management of 37 cases. J. Oral Maxillofac. Surg., 46:376–384, 1988.

aggressive lesion producing pain and loosening of teeth due to resorption of the apices. As described earlier, Chuong and coworkers (1986) divided CGCGs of the jaws into two groups, aggressive and nonaggressive, based on their clinical presentation and behavior as well as on the histopathologic features. Aggressive lesions were described by features such as pain, rapid growth, swelling, root resorption, cortical perforation, and rate of recurrence. Root resorption and cortical involvement are best described in terms of radiographic features. Recurrent lesions are more apt to be found by radiographic follow-up as well.

Radiographic Appearance

The classic radiographic appearance of a CGCG is that of a multilocular lesion anterior to the first molar region in the mandible that may or may not cross the midline. As discussed previously, the lesion may show evidence of expansion, root resorption, and erosion or remodeling of the cortical bone. Perforation of the cortex is rare and is more often a sign of an acute infection or malignant lesion. Some authors have called these lesions soap-bubble radiolucencies. However, this radiographic term is probably better reserved for an ameloblastoma. The CGCG can also displace teeth and cause root divergence. Occasionally, this lesion may be unilocular. Some authors have noted that the root resorption associated with the CGCG is different from that seen with odontogenic cysts (Poyton, 1982). They describe a concave appearance of the root (Fig. 7–3A) and believe this to be an important radiographic distinction. Another radiographically distinct feature described by Stafne (1953) involved the septa or trabeculations traversing the lesion. He reported that these trabeculations were usually less distinct, more variable in thickness, and more irregular in shape than those of an ameloblastoma. Other authors have noted trabecular differences and have described a crenated or scalloped border and curving of the trabeculae. Worth said the margins were less continuous of the CGCG and that internal trabeculae were "wispy." He also thought that the scalloping of the margin—"each scalloped excavation representing a large arc of small circle . . . very suggestive of this particular lesion"—was an important distinction.

Similar radiographic features of the CGCG

have been described in lesions outside of the jaws (Merkow et al, 1985; Wold et al, 1986) but overlap with radiographic features of other giant cell lesions.

Histopathologic Findings

CGCGs are usually described as having ovoid, round, or spindle-shaped fibroblasts that project between giant cells in swirls. Focal areas of herringbone or storiform patterns may also be seen. Endothelial cells are also found within the stroma as well as numerous capillaries. The giant cells are multinucleated and appear like foreign body–type giant cells and tend to cluster. The lesions are nonencapsulated. Foci of woven bone are also present in haphazard patterns. Intravascular and extravascular erythrocytes and hemosiderin may be seen, but there is usually little inflammatory cell infiltrate. Eisenbud and associates (1988) described the features of the CGGG as a less exuberant response than those of an aneurysmal bone cyst with its "larger blood-filled spaces and encompassing osseous septa." It is these overlapping histopathologic features of the traumatic bone cyst, aneurysmal bone cyst, and CGCG that have caused oral pathologists to speculate that these three lesions are variable expressions of the same pathologic process. Table 7–3 suggests a similar mechanistic pathway, which has been synthesized from the numerous articles about these vascular lesions including the A-V malformation.

Treatment

Simple curettage of the lesion to remove all soft tissue and diseased bone has been recommended as treatment for CGCG for many years. More recently, curettage plus peripheral ostectomy using large burs to remove the lesion down to a hard burnished surface of bone has been very successful. Although recurrences do occur, they too are treated easily by curettage. Resection of the mandible or maxilla, even with the so-called aggressive CGCG, is probably not warranted. Radiation therapy has been used for treatment of lesions of the maxilla in conjunction with surgery with excellent results (Chuong et al, 1986). However, as with most benign lesions, radiation therapy is not usually indicated—except for extremely aggressive lesions, which are less amenable to surgery—owing to the potential of radiation to induce malignant transformation.

References

Abrams, B., and Shear, M.: A histological comparison of the giant cells in the central giant cell granuloma of the jaws and the giant cell tumor of bone. J. Oral Pathol., 3:217–223, 1974.

Batsakis, J.G.: Tumors of the Head and Neck, 2nd ed. Baltimore: Williams & Wilkins, 1979, pp. 000.

Chuong, R., Kaban, L.B., Kozakewich, H., and Perez-Atayde, A.: Central giant cell lesions of the jaws: A clinicopathologic study. J. Oral Maxillofac. Surg., 44:708–713, 1986.

Eisenbud, L., Stern, M., Rotherberg, M., and Sachs, S.A.: Central giant cell granuloma of the jaws: Experiences in the management of thirty-seven cases. J. Oral Maxillofac. Surg., 46:376–384, 1988.

Ficarra, G., Kapan, L.B., and Hansen, L.S.: Central giant cell lesions of the mandible and maxilla: A clinicopathologic and cytometric study. Oral Surg., 64:44–49, 1987.

Jaffe, H.L.: Giant-cell reparative granuloma, traumatic bone cyst, and fibrous (fibro-osseous) dysplasia of the jawbones. Oral Surg., 6:159–175, 1953.

Text continued on page 171

Table 7–3. ETIOLOGIC PATHWAY FOR REACTIVE LESIONS

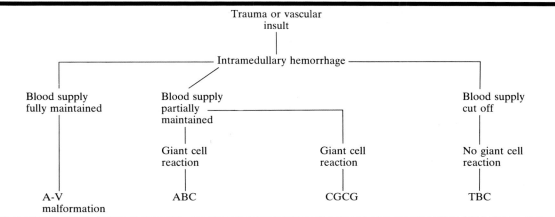

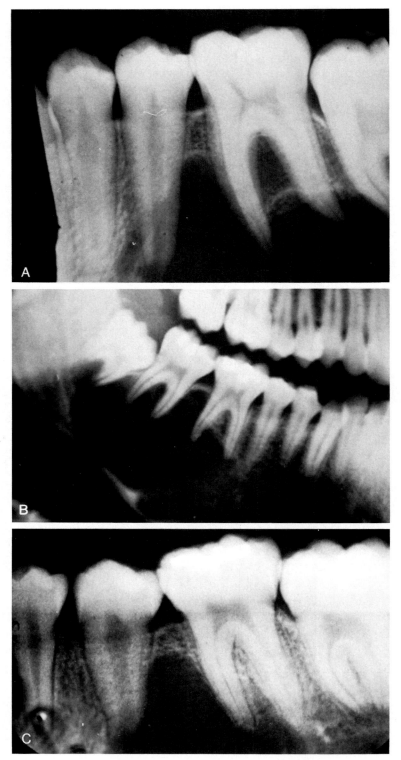

Figure 7–1. *A,* This periapical radiograph of a young adult man demonstrates the classic scalloping of the lesion between the roots of teeth. Note also that there is some evidence of a sclerotic or hyperostotic border along a portion of the lesion but not surrounding it entirely. *B,* A large, traumatic bone cyst in the right mandible. Note that there is some remodeling of the lower cortical border, some scalloping of the superior boundary of the lesion between the root apices, and the suggestion of some expansion of the lesion. *C,* This is a small, well-defined, unilocular radiolucency with no evidence of any cortical outline. The interior contains no radiolucencies. The lesion extends between the root apices but does not resorb teeth. This lesion is consistent with a traumatic bone cyst.

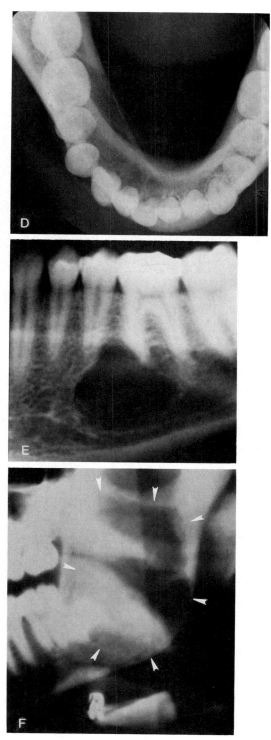

Figure 7–1 *Continued D*, A traumatic bone cyst extending from the canine to the second molar region. Note the slight expansion and thinning of the lingual cortical border. *E*, A typical traumatic bone cyst with some evidence of hyperostosis along the posterior inferior aspect. (Courtesy of Dr. C. Tomich, Indiana University School of Dentistry, Indianapolis, Indiana.) *F*, This illustration and those shown in *G* through *J* represent a single case of a large traumatic bone cyst in a 15-year-old girl. This figure shows a somewhat large, expansile, multilocular lesion in the posterior mandible that has some diffuse or ill-defined borders (*arrows*).

Illustration continued on following page

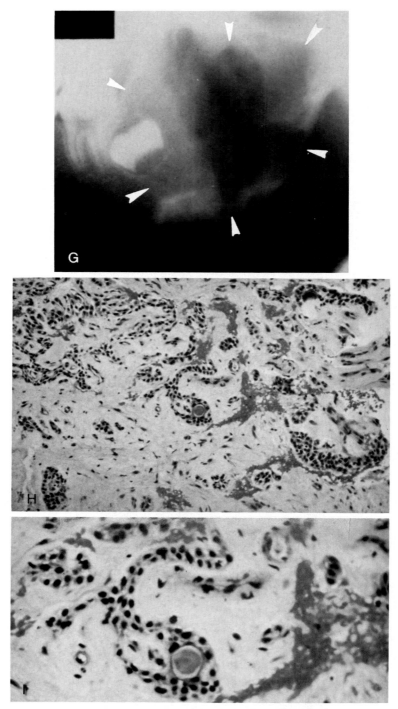

Figure 7–1 *Continued G,* This lateral jaw film reveals the large radiolucent lesion in close proximity to a developing third molar (*arrows*). *H,* A low-power photomicrograph of the tissue in this case reveals a loose, fibrous connective tissue stroma, regions of extravasated blood, and islands of odontogenic-appearing epithelium. The biopsy report identified a traumatic bone cyst and a coexisting odontogenic lesion. The odontogenic lesion was not specified. *I,* A higher power photomicrograph of the lesion in *H.* Note the area of calcification that is suggestive of Liesegang's rings. These changes might be consistent with a calcifying epithelial odontogenic tumor.

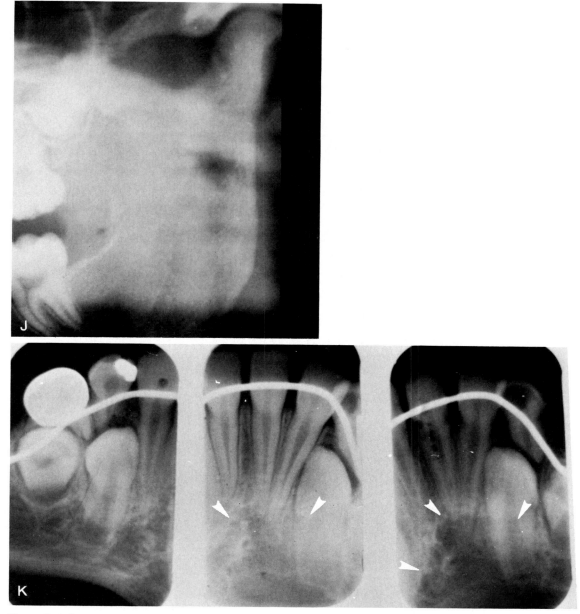

Figure 7–1 *Continued J,* A portion of a panoramic film revealing a completely healed mandible some 12 months after the initial surgical procedure. *K,* These periapical films reveal the presence of a diffuse radiolucency (*ar-rows*) in the anterior mandible of an 8½-year-old girl. The border is not well defined, nor does it have any cortical outline. The progression of the lesion is seen in the next two films (*L* and *M*).

Illustration continued on following page

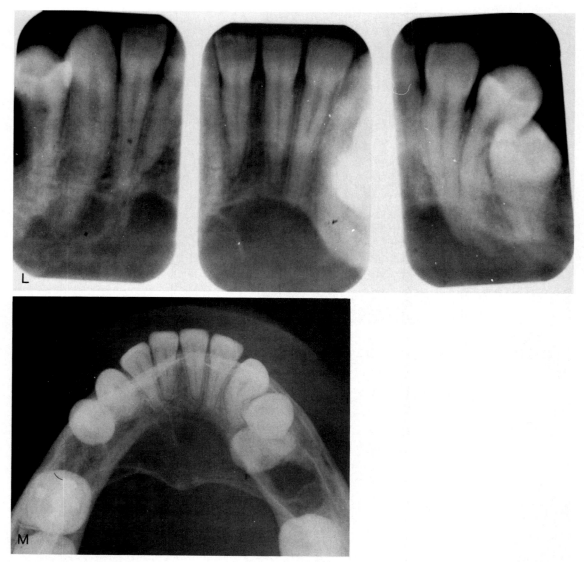

Figure 7–1 *Continued L*, These periapical films reveal a large, well-defined radiolucency in the anterior mandible with some scalloping of the superior border. There is evidence of a cortical outline. *M*, An occlusal film of the same patient at age 15 shows a large, expansile, some-what multilocular radiolucency in the anterior mandible crossing the midline. The differential diagnosis would include a central giant cell granuloma; however, this case documents the slow progression of a traumatic bone cyst during a period of 7 years.

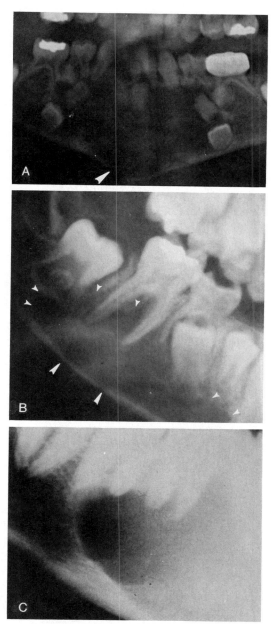

Figure 7–2. *A,* A large, expansile radiolucency in the anterior mandible of a 4½-year-old boy. Note the pathologic fracture along the lower cortical border (*arrow*). Teeth are displaced and roots are resorbed. This lesion proved to be an aneurysmal bone cyst. *B,* Aneurysmal bone cyst in the right mandible of a 9-year-old boy. This lesion has thinned the lower cortical border (*arrows*) and displaced the developing premolar. Its margins are not well delineated, and there is a lack of a cortical outline. *C,* Aneurysmal bone cyst in a lower mandible that appears to scallop between the root apices. Although the radiograph is of poor quality, there appears to be some expansion between the canine and the first premolar. A traumatic bone cyst would not do this. There may also be some root resorption of the second premolar.

Illustration continued on following page

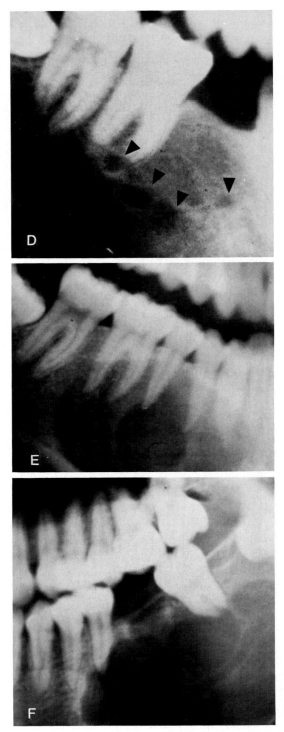

Figure 7–2 *Continued D*, Appearance of the aneurysmal bone cyst seen in *C* 3 years postoperatively. Note: there are some radiolucencies (*arrows*) within a larger radiolucency. This appearance may suggest that a lesion is still present or that the lesion has recurred. *E*, Aneurysmal bone cyst "arising from" or associated with a central ossifying fibroma in a 16-year-old boy. *F*, A panoramic view of a large, slightly multilocular, expansile radiolucency in the left mandible. The lesion has thinned but not perforated the lower cortical border. There is some tooth displacement. (*F* and *J,* From Okuyama, T., Suzuki, H., Umchara, I., et al.: Diagnosis of aneurysmal bone cyst of the mandible. A report of two cases with emphasis on scintigraphic approaches. Clin. Nucl. Med., 10:786–790, 1985.)

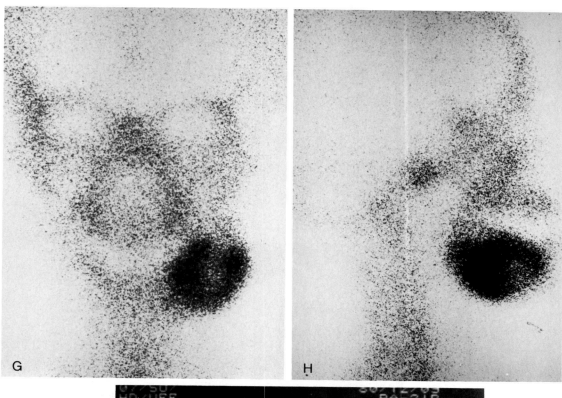

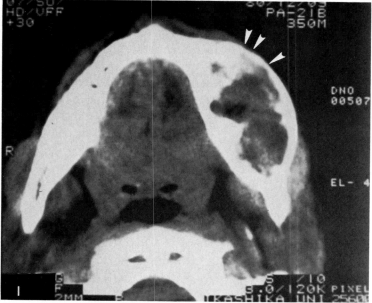

Figure 7–2 *Continued G,* Nuclear scan of an aneurysmal bone cyst using ⁹⁹T methylene diphosphonate. Area of increased uptake is very pronounced. (Courtesy of Dr. T. Okuyama, Tokyo, Japan.) *H,* Radionuclide scan of the case shown in *H* from a lateral perspective. (Courtesy of Dr. T. Okuyama, Tokyo, Japan.) *I,* CT scan at the level of the midramus confirms the expansion and multilocular nature of this aneurysmal bone cyst. Note cortical thinning on the buccal aspect (*arrows*). (Courtesy of Dr. T. Okuyama, Tokyo, Japan.)

Illustration continued on following page

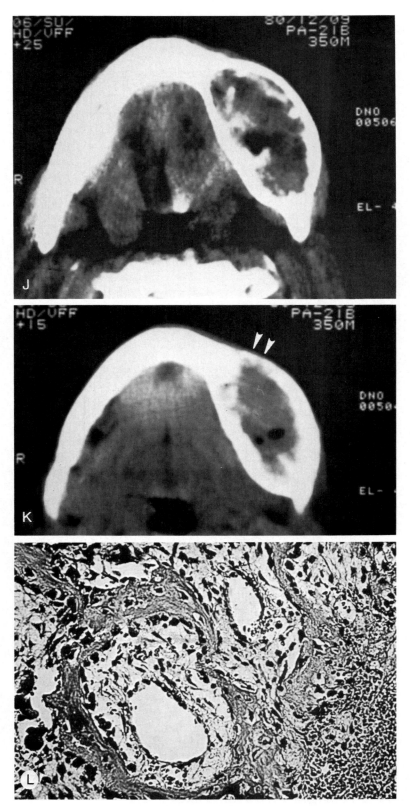

Figure 7–2 *Continued J*, Several bony septa or sequestra are noted within the lesion. They are radiopaque. *K*, This CT scan shows thinning of the cortex nearer the inferior cortical border of the mandible (*arrows*). (Courtesy of Dr. T. Okuyama, Tokyo, Japan.) *L*, Numerous blood-filled spaces in fibrous connective tissue stroma. Some osteoid is also present.

Langland, O.L., Langlais, R.P., and Morris, C.R.: Principles and Practice of Panoramic Radiology. Philadelphia: W.B. Saunders, 1982, p. 293.

Lorenzo, J.D., and Dorfman, H.D.: Giant cell reparative granuloma of short tubular bones of the hands and feet. Am. J. Surg. Pathol., 4:551–563, 1980.

Merkow, R.L., Bansal, M., and Inglis, A.E.: Giant cell reparative granuloma in the hand: Report of three cases and review of the literature. J. Hand Surg., 10A:733–739, 1985.

Mintz, G.A., Abrams, A.M., Carlsen, G.D., Melrose, R.J., and Fister, H.W.: Primary malignant giant cell tumor of the mandible. Report of a case and review of the literature. Oral Surg., 51:164–171, 1981.

Picci, P., Baldini, N., Sudanese, A., Boriani, S., and Campanacci, M.: Giant cell reparative granuloma and other giant cell lesions of the bones of the hands and feet. Skel. Radiol., 15:415–421, 1986.

Poyton, H.G.: Oral Radiology. Baltimore: Williams & Wilkins, 1982, p. 281.

Stafne, E.C.: Value of roentgenograms in diagnosis of tumors of the jaws. Oral Surg., 6:82–92, 1953.

Sturrock, B.D., Marks, R.B., Gross, B.D., and Carr, R.F.: Giant cell tumor of the mandible. J. Oral Maxillofac. Surg., 42:262–267, 1984.

Waldron, C.A., and Shafer, W.G.: The central giant cell reparative granuloma of the jaws: An analysis of 38 cases. Am. J. Clin. Pathol., 65:437–447, 1966.

Wold, L.E., Dobyns, J.H., Swee, R.G., and Dahlin, D.C.: Giant cell reaction (giant cell reparative granuloma) of the small bones of the hands and feet. Am. J. Surg. Pathol., 10:491–496, 1986.

Worth, H.M.: Principles and Practice of Oral Radiologic Interpretation. Chicago: Year Book Medical Publishers, 1963, pp. 497–505.

CENTRAL HEMANGIOMA

Fortunately, hemagiomas arising centrally in the mandible or maxilla are extremely rare. Only 60 cases had been reported up to 1979 (Batsakis, 1979). Several additional cases have been added to the literature since then (Sadowsky et al, 1981; Hayward, 1981; Nelson et al, 1986; Stassi et al, 1984). The central hemangioma is a true vascular neoplasm. Benign forms include angioma, hemangioendothelioma, capillary hemangioma, and cavernous hemangioma. Malignant versions also exist and are known by a wide variety of names. They are extremely rare in the jaws. The central hemangioma appears to be more common in women and is detected usually in the second decade of life (Thoma and Goldman, 1960). Surgical intervention for tooth extraction or biopsy may lead to profound bleeding and even death. **Thorough preoperative evaluation including auscultation, aspiration, and radiographic interpretation is mandatory in patients with any lesion suspected to be of vascular origin.**

Clinical Features

Various clinical features have been reported with the hemangioma including mobile teeth, depressible teeth, spontaneous bleeding around the necks of teeth, expansion, paresthesia, teeth missing in the area, and displaced teeth. Some lesions also exhibit pulsation when palpated or an audible bruit (noise) when auscultated. The area involved may be warm to the touch. Reports seem to indicate a predilection for the mandible (2:1) and for women (Hayward, 1981). The molar region is most often involved, at least in the mandible. A lesion in the maxilla involved a 59-year-old-woman who presented with orbital proptosis and swelling of the eye. This tumor involved a large portion of the maxillary antrum on the left side (Stassi et al, 1984).

Radiographic Appearance

The central hemangioma presents most often as a multilocular or soap-bubble radiolucency but usually has ill-defined and irregular margins. Coarse trabeculae within the lesion are often visible (Fig. 7–4). Some authors describe trabeculae in radiating spicules like the spokes of a wheel (Poyton, 1982; Worth and Stoneman, 1979). This tumor can also exhibit the same sun-burst or sun-ray appearance seen with the osteosarcoma, with trabeculae radiating outward at right angles to the bone. Resorption at the roots of adjacent teeth has been reported by several authors. There are, however, no pathognomonic radiographic features for the central hemangioma. Because it is included in the differential diagnosis of other multilocular lesions, aspiration, auscultation, and careful interpretation of the radiographic features are mandatory before proceeding to biopsy or treatment. If aspiration is positive or if there is a positive finding of pulsation or bruit, arteriography is indicated prior to undertaking any further procedure. Arteriography will delineate the arterial or venous supply to the lesion and helps the surgeon decide which vessels to ligate or tie off prior to removing the lesion (Langland et al, 1982).

Histopathologic Findings

There are several histologic types of central hemagioma. The two most common are the capillary and cavernous types. The capillary type consists of fine capillary loops lined by a single endothelial cell layer. The picture is not unlike that of young granulation tissue (Shafer et al, 1974). The cavernous type consists of many large, thin-walled vessels and sinusoidal, blood-filled spaces. These thin-walled spaces are lined with endothelial cells. One might speculate that the capillary type of hemangioma may give rise to a diffuse, less cystic-appearing lesion radiographically and that the cavernous type might correlate better with a more multilocular appearance.

Treatment

All vascular lesions must be approached carefully and systematically. The potential for uncontrolled hemorrhage and possible death by exsanguination is well documented. Treatment options include radiotherapy, use of sclerosing agents, embolization, and surgical intervention such as curettage and resection. Sclerosing agents promote thrombus formation when injected directly into the lesion (Chin, 1983). If successful, they induce fibrosis of vascular channels, making resection potentially less dangerous. These agents are used in soft tissue hemangiomas and other vascular lesions but usually not in central lesions. Embolization of hemangiomas has been successfully performed using silicone pellets (LaDow and McFall, 1964). Other agents used have included Gelfoam soaked in thrombin and even pieces of muscle. However, injection of these agents into the wrong vessel or their use in an A-V malformation carries with it a serious risk of death.

Radiotherapists consider hemangiomas radiosensitive, and they have thus employed various doses of radiation to obliterate the vascular endothelium and reduce the tumor size. The treatment is not considered curative. Morbidity to other structures such as bone, salivary glands, and possibly thyroid must be considered as well as the potential induction of sarcomatous change. The most common treatment modality is surgical resection. Vessels to the area such as the maxillary, mandibular, or even carotid arteries must often be ligated to control hemorrhage during the procedure. Even bilateral ligation of the external carotid arteries may not be sufficient to prevent hemorrhage because often collateral circulation from an unexpected source may be present. Regardless of the approach, the surgeon must always be prepared to encounter massive bleeding with this and other vascular lesions. A case of spontaneous resolution of a vascular lesion, possibly a hemangioma, was reported following an aspiration procedure (Nelson et al, 1986).

References

Batsakis, J.G.: Tumors of the Head and Neck, 2nd ed. Baltimore: Williams & Wilkins, 1979, pp. 291–296.

Chin, D.C.: Treatment of maxillary hemangioma with a sclerosing agent. Oral Surg., 55:247–249, 1983.

Hayward, J.R.: Central cavernous hemangioma of the mandible: Report of four cases. J. Oral Surg., 39:526–532, 1981.

LaDow, C.S., Henefer, E.P., and McFall, T.A.: Hemangiomas of the mandible. J. Oral Surg., 24:252–259, 1964.

LaDow, C.S., McFall, T.A.: Central hemangioma of the maxilla with von Hippel's disease: Report of a case. J. Oral Surg., 22:252–259, 1964.

Langland, O.L., Langlais, R.P., and Morris, C.R.: Principles and Practice of Panoramic Radiology. Philadelphia: W.B. Saunders, 1982, pp. 299–301.

Nelson, C.L., Tomich, C.E., Buttrum, J.D., and Randolph, G.M.: Spontaneous resolution of a central vascular lesion of the mandible following needle aspiration. J. Oral Maxillofac. Surg., 44:731–734, 1986.

Poyton, H.G.: Oral Radiology. Baltimore: Williams & Wilkins, 1982, pp. 281–284.

Sadowsky, D., Rosenberg, R.D., Kaufman, J., Levine, B.C., and Friedman, J.M.: Central hemangioma of the mandible. Oral Surg., 52:471–477, 1981.

Shafer, W.G., Hine, M.K., and Levy, B.: A Textbook of Oral Pathology, 3rd ed. Philadelphia: W.B. Saunders, 1974, pp. 142–145.

Stassi, M.D., Rao, V.M., and Lowry, L.: Hemangioma of bone arising in the maxilla. Skel. Radiol., 12:187–191, 1984.

Thoma, K.H., and Goldman, H.M.: Oral Pathology, 5th ed. St Louis: C.V. Mosby, 1960, pp. 564–566.

Worth, H.M., and Stoneman, D.W.: Radiology of vascular abnormalities in and about the jaws. Dent. Radiogr. Photog., 52:1–19, 1979.

ARTERIOVENOUS MALFORMATION

The A-V malformation (arteriovenous shunt, fistula, or aneurysm) and the hemangioma have long been considered and are often reported to be the same lesion. In fact, the A-V malformation has also been termed the central hemangioma of bone. However, it is now felt that the hemangioma is a true neoplasm of vascular origin (endothelial proliferation), whereas the A-V malformation can be either a developmental (congenital) or an acquired defect with a normal endothelial maturation that alters the surrounding tissues by hemodynamics (Boyd et al, 1984). Trauma and endocrine disturbances can stimulate or initiate a period of more rapid "growth" or enlargement (Orbach, 1976). Asymptomatic lesions of A-V malformation, present from birth, may not become manifest until puberty or later adult life. The incidence of A-V lesions is low, which is fortunate because there have been **reports of patient deaths by exsanguination following tooth extractions** (Lamberg et al, 1979). Recognition of these defects by their clinical and radiographic features is mandatory for any clinician to prevent such catastrophes. Reports of A-V malformations arising after minor trauma are well documented (Darlow et al,. 1988; Gomes, 1970). They occur in the mandible more often (2:1) than in the maxilla (Lund and Dahlin, 1964). To date only one case has been reported in the maxillary sinus; the patient had had a presenting history of sinus headaches for 20 years. The lesion, however, did not arise within the antrum itself but rather medial to it with secondary expansion.

Clinical Features

As previously mentioned, A-V malformations are more common in the mandible. They also are seen in women twice as often as in men. The peak age incidence reported to date by various authors is the second decade of life (Langland et al, 1982; McCorley and Hall, 1988; Shultz et al, 1988). Presenting symptoms are highly variable and may include spontaneous bleeding from the gingival sulcus, tooth mobility, facial swelling, pulsating or throbbing pain, paresthesia, a bruit (noise) over the involved area on auscultation, an increased warmth over the area, a palpable thrill, tooth displacement, and compressibility of a tooth within its socket followed by a pumping motion of the tooth. Others have reported simply a painless but progressive swelling in an otherwise asymptomatic patient (Van Den Akker et al, 1987). Although some reports claim that the diagnosis is "always clinical," radiography, arteriography, and now magnetic resonance imaging (MRI) or computed tomography (CT) should be performed routinely on these lesions for confirmation of the nature and extent of the suspected vascular anomaly.

Radiographic Appearance

Radiographically, the A-V malformation has no pathognomonic features. However, Worth and Stoneman (1979) have described features of various vascular conditions that should raise

the operator's index of suspicion for such a lesion. A multilocular lesion showing expansion of cortical bone with erosion but no perforation mandates at least the inclusion of vascular lesion within the differential diagnosis. Coupled with some of the clinical features discussed earlier, the prudent operator should perform such tests as auscultation, palpation, aspiration, and CT or MRI. Hudson and coworkers (1985) have achieved good success using these imaging modalities to demonstrate the presence of fluid levels within similar lesions (ABCs). Arteriography employing a contrast agent injected into the region often confirms the presence of the arterial and venous connections (Fig. 7–7B). The extent of the involvement is less easily delineated by the arteriograms.

McCorley and Hall (1988) stated in their review of the literature that, in addition to the multilocular (soap-bubble or honeycombed) appearance, two more common radiographic presentations were a sun-ray appearance and an ill-defined radiolucency. A-V malformations and other vascular lesions can also cause root resorption, cortical expansion, and tooth displacement and have either ill- or well-defined margins.

Histopathologic Findings

A precise histopathologic description of the A-V malformation is difficult to ascertain from reports in the literature. Specimens should show numerous vascular channels, both arterial and venous, with evidence of focal hemorrhage and thrombosis. The vessels are irregular in shape and size. Vascular spaces are lined with normal endothelial cells and filled with blood. Vascular components are surrounded by a dense fibrous connective tissue stroma. No mention of giant cells was found in reports of these lesions.

Treatment

A-V malformations have been treated by curettage, surgical resection, sclerosing agents, irradiation, and embolization of afferent vessels with agents such as Gelfoam (Van Den Akker et al, 1987), ethyl alcohol (McCorley and Hall, 1988), and, more recently, cyanoacrylate (Shultz et al, 1988). Regardless of the treatment employed, the most important aspect of management of these lesions is the control of hemorrhage at the time of aspiration, biopsy, or surgery. Van Den Akker and associates (1987), in their excellent article, cited prophylactic measures for the control of blood flow such as hypotensive anesthesia, hypothermia, and preoperative superselective embolization prior to the ligation of large afferent vessels. However, they also felt that ligation of the external carotid artery—a previously popular therapy—should be abandoned because it fails to affect intraoperative bleeding owing to collateral circulation and because it makes future embolization and arteriography impossible in case of recurrence of the lesion.

References

Boyd, J.B., Mulliken, J.B., Kaban, L.B., Upton III, J., and Murray, J.E.: Skeletal changes associated with vascular malformations. Plast. Reconst. Surg. 74:789–795, 1984.

Darlow, L.D., Murphy, J.B., Berrios, R.J., Park, Y., and Feldman, R.S.: Arteriovenous malformation of the maxillary sinus: An unusual clinical presentation. Oral Surg., 66:21–23, 1988.

Gomes, M.M.: Arteriovenous fistula: Review of 10 years experience at the Mayo Clinic. Mayo Clin. Proc., 45:81–101, 1970.

Hudson, T.M., Hamlin, D.J., and Fitzsimmon, J.R.: Magnetic resonance imaging of fluid levels in an aneurysmal bone cyst and in anticoagulated human blood. Skel. Radiol., 13:267–270, 1985.

Lamberg, M.A., Tasanen, A., and Jaaskelainen, J.: Fatality from central hemangioma of the mandible. J. Oral Surg., 37:578, 1979.

Langland, O.E., Langlais, R.P., and Morris, C.R.: Principles and Practice of Oral Radiology. Philadelphia: W.B. Saunders, 1982, pp. 299–303.

Lund, B.A., and Dahlin, D.C.: Hemangiomas of the mandible and maxilla. J. Oral Surg., 22:234–242, 1964.

McCorley, D.L., and Hall, E.H.: Arteriovenous malformation of the mandible: Report of a case. J. Am. Dent. Assoc., 117:449–451, 1988.

Orbach, S.: Congenital arteriovenous malformation of the face: Report of a case. Oral Surg., 42:2–13, 1976.

Shultz, R.E., Richardson, D.O., Kempf, K.K., Pevsner, P.H., and George, E.D.: Treatment of a central arteriovenous malformation of the mandible with cyanoacrylate: A 4-year follow-up. Oral Surg., 65:267–271, 1988.

Van Den Akker, H.P., Kuiper, L., and Peeters, F.L.M.: Embolization of an arteriovenous malformation of the mandible. J. Oral Maxillofac. Surg., 45:255–260, 1987.

Worth, H.M., and Stoneman, D.W.: Radiology of vascular abnormalities in and about the jaws. Dent. Radiol. Photog., 52:1–19, 23, 1979.

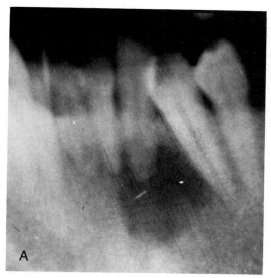

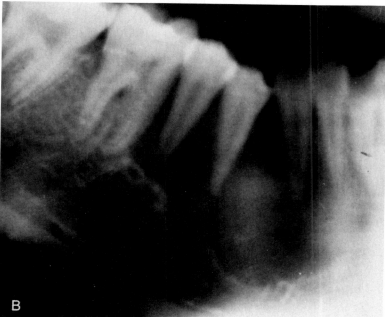

Figure 7–3. *A,* A small, well-defined radiolucency in the canine region with a "cupped out" resorption defect on the apex of the premolar. This was perhaps the only clue to the presence of this central giant cell granuloma because the presenting appearance was not classic. *B,* A large, well-defined radiolucent defect in the posterior mandible. Note the suggestion of locules along the lower aspect of the lesion. There is in addition some tooth displacement. This lesion was a central giant cell granuloma. (Courtesy of Dr. C. Nelson, Indiana University School of Dentistry, Indianapolis, Indiana.)

Illustration continued on following page

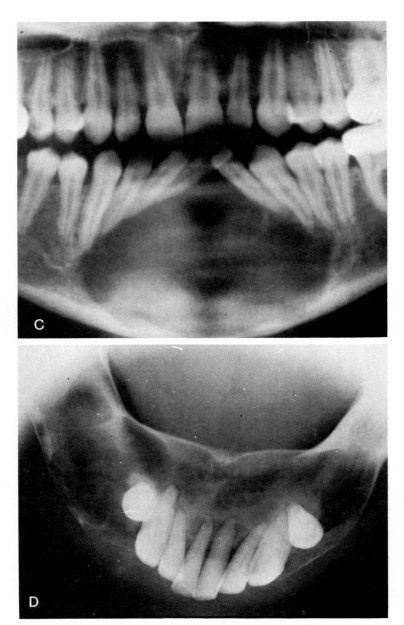

Figure 7–3 *Continued C*, A large, expansile, unilocular radiolucency crossing the midline of the mandible. Note the tooth displacement and probable root resorption of some of the anterior teeth. This lesion is in a good location for a central giant cell granuloma. (Courtesy of Dr. C. Tomich, Indiana University School of Dentistry, Indianapolis, Indiana.) *D*, A large, multilocular, expansile radiolucency in the anterior mandible that is displacing teeth and has remodeled the buccal and lingual cortices. This is almost a classic appearance of the central giant cell granuloma.

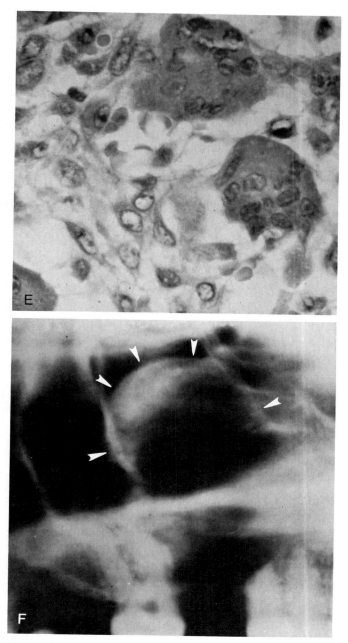

Figure 7–3 *Continued E*, Large multinucleated giant cells in a loose, fibrillar connective tissue stroma. *F*, A large, well-defined **radiopaque** lesion of the right maxillary antrum (*arrowheads*). This lesion was a central giant cell granuloma that arose in the alveolar bone adjacent to the maxillary sinus and then encroached on it. Note the root resorption of the second premolar.

Illustration continued on following page

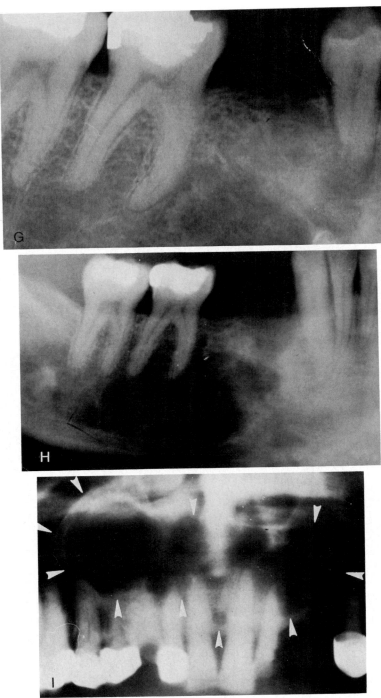

Figure 7–3 *Continued G,* This central giant cell granuloma actually had a peripheral component that presented as a soft tissue swelling distal to the premolar. The lesion is a rather ill-defined radiolucency with an extension around the apex of the premolar. *H,* A panoramic view of the same region reveals a larger, somewhat ill-defined radiolucency adjacent to the apices of the molars. The lesion was a central giant cell granuloma with extension into the oral cavity as a peripheral lesion. The lack of distinct borders may be due in part to the presence of an inflammatory component that was introduced when the lesion reached the oral cavity. *I,* This figure and those in *J* and *K* show a rare presentation of a maxillary central giant cell granuloma (*arrows in I*). (Courtesy of Dr. D. Marlin and Dr. P. Zitterbart, Indiana University School of Dentistry, Indianapolis, Indiana.)

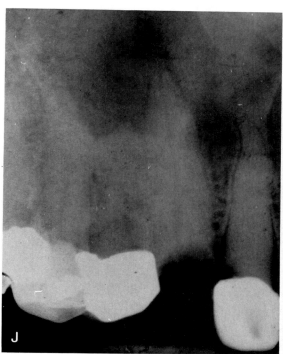

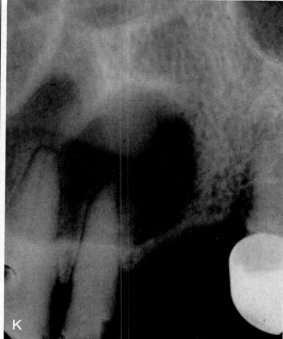

Figure 7–3 *Continued J*, Ill-defined diffuse radiolucency of the anterior maxilla with resorption of the right first premolar apex. *K*, Suggestion of multilocularity of the anterior lesion in the patient's left maxilla.

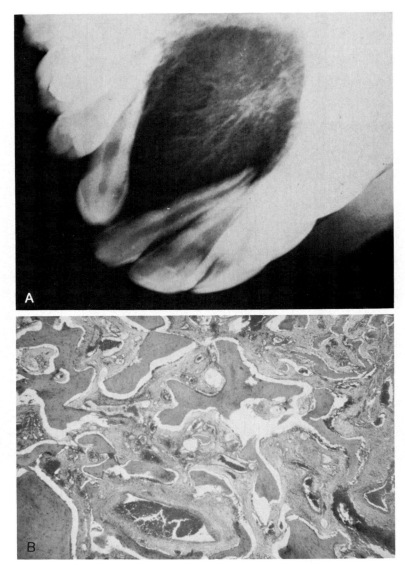

Figure 7–4. A, This large, well-defined radiolucency in the anterior maxilla shows evidence of coarse trabeculae running throughout the lesion. It is expansile and has displaced several teeth. Aspiration of such a lesion with these coarse trabecular patterns is mandatory to prevent severe bleeding, which might lead to exsanguination. B, This low-power view reveals multiple islands of bone in a vascular connective tissue stoma. Numerous vessels are seen within the slide.

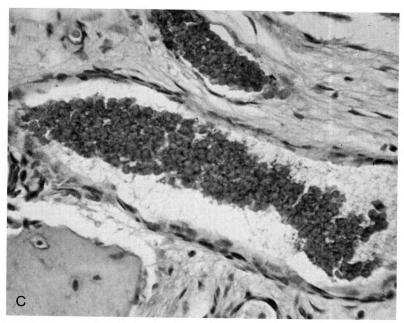

C

Figure 7–4 *Continued C,* This higher-power view of the lesion seen in *A* reveals a large vessel with blood cells accumulated within it. There is a single endothelial cell layer surrounding this vessel, which rests in a young fibrous connective tissue stoma. The lesion was a hemangioma.

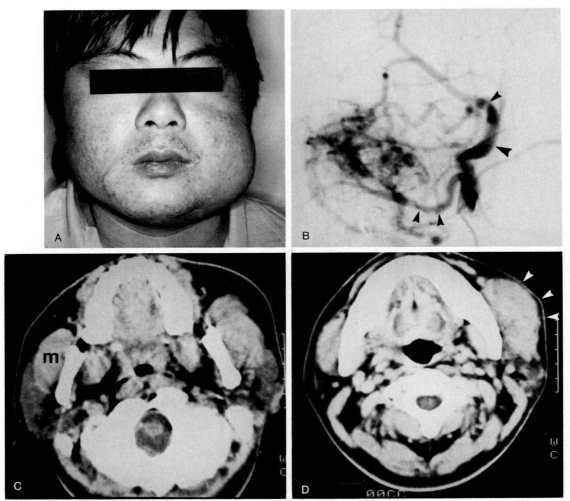

Figure 7–5. *A,* Clinical photograph of a 28-year-old male with a soft tissue hemangioma of the left facial area. (Courtesy of Dr. C. Poon, Taichung Veterans General Hospital, Taiwan, R.O.C.) *B,* Preoperative angiogram of lesion seen in *A. Top arrow* points to maxillary artery. *Top arrows* point to the external carotid artery. *Bottom arrows* point to the facial artery. The lesion seen anterior to these labeled vessels probably represents anastomosing branches of the maxillary artery and facial artery. *C,* CT scan of facial hemangioma that is intimately involved with the masseter muscle on patient's left side. (m = normal masseter muscle mass on right.) *D,* CT scan at a lower level of the face. Note the extreme expansion *(arrows).* No remodeling of the mandible is evident.

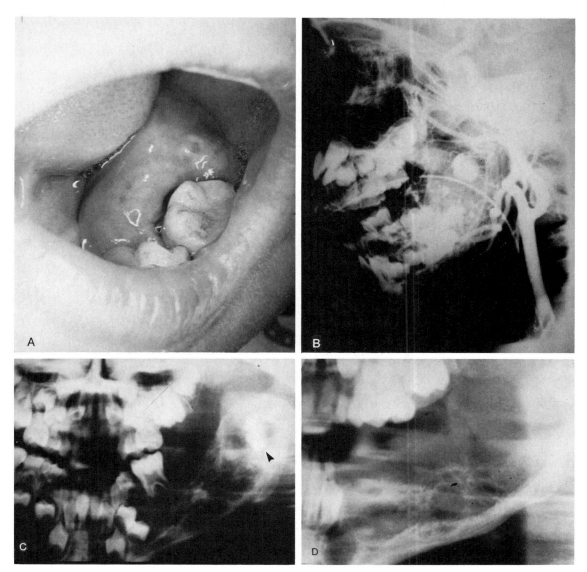

Figure 7–6. *A,* Intraoral presentation of a central hemangioma of bone in a 7-year-old male. (Courtesy of Dr. N. Yin and Dr. C. Poon, Taichung Veterans General Hospital, Taiwan, R.O.C.). *B,* Preoperative angiogram. *C,* Panoramic radiograph reveals a large, expansile, somewhat multilocular lesion that has displaced the developing permanent second molar (*arrow*) as well as the first permanent molar. There has been some destruction of the alveolar crestal bone posterior to the first molar as well. *D,* Postoperative film taken at 12 days. Note the "multilocularity" of the surgery site. This appearance represents irregularities in the lingual cortical plate.

Illustration continued on following page

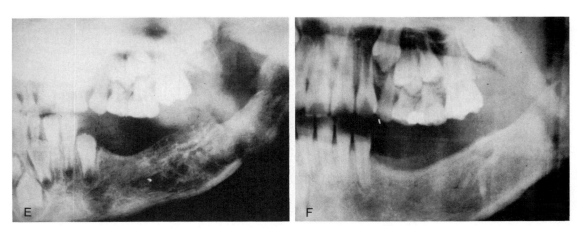

Figure 7–6 *Continued E*, Follow-up film at 7 months. *F*
Follow-up film at 3 years shows complete healing.

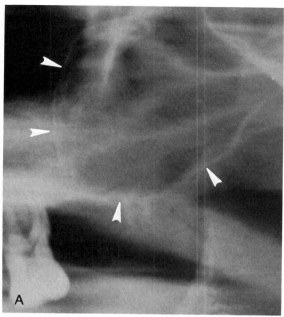

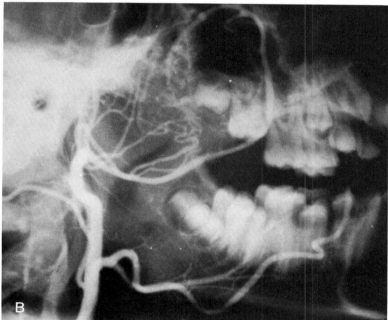

Figure 7–7. *A,* This large, well-defined radiopaque lesion (*arrows*) in the posterior maxilla was encroaching on the maxillary sinus. There are no pathognomonic radiographic features for this lesion. Based on the clinical information, the lesion was suspected to be vascular. *B,* A typical arteriogram of a vascular lesion in the left maxilla reveals numerous small vascular elements within a central portion of the lesion.

Illustration continued on following page

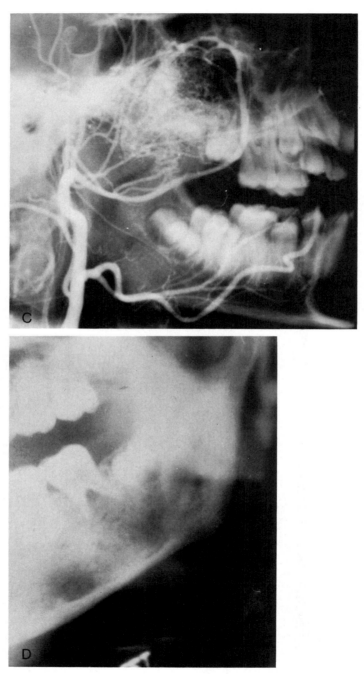

Figure 7–7 *Continued C*, An arteriogram taken slightly later in the examination shows an even higher degree of vascularity and possible anastomoses between the arterial and the venous sides. *D*, A large, somewhat ill-defined radiolucency in the posterior mandible involving the second and third molars. A diffuse lytic lesion that is possibly resorbing the roots of the second molar, the appearance is consistent with an aneurysmal bone cyst.

SOFT TISSUE CALCIFICATIONS

M. VAN DIS

PULP CALCIFICATIONS

LYMPH NODES

SIALOLITHS

TONSILLOLITHS

ANTROLITHS

CALCIFICATIONS IN BLOOD VESSELS

CALCIFICATION OF THE STYLOHYOID LIGAMENT COMPLEX

MYOSITIS OSSIFICANS

Calcification in tissues that normally do not contain such deposits may occur in a variety of disorders, including chronic inflammation or scarring (Table 8–1). The deposition of mineral salts in dead or degenerating tissues is referred to as **dystrophic calcification**. In contrast, **metastatic calcification** is the process by which normal undamaged tissues are calcified by means of a hypercalcemia such as that which occurs in hyperparathyroidism. Mineralization is actually a more correct term for the process, but calcification is the term more commonly used by clinicians. However, the minerals deposited in the tissues may not necessarily be calcium salts exclusively.

PULP CALCIFICATIONS

Clinical Features

A common type of dystrophic calcification is that which occurs in the pulp of teeth. Approximately two-thirds of teeth in young people and up to 90% of mature adult teeth may be affected (Shafer et al, 1983). Either the pulp chamber or the canals may be involved, and there is no apparent predilection for any particular area of the dentition. The calcifications may occur in the form of discrete **pulp stones**. Histologically, these may resemble secondary dentin, or they may be simply masses of calcified material without dentinal tubules. The stones

187

Table 8–1. RADIOGRAPHIC FEATURES OF SOFT TISSUE CALCIFICATIONS

Soft Tissue Calcification	Radiographic Features
Pulp calcification	Uniformly dense, round masses in pulp chamber or wispy calcification in canals
Lymph node	Nonuniformly dense, irregular outline Single or multiple
Sialolith	Uniformly dense if visible; may be lamellar Usually smooth outline Round to elongated Single or multiple
Tonsillolith	Uniformly dense Fairly small (several mm) Single or multiple
Antrolith	Uniformly dense; may have more opaque outline Various sizes and shapes Single or multiple
Calcified blood vessels	Parallel opaque lines (outlining a tube) or irregular, uniformly dense patches or masses
Phlebolith	Circular Lamellar Relatively small (several mm) Multiple
Stylohyoid ligament complex	Various shapes and sizes Various densities Unilateral or bilateral
Myositis ossificans	Ranges from wisps to mature trabecular pattern Separated from periosteum by radiolucent zone Shows up on ultrasound, CT, and nuclear medicine scans

may be attached to the walls of the pulp chamber, or they may lie free in the pulp space. **Diffuse calcifications**, amorphous aggregates of material, are frequently seen in the root canals.

The etiology of pulp calcification is unknown. The finding is not associated with any clinical signs or symptoms, and there does not appear to be an association with pulpal inflammation, the presence of dental restoration, or any systemic diseases (Shafer et al, 1983).

Radiographic Appearance

Pulp calcifications may not be large or dense enough to be seen on radiographs. However, if they are visible, they may appear in the form of round masses within the chambers, or they may be seen as "strings" of opaque material in the chambers or canals (Fig. 8–1A and B).

Treatment

Pulp calcifications appear to be incidental findings without any clinical significance, and no treatment is needed. However, should the affected tooth require endodontic therapy, difficulty may be encountered in extirpating the pulp if large or numerous calcifications are present because they obstruct access to the canals.

References

Shafer, W.G., Hine, M.K., and Levy, B.M.: A Textbook of Oral Pathology, 4th ed. Philadelphia: W.B. Saunders, 1983, pp. 325–328.

LYMPH NODES

Clinical Features

A calcified lymph node usually does not cause any symptoms for the patient, but the clinician may be able to detect it on palpation. Careful questioning of the patient may elicit a history of chronic inflammation in the area, such as a tuberculous infection (Wright, 1988). Patients who have been treated for lymphoma may have calcified nodes; more rarely, patients with untreated lymphomas may have lymph node calcification (Williams and Cherryman, 1987).

A single node may be calcified, or several nodes may be involved to the extent that an entire lymph node chain may be affected. Common sites in which a dentist may discover calcified lymph nodes include the submandibular, submental, preauricular, and cervical areas.

Radiographic Appearance

A calcified lymph node usually appears on radiographs as a distinct, irregularly shaped opacity; however, areas of radiolucency may be seen within the lesion as well. The irregular shape is a radiographic hallmark and may be described as cauliflower-like. Calcified lymph nodes are often noted on panoramic films, where they may appear below the inferior border of the mandible and near the mandibular angle (Fig. 8–2 *A* and *B*). Consequently, they need to be differentiated from a sialolith or stone in the submandibular gland or duct. Calcified nodes are often multiple, whereas a submandibular sialolith is most frequently solitary. Calcified lymph nodes also may be seen near the posterior border of the ramus in the region of the cervical spine.

Treatment

No treatment is needed for a calcified lymph node other than notation of its presence, determination of any precipitating factors for its presence, and periodic radiographic observation.

References

Williams, M.P., and Cherryman, G.R.: Lymph-node calcification in Lennert's lymphoma. Br. J. Radiol., 60:1131–1132, 1987.
Wright, S.M.: Massive calcification following tuberculosis. Oral Surg. Oral Med. Oral Pathol., 65:262–263, 1988.

SIALOLITHS

Clinical Features

A **sialolith** (salivary stone) or salivary gland **calculus** is an aggregation of calcified material within the ducts or glandular tissue of salivary glands. It is the one of the most frequent disorders of salivary glands, second only to mumps (viral parotitis). These calcifications form in patients any time from the first decade of life on, with the peak incidence occurring between the fourth and the sixth decades. Men are affected twice as often as women (Rabinov and Weber, 1985).

The submandibular gland is the most frequently affected major salivary gland (approximately 80%), followed by the parotid gland (19%) and the sublingual gland (1%) (Rabinov and Weber, 1985). Sialoliths may also occur in the minor salivary glands, primarily in the upper lip and buccal mucosa (Jensen et al, 1979). Blandin's glands or the anterior lingual glands have also been reported to contain sialoliths (Tanda et al, 1988). Stones in the submandibular gland tend to form near the hilum of the gland or in the proximal portion of Wharton's duct. Parotid calculi are most frequently located in Stenson's duct and are usually smaller than submandibular sialoliths. The parotid gland is more likely to develop multiple stones or calculi than the submandibular gland (Rabinov and Weber, 1985).

The pathogenesis of salivary gland calculi appears to be related to the pH level of the saliva (a more alkaline pH favors calculus formation), mucus content of the saliva, stasis of flow, physical course of the duct (Rabinov and Weber, 1985), and the formation of eosinophilic crystalloids in the ducts (Takeda, 1986). The stones are formed in a lamellar fashion, usually with layers of organic debris caught between layers of calcium phosphates and carbonates. Stones vary greatly in size and shape; they may be relatively smooth and cylindrical, or pointed on the ends, or very irregular and lumpy.

Patients with sialolithiasis may be totally asymptomatic, or they may develop an obstructive sialadenitis characterized by pain and periodic swelling, especially around mealtime when salivary flow is stimulated. The swelling may subside in an hour or two or may persist for several hours, or even days or weeks. Such a gland often becomes secondarily infected owing to stasis of flow and retrograde bacterial involvement.

Radiographic Appearance

Sialoliths may be discovered on routine films in asymptomatic patients. Submandibular sialoliths may appear on a periapical film as a radiopacity superimposed over the alveolar bone and possibly the roots of mandibular teeth. They are frequently elongated in shape. Submandibular sialoliths may be difficult to see on panoramic films because most of Wharton's duct is not within the focal trough (Fig. 8–3 *A–D*). However, if a sialolith is suspected, adjunctive views such as a mandibular occlusal film will frequently detect the stone. Parotid sialoliths may be seen on a panoramic film superimposed over the ramus.

The radiodensity of sialoliths varies depending on the mineral content; however, approximately one-third of sialoliths are radiolucent and have been termed mucous plugs (Rabinov and Weber, 1985; Langlais and Kasle, 1975). Sialography, the injection of radiopaque contrast medium into the duct system of a major salivary gland, is useful in the assessment of sialolithiasis and its sequelae (Fig. 8–4). Sialography may also provide additional information when one needs to determine whether a radiopacity is within a salivary gland or external to it. Computed tomography (CT) is superior to sialography alone in the assessment of space-occupying lesions of salivary glands; however, it may be used in conjunction with sialography (Van Den Akker, 1988).

Treatment

Sialoliths that cause obstructive symptoms in a patient should be removed. If the stone is located near a duct orifice, it is possible to remove the obstruction without removing the salivary gland. However, if the stone is located deeper within the duct or gland, or if the gland shows signs of chronic inflammation with loss of function clinically and on sialographic examination, the entire gland may need to be sacrificed. The submandibular gland is often removed through an external incision, and the main duct is ligated and left in place. However, recurrent calculi have occasionally been discovered in such a residual duct (Patton, 1987). Lithotripsy, the use of high-energy shock waves to disintegrate stones, especially of the kidney, has been successfully employed for the treatment of salivary gland stones (Marmary, 1986).

References

Jensen, J.L., Howell, F.V., Rick, G.M., and Correll, R.W.: Minor salivary gland calculi. Oral Surg. Oral Med. Oral Pathol., 47:44–50, 1979.

Langlais, R.P., and Kasle, M.J.: Sialolithiasis: The radiolucent ones. Oral Surg., 40(5):686–690, 1975.

Marmary, Y.: A novel and non-invasive method for the removal of salivary gland stones. Int. J. Oral Maxillofac. Surg., 15:585–587, 1986.

Patton, D.W.: Recurrent calculus formation following removal of the submandibular salivary gland. Br J. Oral Maxillofac. Surg., 25:15–20, 1987.

Rabinov, K., and Weber, A.L.: Radiology of the Salivary Glands. Boston: G.K. Hall, 1985, pp. 153–156.

Takeda, Y.: Crystalloids with calcareous deposition in the parotid gland: One of the possible causes of development of salivary calculi. J. Oral Pathol., 15:459–561, 1986.

Tanda, N., Echigo, S., and Teshima, T.: Sialolithiasis of a Blandin's gland duct. Int. J. Oral Maxillofac. Surg., 17:78–80, 1988.

Van Den Akker, H.P.: Diagnostic imaging in salivary gland disease. Oral Surg. Oral Med. Oral Pathol., 66:625–637, 1988.

TONSILLOLITHS

Clinical Features

Retention of bacterial debris in tonsillar crypts may give rise to tonsillar concretions or **tonsilloliths**. The affected patient is usually a young adult with a long history of recurrent sore throat. The patient may be asymptomatic or may complain of persistent throat irritation, foul taste and odor, otalgia, or foreign body sensation (Pruet and Duplan, 1987). It may be possible to see a white or yellowish object within a tonsillar crypt during a clinical examination; however, the tonsillolith may be located deeper within the tissues and may not be visible during a routine examination.

The mineralized material in tonsilloliths has been reported to be primarily calcium hydroxyapatite and calcium carbonate apatite. Fragments of vegetable matter and colonies of gram-positive bacteria and *Leptothrix buccalis* may form the nidus for the concretions (Pruet and Duplan, 1987).

Radiographic Appearance

Tonsilloliths may be discovered on routine films in asymptomatic patients. Aspestrand and Kolbenstvedt (1987) found tonsillar calcifications in 16% of 100 patients who received CT scans of the oropharyngeal region. Lateral projections or panoramic films may demonstrate small opaque masses in soft tissue near the anterior border of the oropharyngeal airway space (Fig. 8–5). The lesions may be single or multiple, ranging in size from a few millimeters to several centimeters in diameter. Axial CT sections may demonstrate these lesions and may provide additional information when differentiation among calcification of the lymph nodes, salivary glands, or tonsillar crypts is difficult (Aspestrand and Kolbenstvedt, 1987).

Treatment

Surgical removal of a tonsillolith may be necessary to alleviate symptoms or if a definitive diagnosis cannot be reached in any other way. Removal of the tonsillolith may require only manual expression from the crypt with gentle pressure with the patient under anesthesia, or incision may be necessary to expose the concretion. Tonsillectomy is indicated only if recurrent tonsillitis is a problem.

References

Aspestrand, F., and Kolbenstvedt, A.: Calcifications of the palatine tonsillary region: CT demonstration. Radiology 165:479–480, 1987.

Pruet, C.W., and Duplan, D.A.: Tonsil concretions and tonsilloliths. Otolaryngol. Clin. North Am., 20:305–309, 1987.

ANTROLITHS

Clinical Features

A calcified mass in the maxillary sinus or antrum is referred to as an **antrolith**. The calcification usually develops in a chronically inflamed area in which degenerating tissues or foreign bodies such as root tips, bone fragments, or other foreign objects are located. A foreign body may become completely encrusted with calcified material. In many cases, the patient is asymptomatic and is unaware of the presence of an antrolith. If symptoms are present, they are usually identical to those of maxillary sinusitis (see Chapter 9).

Radiographic Appearance

Antroliths are frequently discovered as an incidental finding on dental films. They may take on a variety of shapes, sizes, and densities depending on the degree of calcification present. However, they most likely have a greater density than the soft shadow of a pseudocyst, for example. Antroliths usually have a rather homogeneous character; however, they may have a more radiopaque rim or shell (Blaschke and Brady, 1979) (Fig. 8–6 A and B). It is recommended that an object suspected to be an antrolith on a panoramic film be evaluated with an additional view such as a Waters' projection to verify its presence, help locate it, and eliminate any possible interference from superimposed structures such as the nasal conchae, hard palate, or zygomatic processes.

Treatment

Surgical removal is the treatment of choice for a symptomatic antrolith.

Reference

Blaschke, D.D., and Brady, F.A.: The maxillary antrolith. Oral Surg. Oral Med. Oral Pathol., 48:187–189, 1979.

CALCIFICATIONS IN BLOOD VESSELS

Clinical Features

Calcification of blood vessel walls is associated with diseases such as arteriosclerosis, atherosclerosis, hyperparathyroidism, diabetes mellitus, end-stage renal disease, and encephalotrigeminal angiomatosis (Sturge-Weber disease). Encephalotrigeminal angiomatosis is a congenital disorder affecting the neural and vascular tissues as well as the skin. Facial, oral mucosal, and leptomeningeal angiomatoses are characteristic of the disorder. Facial lesions are visible as red-purple discolorations, sometimes referred to as **port-wine stain** or **nevus flammeus**. Mucosal lesions are almost always unilateral, following a trigeminal distribution. The leptomeningeal angiomatosis does not cause any clinical symptoms. However, mental retardation or epilepsy may result from brain involvement (Shklar and McCarthy, 1976). Calcification of cranial blood vessels may occur in this disease.

Hypercalcemia, such as that which occurs in hyperparathyroidism and renal osteodystrophy, may cause deposition of calcium salts in the medial layer of arteries, including those that sustain the maxillofacial regions. Dystrophic calcification occurs in the intimal layers of arteries in the advanced stages of atherosclerosis. No specific symptoms are associated with the calcification of blood vessels.

A **phlebolith** is a calcified vascular thrombus that is most frequently associated with a hemangioma not contained within bone. Again, there are no specific symptoms for phleboliths.

Radiographic Appearance

The cranial lesions of encephalotrigeminal angiomatosis may be visible on skull films as pairs of parallel radiopaque lines. These "railroad tracks" or "tram-like calcifications" are evidence of calcification in the medial layer of the blood vessels (Fig. 8–7A).

In patients with arteriosclerosis, renal disease or renal transplant, primary or secondary hyperparathyroidism, or diabetes mellitus

Text continued on page 198

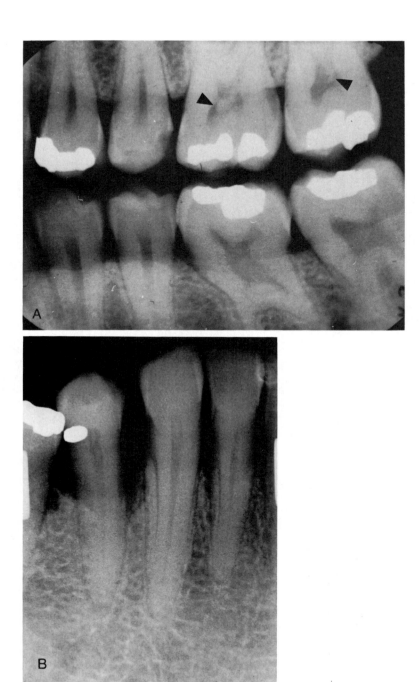

Figure 8–1. *A*,The round masses in the pulp chambers (*arrows*) of the maxillary first and second molars are typical of pulp stones. Note the unusual shape of the pulp chamber and the roots of the mandibular first molar. *B*, Dystrophic calcifications in anterior pulp chambers appearing as "strings."

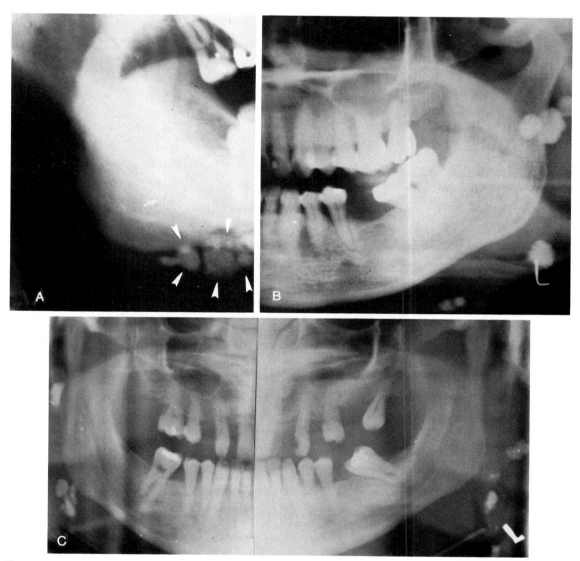

Figure 8–2. *A,* The irregular, cauliflower-like appearance of this radiopacity (*arrows*) is characteristic of a calcified lymph node. *B,* This film shows multiple irregular opacities consistent with the radiographic appearance of calcified lymph nodes. *C,* Bilateral chains of calcified lymph nodes.

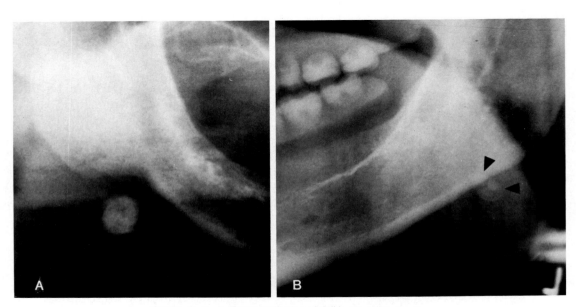

Figure 8–3. *A,* Submandibular sialolith as seen on a panoramic radiograph. *B,* Sialolith (*arrowheads*) partially superimposed over mandibular cortex.

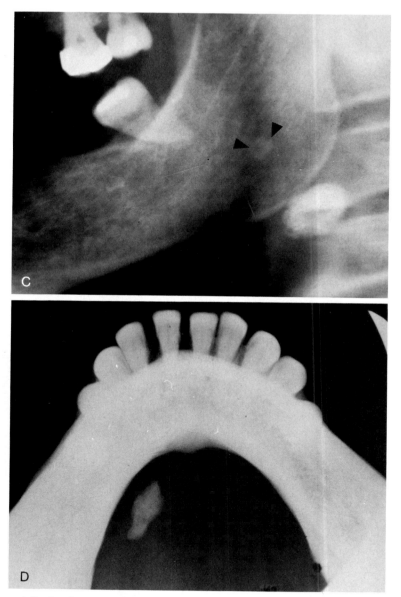

Figure 8–3 *Continued C,* Smaller radiopacity (*arrowheads*) could be a sialolith. The presence of more than one opacity in this film might call for a sialogram to differentiate them from calcified lymph nodes. *D,* Occlusal film shows that the sialolith is present in Wharton's duct.

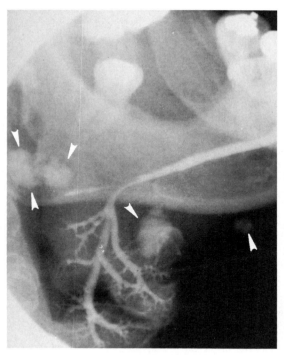

Figure 8–4. The opacities (*arrowheads*) at the inferior border of the mandible on the panoramic film proved to be lymph nodes and not sialoliths on sialography. Dilation of the secondary and tertiary ducts is a radiographic sign of chronic inflammation in the gland.

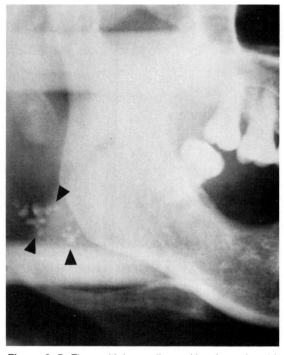

Figure 8–5. The multiple small opacities (*arrowheads*) seen at the anterior edge of the airway space are consistent with the radiographic appearance of tonsilloliths.

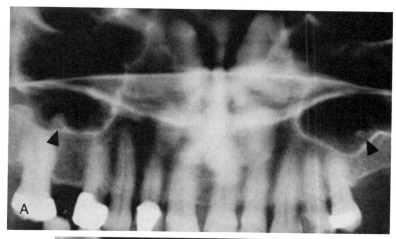

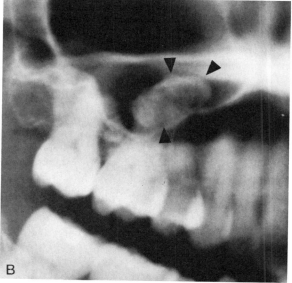

Figure 8–6. *A*, The small opacities on the floors of the maxillary sinuses are most likely to be antroliths (*arrowheads*). *B*, This antrolith (*arrowheads*) has a more radi-opaque shell as described by Blaschke and Brady. The patient reported symptoms of congestion in that sinus.

opaque parallel lines or ring-like structures may be visible on radiographs of the head and neck region (Miles and Craig, 1983). As in encephalotrigeminal angiomatosis, this type of radiographic evidence is typical of calcification of the medial layer of the vessel, usually the carotid and facial arteries, and may be seen on panoramic or intraoral films (Fig. 8–7*B*–*E*). However, plaque-like radiopaque patches outside the jaws may also be seen on radiographs; these may represent calcifications of the intima of the vessels (Fig. 8–7*F*). Some clinicians use the degree of calcification of blood vessels as a measure of disease progress and prognosis for patients with hyperparathyroidism secondary to renal dialysis or transplantation (Miles et al, 1983).

Phleboliths frequently are seen as multiple, round radiopacities no more than 5 to 6 mm in diameter. They often have radiolucent centers and target-like, concentric rings (Poyton, 1982; Langland et al, 1989) (Fig. 8–8 *A* and *B*). Treatment is usually not prescribed for the phlebolith per se, but the associated hemangioma may require treatment. If a hemangioma has not been diagnosed, the presence of phleboliths should alert the clinician that a vascular anomaly may be present that requires further investigation.

References

Langland, O.E., Langlais, R.P., McDavid, W.D., and DelBalso, A.M.: Panoramic Radiology, 2nd ed. Philadelphia: Lea & Febiger, 1989, p. 328.

Miles, D.A., and Craig, R.M.: The calcified facial artery. Oral Surg. Oral Med. Oral Pathol., 55:214–219, 1983.

Miles, D.A., Craig, R.M., Langlais, R.P., and Wadsworth, W.C.: Facial artery calcification: A case report of its clinical significance. J. Can. Dent. Assoc., 49:200–202, 1983.

Poyton, H.G.: Oral Radiology. Baltimore: Williams & Wilkins, 1982, p. 284.

Shklar, G., and McCarthy, P.L.: The Oral Manifestations of Systemic Disease. Boston: Butterworths, 1976, p. 265.

CALCIFICATION OF THE STYLOHYOID LIGAMENT COMPLEX

Clinical Features

Calcification of the stylohyoid ligament complex appears to be relatively common, although the reported incidence ranges from approximately 1 to 80% (Gossman and Tarsitano, 1977; Ruprecht et al, 1988). Although the etiology of the condition is not known, some authors suggest that it may be linked with aging (Keur et al, 1986). Others feel it is a developmental anomaly in which the embryonic cartilage remnants in the ceratohyal portion of the complex develop into bone (Goldstein and Scopp, 1973). In support of the developmental theory, Camarda and coworkers (1989b) found an incidence of ossification of the ligament complex in adolescents and young adults of approximately 40%. It should be noted that the term ossification may be preferable to calcification in this instance because histologically the process is a hyperplasia of the styloid process or a metaplasia of the stylohyoid fibrocartilage into osseous tissue (Camarda et al, 1989a).

Elongation of the styloid process or calcification of the stylohyoid ligament complex may give rise to clinical symptoms of facial pain, throat discomfort, otalgia, dysphagia, headache, or vertigo (Monsour and Young, 1986; Chase et al, 1986). When symptoms are present, the condition is referred to in a variety of ways, including Eagle's syndrome, elongated styloid process syndrome, styloid syndrome, styloid-stylohyoid syndrome, styloid process–carotid artery syndrome, or pseudostyloid syndrome (Langlais et al, 1986; Camarda et al, 1989a). Symptoms are thought to be caused by pressure or impingement on the internal or external carotid musculature (Chase et al, 1986).

When Eagle first described the symptoms just listed, the patients had had recent tonsillectomies and the elongated processes could be palpated in the tonsillar fossae. He proposed that trauma from the tonsillectomy stimulated overgrowth of the styloid process, causing the symptoms of pain and dysphagia (Eagle, 1937). Camarda et al (1989a) proposed that a diagnosis of Eagle's syndrome be reserved for patients who are symptomatic and have clinical evidence of an elongated styloid process (by palpation), radiographic evidence of styloid process elongation or ossification of the stylohyoid ligament complex, and a history of pharyngeal trauma such as a tonsillectomy. The authors further proposed that patients who are symptomatic and have radiographic evidence of ossification of the ligament complex at a young age but no history of trauma be diagnosed as having stylohyoid syndrome.

Furthermore, they proposed that patients who have the same pharyngeal or facial symptoms and are over 40 years of age but have *no* radiographic evidence of ossification be diagnosed as having pseudostylohyoid syndrome.

Radiographic Appearance

Dental practitioners are most likely to see calcification or ossification of the stylohyoid ligament complex on panoramic radiographs; however, these signs may be seen on virtually any extraoral radiograph of the maxillofacial region (Fig. 8–9 *A–D*). Tomographs taken with the patient's mouth open may also be useful in assessing the impingement of the stylohyoid ligament complex on adjacent structures (Chase et al, 1986). Computed tomographic and magnetic resonance scans have seldom been used in the diagnosis of this condition (Camarda et al, 1989b).

The normal length of the styloid process is usually considered to be approximately 25 to 30 mm (Langlais et al, 1986). However, because of the magnification inherent in the panoramic image, some authors have considered anything over 40 mm to be elongated (Monsour and Young, 1986), whereas others have considered lengths greater than 30 mm elongated (Keur et al, 1986). The styloid process and ossification of the ligament complex may take on a variety of radiographic appearances. Langlais and associates (1986) and Monsour and Young (1986) described some of these variations in terms of morphology and pattern of calcification. Categories include elongated, bent, segmented, pseudoarticulated, partially calcified, completely calcified, and nodular.

Treatment

Chase and colleagues (1986) have described various treatments for symptomatic patients with elongated and calcified stylohyoid ligament complexes. Asymptomatic patients require no treatment. Nonsurgical approaches to the problem include transpharyngeal injection of steroids and lidocaine in post-tonsillectomy patients with symptoms, or manual fracture of the elongated process after appropriate local anesthesia. Surgical approaches may be extraoral or transpharyngeal. Extraoral approaches are preferred because they provide better visualization and access to the area, but an intraoral approach may be used if the process is palpable in the tonsillar fossa.

References

Camarda, A.J., Deschamps, C., and Forest, D.: I. Stylohyoid chain ossification: A discussion of etiology. Oral Surg. Oral Med. Oral Pathol., 67:508–514, 1989a.

Camarda, A.J., Deschamps, C., and Forest, D.: II. Stylohyoid chain ossification: A discussion of etiology. Oral Surg. Oral Med. Oral Pathol., 67:515–520, 1989b.

Chase, D.C., Zarmen, A., Bigelow, W.C., and McCoy, J.M.: Eagle's syndrome: A comparison of intraoral versus extraoral surgical approaches. Oral Surg. Oral Med. Oral Pathol., 62:625–629, 1986.

Eagle, W.W.: Elongated styloid process: A report of two cases. Arch. Otolaryngol., 25:584–587, 1937.

Goldstein, G.R., and Scopp, I.W.: Radiographic interpretation of calcified stylomandibular and stylohyoid ligaments. J. Prosthet. Dent., 30:330–334, 1973.

Gossman, J.R., and Tarsitano, J.J.: The styloid-stylohyoid syndrome. J. Oral Surg., 35:555–560, 1977.

Keur, J.J., Campbell, J.P.S., McCarthy, J.F., and Ralph, W.J.: The clinical significance of the elongated styloid process. Oral Surg. Oral Med. Oral Pathol., 61:399–404, 1986.

Langlais, R.P., Miles, D.A., and Van Dis, M.L.: Elongation and mineralized stylohyoid ligament complex: A proposed classification and report of a case of Eagle's syndrome. Oral Surg. Oral Med. Oral Pathol., 61:527–532, 1986.

Monsour, P.A., and Young, W.G.: Variability of the styloid process and styloid ligament in panoramic radiographs. Oral Surg. Oral Med. Oral Pathol., 61:522–526, 1986.

Ruprecht, A., Sastry, K.A.R.H., Gerard, P., and Mohammad, A.R.: Variation in the ossification of the stylohyoid process and ligament. Dentomaxillofac. Radiol., 17:61–66, 1988.

MYOSITIS OSSIFICANS

Clinical Features

There are two basic types of ossification in the skeletal musculature: that which results from trauma and a rare, inherited disorder of connective tissue that leads to progressively ossified soft tissues. Trauma to soft tissues, particularly skeletal muscle, may lead to ossification at the site of injury. The condition is referred to as **traumatic myositis ossificans**. However, this may be a misnomer in that the muscle fibers themselves are not involved, and the lesion is not inflammatory in nature (Connor, 1983). Other names for the condition include **myositis ossificans traumatica, traumatic ossifying myo-osteitis**, and **heterotopic bone formation** (Connor, 1983).

Traumatic myositis ossificans is primarily a disease of young adults and has a male predilection. The extremities are common areas of involvement, as are the muscles of mastication, especially the masseter muscle. Ossification of soft tissue should be a diagnostic consideration if pain, swelling, and local tenderness persist following an injury. Both active and passive movement may be restricted, and as the lesion matures, a hard, palpable mass may be discerned. If the lesion is large enough or situated in a particular way, there may be compression of blood vessels or nerves in the area.

Several theories have been proposed to explain the cause of the ossification. Older theories included ossification of a hematoma, activation of periosteal remnants present in the muscle, displacement of osteoblasts into the muscle, metaplasia of pleuripotential intramuscular connective tissue, and metaplasia of fibrocartilage (often present in tendons) (Plezia et al, 1977; Connor, 1983). However, it now appears that the origin of the calcification is a group of osteogenic precursor cells present in skeletal muscle connective tissue that are induced to generate bone by the trauma (Connor, 1983).

Histologically, the lesion may resemble an osteogenic sarcoma. It consists of a focus of rapidly proliferating fibroblasts with hemorrhage and necrosis of muscle tissue. This core is surrounded by osteoblasts and immature bone, and the periphery is made up of mature trabecular bone, which is separated from the connective tissue that envelops the muscle (Salzman et al, 1987).

The inherited connective tissue disorder is known as **fibrodysplasia ossificans progressiva**. It has an autosomal dominant mode of transmission and affects men and women equally. The disease often presents in the first few years of life. Signs and symptoms include skeletal malformations affecting areas such as the thumb, big toe, femoral neck, and cervical vertebrae, and ectopic ossifications that may present as localized soft tissue swellings accompanied by heat, tenderness, and fever. Commonly affected areas include the back and neck. The disease often leads to irreversible limitation of movement, and skeletal deformities secondary to immobility may be seen. Cervical stiffness and inability to open the mouth may be seen in this disease (Stocks and Mills, 1988; Nunnelly and Yussen, 1986).

Radiographic Appearance

There is usually no radiographic evidence of calcification for several weeks in traumatic myositis ossificans. The first signs on plain radiographs are wispy strands similar in appearance to cotton candy. A periosteal reaction may be present, but the calcification in the muscle tissue is distinctly separated from the periosteum by a radiolucent zone. As the lesion matures, lacy patterns of new bone appear in about 6 to 8 weeks. The lesion appears well trabeculated in 5 to 6 months.

It has been reported that ultrasound may provide very early information about this condition, before the radiographic appearance of calcifications (Kirkpatrick et al, 1987). Radionuclide scans, both with ^{99m}Tc-methylene diphosphonate and with ^{67}Ga, reveal areas of increased isotope activity in the area of myositis ossificans (Edeling, 1986). These scans may provide early information for diagnosis and can be used to help determine when treatment should be carried out. CT may be used to determine the size, density, maturity, and location of the lesion, to differentiate the lesion from other conditions such as sarcoma, and to plan resection (Kirkpatrick et al, 1987; Salzman et al, 1987).

The radiographic features of fibrodysplasia ossificans progressiva include the skeletal deformities and ectopic ossifications. Another sign in the maxillofacial region may be that of a broad, flat condyle (Renton et al, 1982). CT may be beneficial in the early diagnosis of the disorder. To date, there has been no report of the use of MRI in the detection of this disorder (Stocks and Mills, 1988).

Treatment

Surgery is usually indicated for traumatic myositis ossificans; however, it should be deferred until the lesion is mature, as evaluated by radiographs and isotope scans. Early excision may lead to locally extensive recurrent ossification (Connor, 1983).

The management of fibrodysplasia ossificans progressiva is very difficult. Corticosteroids have been used for many years without objective benefit. Excision of ectopic bone usually results in recurrence in a short period of time. Patients should be advised to avoid possible precipitating factors such as local trauma, intramuscular injection, and excision of ectopic bone. Dental treatment should be as atraumatic as possible to avoid injury to the maxillofacial musculature. Measures should be taken to help patients cope with the disabilities, such as psychologic and genetic counseling (Connor, 1983).

References

Connor, J.M.: Soft Tissue Ossification. Berlin: Springer-Verlag, 1983, pp. 17–24, 70–71.

Edeling, C.: ^{99m}Tc-methylene diphosphonate and ^{67}Ga uptake in myositis ossificans. Eur. J. Nucl. Med., 12:311–312, 1986.

Kirkpatrick, J.S., Koman, L.A., and Robere, G.D.: The role of ultrasound in the early diagnosis of myositis ossificans. Am. J. Sports Med., 15:79–81, 1987.

Nunnelly, J.F., and Yussen, P.S.: Computed tomographic findings in patients with limited jaw movement due to myositis ossificans progressiva. J. Oral Maxillofac. Surg., 44:818–821, 1986.

Plezia, R.A., Mintz, S.M., and Calligaro, P.: Myositis ossificans traumatica of the masseter muscle. Oral Surg. Oral Med. Oral Pathol., 44:351–357, 1977.

Renton, P., Parkin, S.F., and Stamp, T.C.B.: Abnormal temporomandibular joints in fibrodysplasia ossificans progressiva. Br. J. Oral Surg., 20:31–38, 1982.

Salzman, L., Lee, V.W., and Grant, P.: Gallium uptake in myositis ossificans: Potential pitfalls in diagnosis. Clin. Nucl. Med., 12:308–318, 1987.

Stocks, P., and Mills, P.: Fibrodysplasia ossificans progressiva: A case study. Radiography 54:61–65, 1988.

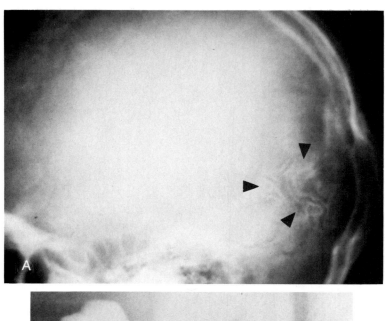

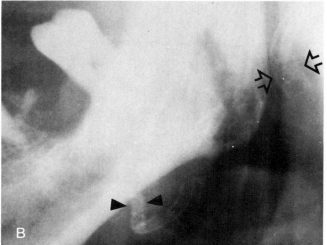

Figure 8–7. *A*, Calcification of cranial vessels (*arrowheads*) in Sturge-Weber disease. *B*, Calcifications of the medial layers of the facial artery (*arrowheads*) and the external carotid artery (*open arrows*).

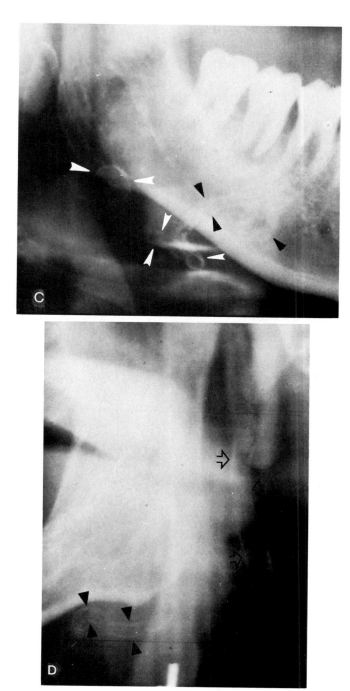

Figure 8–7 *Continued C,* Another example of a calcified facial artery. *Arrowheads* outline vessels. *D,* Calcified facial (*arrowheads*) and carotid (*open arrows*) arteries of an elderly diabetic.

Illustration continued on following page

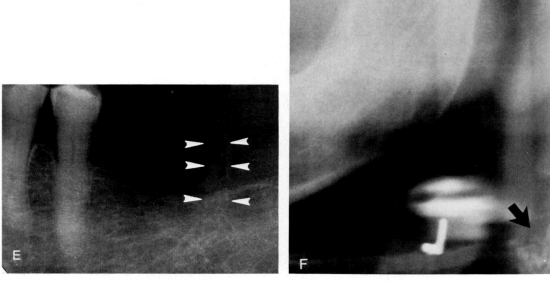

Figure 8–7 *Continued E,* Example of intraoral film with calcified vessel (*arrowheads*). *F,* Plaque-like calcifications (*arrow*) in intima of vessels.

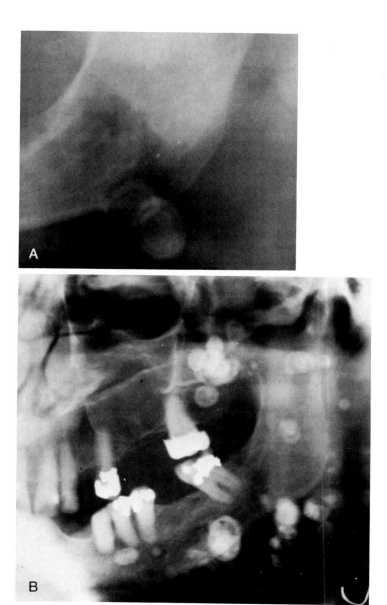

Figure 8–8. *A*, Concentric rings of two phleboliths. *B*, The multiple, target-like lesions are phleboliths associated with a soft tissue hemangioma.

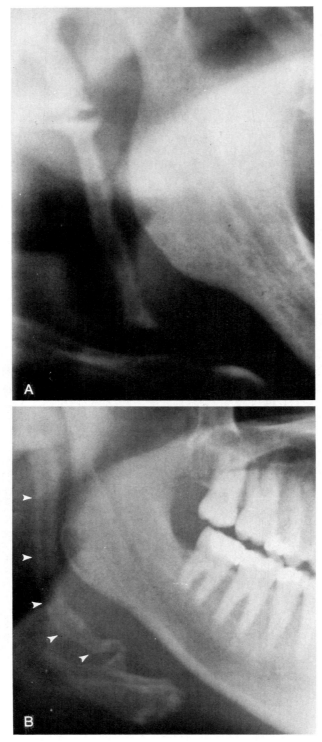

Figure 8–9. Elongated and calcified stylohyoid ligament complexes may take on a variety of shapes and sizes. A, This film shows a complex with corticated borders and a pseudojoint. B, This complex reaches down to the hyoid bone (*arrows*).

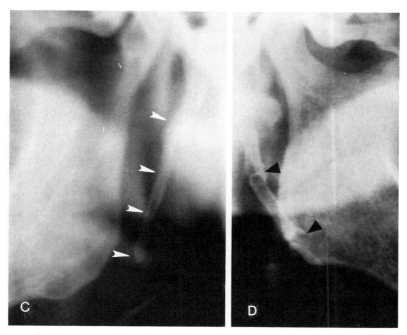

Figure 8–9 *Continued C*, This process (*arrowheads*) is more slender and tapered, *D*, A segmented type of elongated, calcified stylohyoid process (*arrowheads* indicate junction of segments).

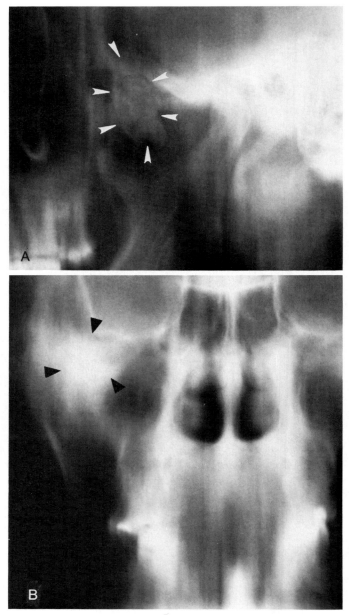

Figure 8–10. Myositis ossificans in the facial tissues of a patient. A, The lesion (arrows) is located superior to the coronoid process and coronoid notch. B, The tomogram reveals the lesion (arrows) lateral to the maxillary sinus and inferior to the patient's right orbit.

THE MAXILLARY SINUS

M. VAN DIS

The maxillary sinus, the largest of the paranasal sinuses, is an air-filled cavity lined by mucosa containing ciliated, pseudostratified columnar epithelium and goblet cells. In a healthy sinus, the seromucinous glands are found mostly in the vicinity of the ostium, although there are a few scattered throughout the mucosa. The medial wall of the sinus coincides with the lateral wall of the nasal fossa; the lateral wall is formed by the infratemporal portion of the maxilla, the superior aspect abuts the floor of the orbit, and the inferior aspect usually lies in the alveolar process of the maxilla, about 0.5 to 1.0 cm below the level of the nasal cavity floor. The floor of the sinus may be situated above the apices of the posterior maxillary teeth, or it may extend farther into the alveolar process between the roots of the teeth. The roots of the teeth may produce conical elevations on the floor. Because of the proximity of the sinus to the dental structures, it is important for the practitioner to recognize the normal anatomy of the maxillary sinus on dental and maxillofacial radiographs. In addition, disorders of the sinus may create symptoms that the patient interprets as dental pain, and conversely, dental diseases may influence the health of the sinus. Many diseases affecting the maxillary sinuses lead to changes that can be seen radiographically, and a practitioner's ability to interpret these changes is vital for the accurate diagnosis and treatment of the patient's condition (Table 9–1).

Table 9–1. RADIOGRAPHIC VISUALIZATION AND PATHOLOGIC CORRELATION OF ABNORMALITIES OF THE MAXILLARY SINUS

Radiographic Appearance	Pathologic Correlation
Thickened mucosal lining	Inflammation
Halo effect	Periosteal reaction to odontogenic inflammation
Air-fluid level	Accumulation of fluids from acute inflammation or trauma
Opacification	Inflammation Accumulation of fluids Mucocele Tumor formation
Homogeneous, dome-shaped opacity	Antral pseudocyst Mucous retention cyst Tumor formation Polyp formation
Sclerosis of sinus walls	Chronic inflammation
Erosion of sinus walls	Inflammation Polyps Mucocele Tumor (malignant) formation
Discontinuous bony segments Overlapping bony segments Displaced bony segments	Fracture (trauma)

RADIOGRAPHIC VISUALIZATION OF THE MAXILLARY SINUSES

Proper visualization of the maxillary sinuses is critical for interpretation of radiographic signs. An occipitomental view, first described by Waters and Waldron in 1915, was primarily designed for visualization of the maxillary sinuses. When making this film, the patient's head is tipped upward at an angle of approximately 40 degrees to avoid superimposing the dense petrous portion of the temporal bone over the inferior aspect of the sinuses (Fig. 9–1). Traditionally, this projection has been referred to as the **Waters view**. This projection allows a relatively clear view of the superior, lateral, and medial aspects of the sinus (Fig. 9–2). However, the most posteroinferior part of the sinus may be obscured by the alveolar process and posterior teeth. Therefore, additional views are recommended when evaluating the maxillary sinuses. A **panoramic** radiograph provides good visualization of the anterior, lateral, and inferior aspects of the maxillary sinuses, although some structures such as the nasal conchae and zygomatic arches are often superimposed over the antra, obscuring some information (Fig. 9–3). A **lateral projection** (Fig. 9–4) allows a view of the anterior and posterior walls; however, both sinuses are superimposed over each other. Because a good deal of sinus pathosis is unilateral, a view that allows comparison of both antra provides more information. A **submentovertex (basilar** or **basal) view** (Fig. 9–5) allows visualization primarily of the medial, lateral, and posterior aspects of the maxillary sinuses. A **Caldwell view** (Fig. 9–6) provides a slightly different view of the superior and medial aspects of the antra than a Waters view. **Tomograms** (Fig. 9–7) allow examination of cross sections of the area in frontal, lateral, or basal views, and **computed tomography (CT)** in both axial and coronal planes is very useful in demonstrating the sinuses and adjacent tissues (Fig. 9–8). **Radioisotope (nuclear) scans** may provide information about the metabolic activity in the sinuses (Fig. 9–9). **Ultrasonography** may be beneficial in differentiating among fluids, inflamed mucosa, and solid tumors (Fouad et al, 1984), but it is usually not sufficient to provide a diagnosis of sinusitis (Shapiro et al, 1986). Injection of a **contrast medium** into the sinus may help to delineate the antral architecture (Fig. 9–10) (Dodd and Jing, 1977; Carter, 1982).

References

Carter, B.L.: Computed tomography. *In* Valvassori, G.E., Potter, G.D., Hanafee, W.N., Carter, B.L., and Buckingham, R.A. (eds.): Radiology of the Ear, Nose and Throat. Philadelphia: W.B. Saunders, 1982, p. 214.

Text continued on page 215

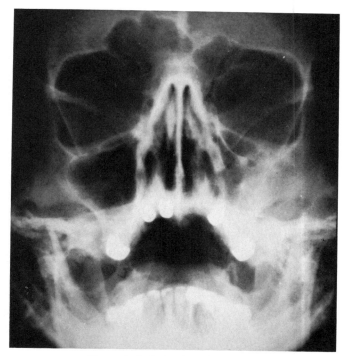

Figure 9–1. A standard Waters view.

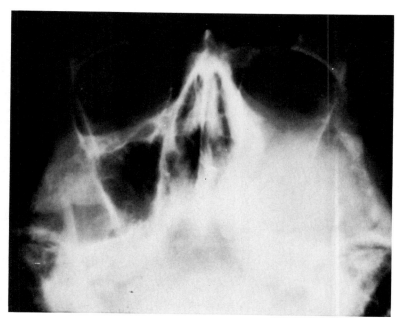

Figure 9–2. A standard Waters view outlining the medial, lateral, and superior aspects of the antrum. Note, however, that the inferior portion is obscured by the superimposition of the petrous portion of the temporal bone. The opposite opacified antrum contains a squamous cell carcinoma that invades the sinus and orbit as well as the maxilla.

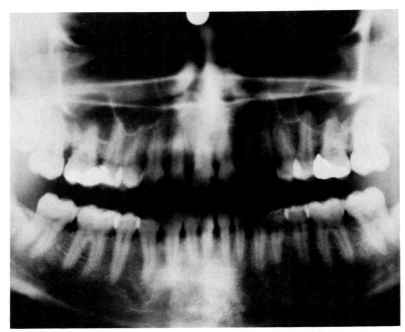

Figure 9–3. This panoramic view details nicely the inferior portion of both maxillary antra. Both sinuses are multiloc- ular and are in close proximity to the apices of the maxillary teeth.

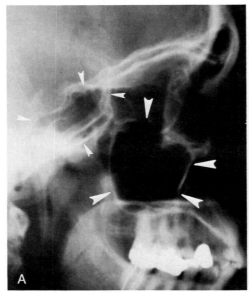
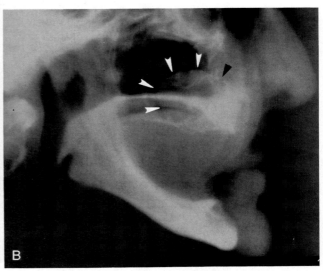

Figure 9–4. *A*, A standard lateral skull view detailing the maxillary sinus, frontal sinus (*large arrowheads*), and sphenoid sinus (*small arrowheads*). *B*, A lateral skull view of the maxillary sinus with reduced kilovoltage and ex- posure time to delineate the soft tissue including the mass in the right maxillary sinus (*arrowheads*).

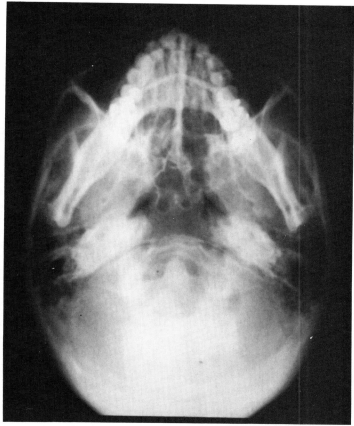

Figure 9–5. A submentovertex or basilar view. The sphenoid sinuses visualized here are multilocular and lie equidistant between the condylar heads posterior to the hard palatal region. The ethmoid sinuses are anterior to the sphenoidal sinuses.

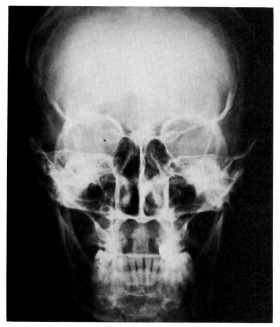

Figure 9–6. A typical Caldwell view.

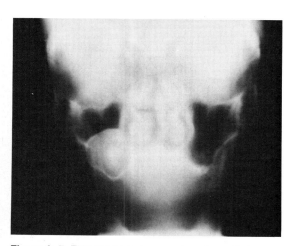

Figure 9–7. This image is a coronal section with tomography used to outline the lesion in the right maxillary sinus, as also seen in the lateral view in Figure 9–4 *B*. The lesion was an odontogenic cyst.

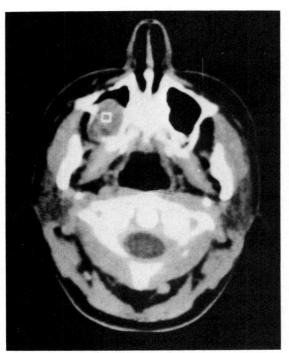

Figure 9–8. A CT scan of the maxillary sinuses at about the level of the midramus region of the mandible. The right maxillary sinus contains a large cyst, which the cursor of the computer console shows as a square.

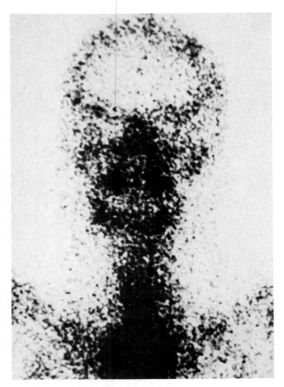

Figure 9–9. A nuclear scan of a patient with maxillary sinus disease. Note the dark uptake in the region of the sinuses. Although very sensitive to changes in bone, this type of imaging is not specific for the disease process.

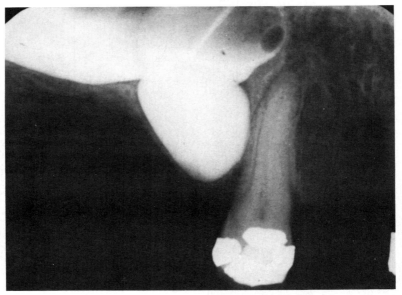

Figure 9–10. Contrast medium expressed into a radiolucent region of the upper maxilla finds its way into the maxillary antrum. The small lucency at the anterior edge delineates a void in the dye. The lesion suspected of being a residual cyst was actually a loculus of the maxillary antrum.

Dodd, G.D., and Jing, B.S.: Radiology of the Nose, Paranasal Sinuses and Nasopharynx. Baltimore: Williams & Wilkins, 1977, p. 77.

Fouad, H., Khalifa, M.C., Labib, T., El-Hoshy, Z., and El Assy, A.E.H.: Diagnostic ultrasonography in maxillary sinus disease. J. Laryngol. Otol., 98:887–894, 1984.

Shapiro, G.G., Furukawa, C.T., Pierson, W.E., Gilbertson, E., and Bierman, C.W.: Comparison of maxillary sinus radiology and ultrasound for diagnosis of sinusitis. J. Allerg. Clin. Immunol., 77:59–64, 1986.

Waters, C.A., and Waldron, C.W.: Roentgenology of accessory nasal sinuses describing a modification of the occipitofrontal position. Am. J. Roentgenol., 2:633–639, 1915.

INFLAMMATION IN THE SINUS

Inflammation of Odontogenic Origin

Clinical Features

Owing to the close proximity of the apices of the maxillary posterior teeth to the mucosal lining on the floor of the sinus, inflammatory changes in the periodontium or alveolar bone may affect the maxillary sinus. For example, inflammation associated with pronounced periodontal disease in the maxillary posterior area may cause a hyperplastic reaction in the mucosa lining the sinus floor. In a healthy state, the mucosa is very thin, not more than 3 mm (Dolan and Smoker, 1983). The insult of periodontal inflammation is usually widespread enough to affect a fairly large area of the mucosa on the sinus floor. On the other hand, a single tooth with chronic periapical periodontitis may produce a very localized inflammatory response in the mucosal lining adjacent to that tooth. This has been called **periapical mucositis** (Langland et al, 1989). These hyperplastic conditions are most often asymptomatic and usually resolve by themselves when the dental or periodontal problem is treated.

A periapical cyst or granuloma may produce an expanding lesion that causes an inward bulge of the sinus floor or may even perforate the floor. In such a case, the displaced periosteum may generate a new area of floor, maintaining the bulged shape. The lesion should resolve with appropriate treatment of the offending tooth.

Radiographic Appearance

Generalized sinus mucosal hyperplasia from periodontitis produces a radiopaque band that follows the contours of the sinus walls or floor (Fig. 9–11 *A* and *B*). Localized periapical mucositis produces only a localized thickening of the mucosal lining adjacent to the offending tooth (Fig. 9–12 *A* and *B*). A periapical lesion that bulges into the antrum under a displaced periosteum produces the characteristic periapical radiolucency surrounded by a thin opaque line of new bone (Fig. 9–13 *A* and *B*). This radiographic appearance has been called the **halo effect** (Langland et al, 1989).

Inflammation of Nonodontogenic Origin

Clinical Features

In many instances, signs of inflammatory change in the maxillary sinuses are not associated with dental disease. **Acute maxillary sinusitis** is often caused by extension of an inflammatory process from the nasal cavity after an upper respiratory infection. The condition is usually accompanied by a mucopurulent rhinorrhea, pain, and pressure tenderness in the area. Sinusitis does not cause swelling over the cheek (Ludman, 1981). The maxillary posterior teeth below the affected sinus may be sensitive to percussion, or the patient may experience a dull ache and attribute it to a toothache. **Chronic sinusitis** may ensue if the initial infection does not resolve, and the patient may experience recurrent episodes of discomfort. **Allergic sinusitis** is a local response in the upper respiratory tract to irritating allergens. Allergic and infectious sinusitis may coexist (Dodd and Jing, 1977). **Granulomatous sinusitis** can be the result of fungal infections in the sinus such as mucormycosis, aspergillosis, or histoplasmosis. Syphilis, tuberculosis, or sacroid may cause similar reactions (Potter, 1982). Patients with sinusitis of any kind should be referred to their physician or otolaryngologist for treatment.

Radiographic Appearance

One of the radiographic signs of inflammation in the sinus is thickening of the mucosa. The mucosa may become very hyperplastic, to the point where it almost fills the entire sinus (Fig. 9–14). Hyperplasia on the lateral or medial walls of the sinus may contribute to a radiographic appearance of an opaque or "cloudy" sinus on a periapical or panoramic film (Fig. 9–15); a cloudy sinus on a radiograph may mean that the anterior or posterior mucous membranes are hyperplastic (Fig. 9–16). This radiographic change may be seen in chronic sinusitis, allergic sinusitis, or granulomatous sinusitis. A diffuse soft tissue change within and adjacent to the sinuses is visible with CT (Carter, 1982). However, the clinician should be aware that **almost any lesion of the sinus**—including cysts or tumors (both benign and malignant)—**will appear radiopaque** because it arises in or encroaches on an air space that is a radiolucent area when healthy.

The mucosa may also become irregular or lobulated in appearance, particularly in patients with allergic sinusitis (Dodd and Jing, 1977). Multiple smooth, rounded, opaque shadows on the walls of the sinus may indicate polyp formation (Fig. 9–17). Polypoid hyperplasia may occur in a localized area, or it may appear throughout the sinus lining. The condition is frequently associated with allergic sinusitis and generalized thickening of the mucosa; it may also be seen in patients with granulomatous sinusitis (Potter, 1982). On CT scans, polyps may appear as well-circumscribed, round soft tissue lesions that protrude into air spaces and the walls of the sinus without extending deeply into them (Hasso, 1984).

Another radiographic sign of inflammation is an air-fluid level in the maxillary sinus. When the line of demarcation between the air in the sinus and the antral floor is straight and horizontal, a diagnosis of fluid retention in the sinus should be considered (Fig. 9–18). The most common fluids found in the maxillary sinus are blood products resulting from trauma or surgery or pus that accumulates in acute sinusitis. The presence of fluid in the sinus may be confirmed by taking an additional radiograph with the patient's head tipped to one side. If fluid is present, it will follow gravity and find a new level in the sinus. Comparison of the two films should confirm the diagnosis. If the fluid is quite viscous, however, it may take a few minutes to reach its new level, so adequate time should be allowed before the second film is exposed. Caution should also be exercised in viewing panoramic films because the shadow of the dorsum of the tongue may be superimposed over the sinus, creating the illusion of a fluid level (Fig. 9–19).

Complete opacification of the sinus is a radiographic sign that may indicate that the sinus is completely filled with hyperplastic tissue, secretions, polyps, or any combination thereof (Fig. 9–20). This may occur in any inflammatory condition.

The bony outline of the walls of the sinus is usually unchanged in acute sinusitis. However, in chronic sinusitis sclerotic changes may cause the walls to appear denser and thicker than normal, especially the lateral walls (Potter, 1982). In allergic sinusitis the walls may erode and may appear rarefied on a radiograph. Polypoid hyperplasia may cause displacement or destruction of the sinus walls (Dodd and Jing, 1977) (Fig. 9–21).

References

Carter, B.L.: Computed tomography. *In* Valvassori, G.E., Potter, G.D., Hanafee, W.N., Carter, B.L., and Buckingham, R.A. (eds.): Radiology of the Ear, Nose and Throat. Philadelphia: W.B. Saunders, 1982, pp. 214, 229.

Dodd, G.D., and Jing, B.S.: Radiology of the Nose, Paranasal Sinuses and Nasopharynx. Baltimore: Williams & Wilkins, 1977, pp. 114–116.

Dolan, K.D., and Smoker, W.R.K.: Paranasal sinus radiology, part 4A: Maxillary sinuses. Head Neck Surg., 5:345–362, 1983.

Hasso, A.N.: CT of tumors and tumor-like conditions of the paranasal sinuses. Radiol. Clin. North Am., 22:119–130, 1984.

Langland, O.E., Langlais, R.P., McDavid, W.D., and Del Balso, A.M.: Panoramic Radiology, 2nd ed. Philadelphia: Lea & Febiger, 1989, p. 406.

Ludman, H.: Paranasal sinus diseases. Br. Med. J., 282:1054–1057, 1981.

Potter, G.D.: Radiology of the paranasal sinuses and facial bones. *In* Valvassori, G.E., Potter, G.D., Hanafee, W.N., Carter, B.L., and Buckingham, R.A. (eds.): Radiology of the Ear, Nose and Throat. Philadelphia: W.B. Saunders, 1982, pp. 185, 191–192.

CYSTS AND CYST-LIKE CONDITIONS OF THE SINUS MUCOSA

Clinical Features

An accumulation of fluid beneath the periosteum of the sinus mucosa may lift it away from the wall or floor and give rise to a dome-shaped lesion. Such a lesion has been called an **antral pseudocyst (mucosal cyst, serous cyst, nonsecreting cyst).** Gardner (1984) argued that the term pseudocyst is appropriate in that this lesion lacks an epithelial lining. The source of the fluid has been attributed to an inflammatory exudate, possibly from bacterial toxins in the sinus mucosa, or from odontogenic sources (Gardner, 1984). Figure 9–22A depicts a possible antral pseudocyst.

An **antral retention cyst (mucous retention cyst)** is the result of partial blockage of a seromucinous gland duct. The blockage may result from sinus infection, allergy, or an odontogenic cause (Allard et al, 1981). The obstruction causes dilatation of the duct, and therefore the lesion is lined with epithelium and is a cyst by definition (Gardner, 1984). The seromucinous glands are normally most numerous around the ostium of the sinus; however, the glands may proliferate throughout the mucosa in chronic inflammation, and they are frequently found in sinus polyps. The term mucocele has been used inappropriately to describe either the pseudocyst or the retention cyst. The mucocele is distinctly different and shows more aggressive behavior than does a pseudocyst or retention cyst. Patients are frequently unaware that they have a pseudocyst or retention cyst. These lesions most often resolve without any intervention.

A **mucocele** in a sinus is caused by blockage of the ostium and is an expansile destructive lesion lined by epithelium and filled with mucoid secretions. It occurs most commonly in the frontal and ethmoidal sinuses and is a rare lesion in the maxillary antra. Blockage of the ostium may be caused by a number of factors, including trauma, surgery, inflammation, polyps, or tumors (Dodd and Jing, 1977). If the ostium is blocked and the sinus fills with a suppurative exudate, it is called a **pyocele** or **empyema**. Ocular signs of blockage may include periorbital swelling, epiphora, or proptosis (Ormerod et al, 1987).

Radiographic Appearance

Dome-shaped, homogeneous radiopacities at the base of the maxillary sinuses are frequently seen on dental radiographs, and it has been stated that they are best seen on panoramic films (Allard et al, 1981). This appearance is characteristic of an antral pseudocyst (Fig. 9–22 B). Some retention cysts are too small to be evident radiographically, but they occasionally grow large enough to produce a rounded opacity in the sinus (Gardner, 1984). In these instances, they resemble pseudocysts (Figs. 9–23 A–C). When making a differential diagnosis, one should consider that pseudocysts occur more frequently than retention cysts that are visible radiographically (Gard-

ner, 1984). Other lesions such as odontogenic cysts, benign tumors, or early malignant tumors may also be dome-shaped lesions (Dolan and Smoker, 1983).

The radiographic appearance of an antral mucocele or pyocele in its early stages is that of a uniformly cloudy or opaque sinus with normal bony walls. (This is also the appearance of generalized inflammation in the mucosal lining due to sinusitis.) Less dense or radiolucent areas may be apparent within the opacity (Atherino and Atherino, 1984). However, as the pressure increases and the mucocele enlarges, the sinus walls erode and may eventually perforate (Gardner and Gullane, 1986). Destruction of the bony walls of the sinus and radiolucencies in an opaque sinus are also signs of malignancy, and therefore all conditions that have such radiographic appearances should be investigated further.

References

Allard, R.H.B., van der Kwast, W.A.M., and van der Waal, I.: Mucosal antral cysts. Oral Surg., 51:2–9, 1981.

Atherino, C.C.T., and Atherino, T.C.A.: Maxillary sinus mucopyoceles. Arch. Otolaryngol., 110:200–202, 1984.

Dodd, G.D., and Jing, B.S.: Radiology of the nose, paranasal sinuses, and nasopharynx. Baltimore: Williams & Wilkins, 1977, p. 124.

Dolan, K.D., and Smoker, W.R.K.: Paranasal sinus radiology, part 4A: Maxillary sinuses. Head Neck Surg., 5:345–362, 1983.

Gardner, D.G.: Pseudocysts and retention cysts of the maxillary sinus. Oral Surg. Oral Med. Oral Pathol., 58:561–567, 1984.

Gardner, D.G., and Gullane, P.J.: Mucoceles of the maxillary sinus. Oral Surg. Oral Med. Oral Pathol., 62:538–543, 1986.

Ormerod, L.D., Weber, A.L., Rauch, S.D., and Feldon, S.E.: Ophthalmic manifestations of maxillary sinus mucoceles. Ophthalmology 94:1013–1019, 1987.

OTHER CONDITIONS AFFECTING THE MAXILLARY SINUS

Clinical Features

Virtually any pathologic process that occurs in the maxillofacial complex can affect the maxillary sinus. Any **odontogenic cyst** in the maxilla may expand so that it displaces the walls or floor of the sinus. For example, the odontogenic keratocyst has great potential for expansion. Although it occurs more frequently in the mandible, the keratocyst does occur in the maxilla (Haring and Van Dis, 1988). A periapical cyst or residual odontogenic cyst in the posterior maxillary area may also expand against the floor of the sinus.

Benign tumors may originate in or invade the maxillary sinus. Primary benign tumors usually arise from the mucosa or bony walls and may include lesions such as papillomas, adenomas, angiofibromas, or hemangiomas. Secondary tumors such as **odontogenic tumors** arise outside the sinus but may invade the antrum. For example, the ameloblastoma, a locally aggressive odontogenic tumor, is relatively uncommon in the maxilla. However, it occasionally is present in the upper jaw and may expand at the expense of the maxillary sinus. Odontomas have also been reported to occur in the maxillary sinus (Reuben, 1983; Shatz and Calderson, 1987). **Fibro-osseous lesions** such as the cemento-ossifying fibroma or fibrous dysplasia may occur in the maxilla and involve the sinus (Goaz and White, 1987).

Malignant tumors are also seen in the antra. Primary malignancies include carcinomas, adenocarcinomas, sarcomas, and malignant lymphomas. Secondary lesions may extend directly into the sinus, originating from areas such as the nasopharynx, nasal cavity, or oral cavity. Metastatic lesions from the breast, lung, kidney, or prostate may also involve the sinus. Any suspected lesion in the sinus that cannot be related to an inflammatory condition should be referred to an oral surgeon for biopsy and subsequent microscopic evaluation by an oral pathologist.

Radiographic Appearance

Care must be taken not to mistake a lesion within the sinus for a lesion that is expanding against the sinus floor. An external expansile lesion usually has a thin radiopaque outline representing the displaced sinus wall (Fig. 9–24 A–D), and a lesion inside the sinus, such as a pseudocyst, does not have a bony outline (Fig. 9–25). CT is useful in the evaluation of such lesions (Hasso, 1984).

Lesions that arise outside the sinus generally have the same type of appearance that they would have elsewhere in the jaws. For example, the ameloblastoma seen in Figure 9–26 A–C has the characteristic multilocular appearance. It destroyed the floor of the sinus and grew up into the antrum. In Tsaknis and Nelson's study (1980), maxillary ameloblastomas were accompanied by antral cloudiness

and a thickened mucosa. The cemento-ossifying fibroma seen in Figure 9–27 appears to have obliterated the sinus floor and to have grown into the antrum as a mass. With CT, the lesion may appear as a diffusely dense entity with bony expansion and margination (Hasso, 1984). CT may also show increased density in such an area.

Radiographic signs of malignancy are relatively nonspecific and include opacity of the sinus, a soft tissue mass in the sinus, sclerosis or erosion of the walls, or destruction of the walls (Fig. 9–28). These changes may be seen on plain films or CT scans. Eddleston and Johnson (1983) found that conventional imaging compared favorably with CT in the initial assessment of disease, but CT proved most useful in assessing extension into the orbit, infratemporal fossa, and cranial cavity. Disruption of fascial planes beyond the sinus walls is the most characteristic CT sign of malignancy (Hasso, 1984). Magnetic resonance imaging is also effective in the evaluation of neoplasia, particularly in assessing the aggressiveness of some tumors (Shapiro and Som, 1989).

References

Eddleston, B., and Johnson, R.J.: A comparison of conventional radiographic imaging and computed tomography in malignant disease of the paranasal sinuses and the post-nasal space. Clin. Radiol., 34:161–172, 1983.

Goaz, P., and White, S.C.: Oral Radiology: Principles and Interpretation, 2nd ed. St. Louis: C.V. Mosby, 1987, p. 697.

Haring, J.I., and Van Dis, M.L.: Odontogenic keratocysts: A clinical, radiographic and histopathologic study. Oral Surg. Oral Med. Oral Pathol., 66:145–153, 1988.

Hasso, A.N.: CT of tumors and tumor-like conditions of the paranasal sinuses. Radiol. Clin. North Am., 22:119–130, 1984.

Reuben, B.: Odontoma of the maxillary sinus—a case report. Quint. Int., 14:287–290, 1983.

Shapiro, M.D., and Som, P.M.: MRI of the paranasal sinuses and nasal cavity. Radiol. Clin. North Am., 27:447–475, 1989.

Shatz, A., and Calderson, S.: Complex odontoma in the maxillary sinus: An unusual presentation. Ann. Dent., 46:38–40, 1987.

Tsaknis, P.J., and Nelson, J.F.: The maxillary ameloblastoma: An analysis of 24 cases. J. Oral Surg., 38:336–342, 1980.

TRAUMA

Trauma to the area of the maxillary sinus may be the result of simple surgical problems, such as displacing a root tip from a maxillary

Text continued on page 233

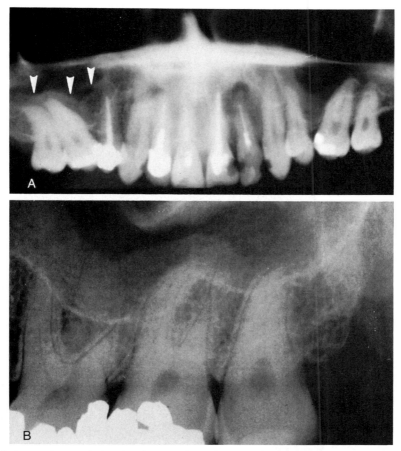

Figure 9–11. *A,* Moderate changes in the alveolar crestal bone levels consistent with periodontitis have stimulated a thickened mucosa along the antral floor (*arrowheads*).

B, An intraoral periapical radiograph shows thickening of the antral floor in response to mild periodontal changes.

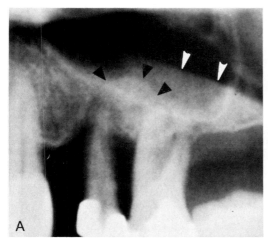

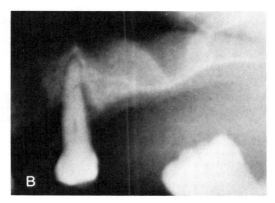

Figure 9–12. *A,* Gross changes of the periodontium surrounding the premolar have led to a localized thickening (*black arrowheads*). The additional opacity (*white arrowheads*) is due to the superimposition of the soft tissue of the tongue on a panoramic radiograph. *B,* Another region of periapical mucositis associated with a periodontally involved premolar.

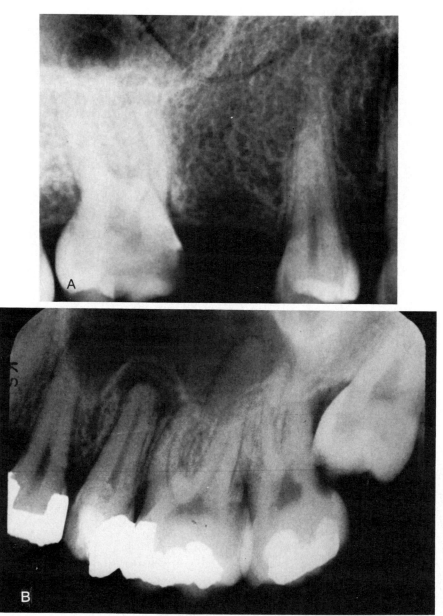

Figure 9–13. *A*, Thin cortical outline of periapical lesion produces a halo effect. *B*, The death of the pulp of the second premolar has led to an apical periodontitis and elevation of the antral floor, which produces a periapical halo. Note also in this film the severe resorption beneath the dentinoenamel junction on the second molar from the impacted third molar.

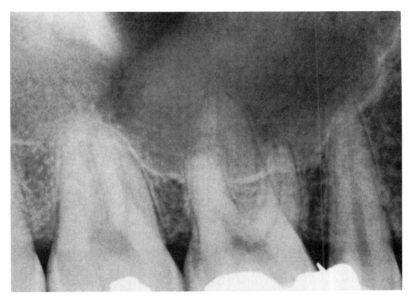

Figure 9–14. An opacified or cloudy sinus not associated with a dental etiology. Only a small area of radiolucency near the superior edge of the film denotes a well-aerated portion of the antrum.

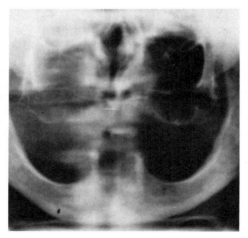

Figure 9–15. A totally opacified right maxillary antrum due to a sinus lesion.

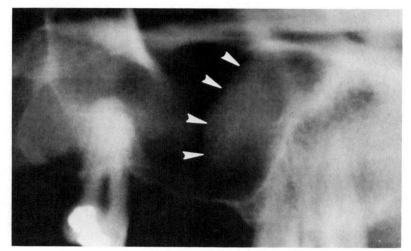

Figure 9–16. Thickening of the sinus membrane along the anterior wall (*arrowheads*).

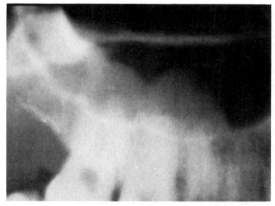

Figure 9–17. Multiple elevations arising from the sinus floor consistent with antral polyps.

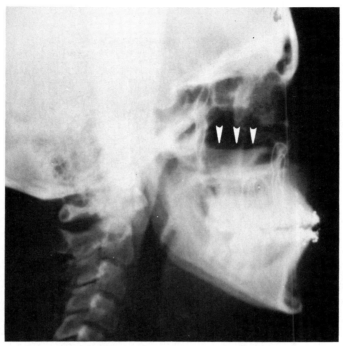

Figure 9–18. Lateral cephalometric radiograph following orthognathic surgery demonstrates a fluid level (*arrowheads*).

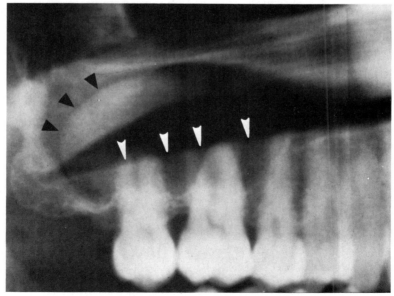

Figure 9–19. The mucous retention cyst (*black arrowheads*) filling most of the right maxillary antrum has the oropharyngeal airway superimposed through its entire width. The dorsum of the tongue (*white arrowheads*) is seen in the lower region.

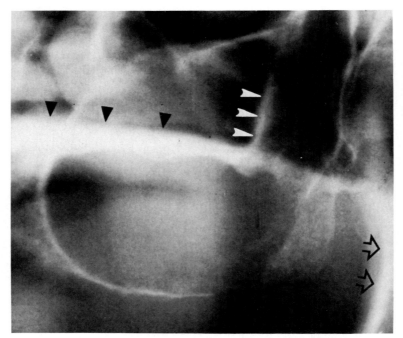

Figure 9–20. Expansion and opacification of the entire left maxillary sinus. *Open black arrows* demonstrate the external oblique ridge. *White arrowheads* demonstrate the anterior border of the zygoma. *Black arrowheads* represent the hard palate.

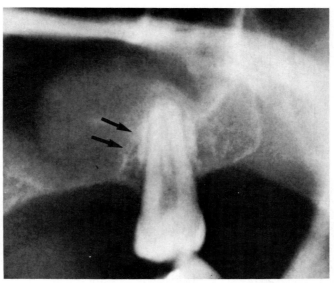

Figure 9–21. Polyploid hyperplasia causing destruction of a portion of the inferior border or wall of the maxillary sinus (*arrows*).

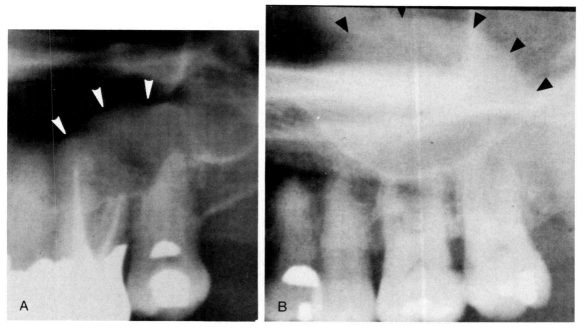

Figure 9–22. *A*, An antral pseudocyst (*arrowheads*). *B*, A mucous retention cyst or antral pseudocyst (*arrowheads*). This lesion has undergone extensive proliferation.

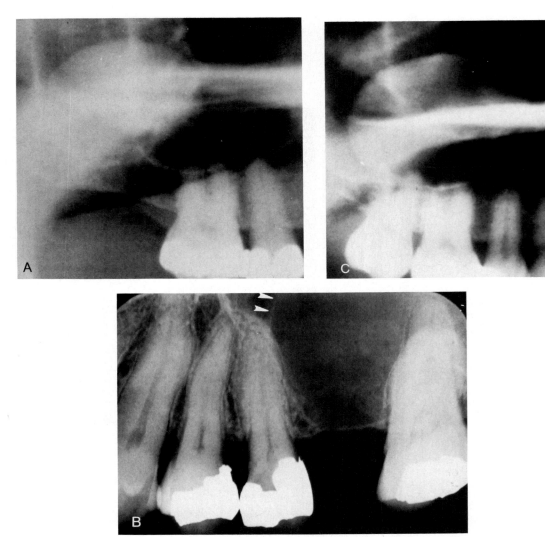

Figure 9–23. *A*, A large antral pseudocyst in the posterior portion of the right maxillary antrum on a panoramic film. *B*, The inferior aspect of this left maxillary antrum is almost entirely filled by an opaque lesion. The border of the lesion can be seen near the apex of the second premolar (*arrowheads*). More detailed imaging of the area is required for an accurate diagnosis. *C*, Another very large antral pseudocyst.

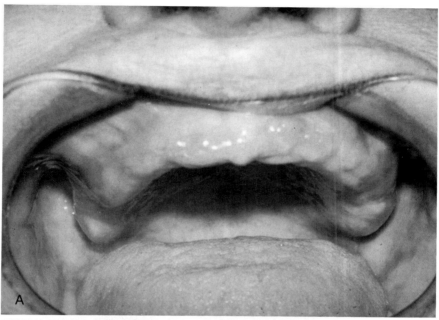

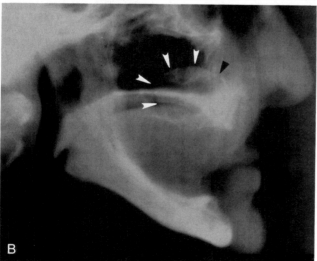

Figure 9–24. *A,* A large expansion in the mucobuccal fold area in the region of the premolars in a 58-year-old woman. *B,* A large, well-defined, somewhat round radi-opacity in the right maxillary antrum (*arrowheads*). This lesion shows evidence of a sclerotic or cortical border. Expansion of the inferior aspect is present.

Illustration continued on following page

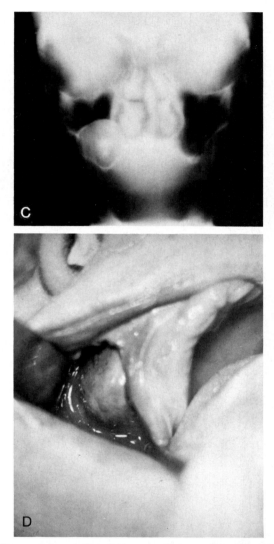

Figure 9–24 *Continued C,* Tomography of the right maxillary antrum in this case reveals a well-defined, expansile radiopacity with a sclerotic or hyperostotic border. Note the loss of definition of the lateral wall of the sinus. Compare this with the patient's left side, where this lateral wall is concave in the inferior aspect. The central opacity within this lesion, although it appeared tooth-like, was not odontogenic. *D,* Surgical exposure of the cyst invading the right maxillary antrum. The cyst was of odontogenic origin and had expanded into the right sinus.

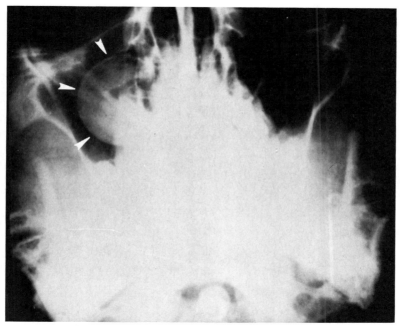

Figure 9–25. Large, expansile radiopaque lesion in the right maxillary antrum with cortical outline (*arrowheads*). This bony outline precludes lesions such as an antral pseudocyst or mucous retention cyst.

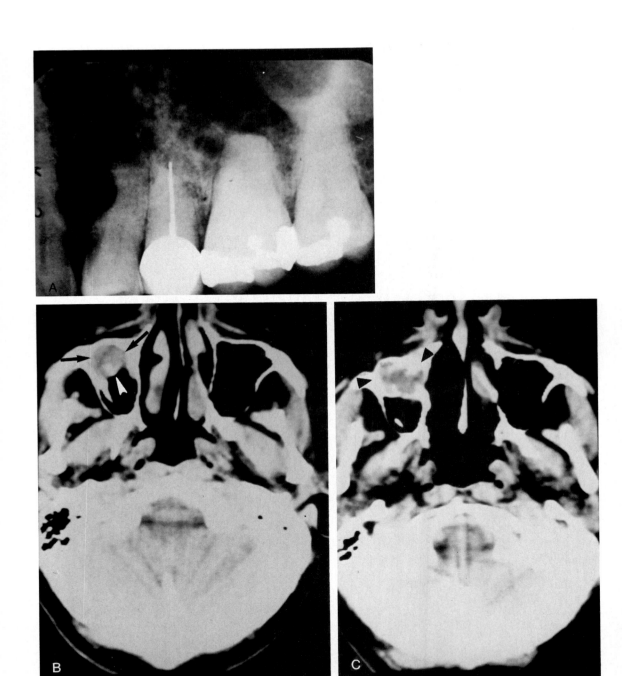

Figure 9–26. *A,* A multilocular lesion in the left maxillary sinus region has destroyed any evidence of the cortical floor of the antrum. Note that there is root resorption of the two premolars and palatal root of the first molar. This lesion was an ameloblastoma. *B,* Although multilocularity is not evident in this CT view, the large mass can be seen in the patient's left anterior maxillary sinus region (*arrows*). *C,* A CT view in a slightly more inferior position demonstrates a suggestion of bony walls creating locules within the left antrum. The lesion is outlined by *arrowheads.*

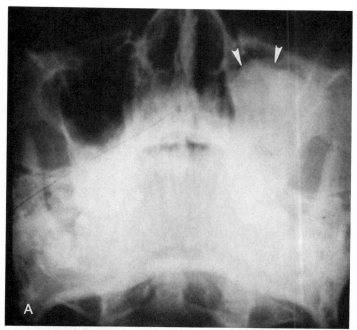

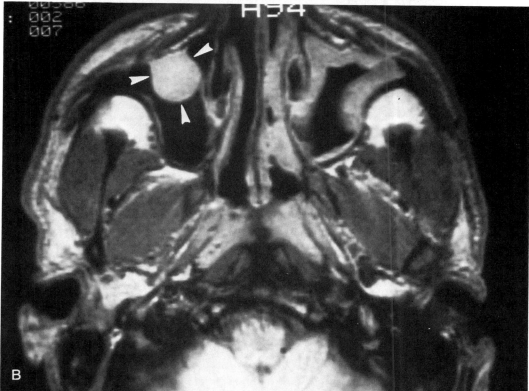

Figure 9–27. *A,* A large radiopaque mass appears in the patient's left maxillary sinus. The lesion has not quite filled the entire antrum (*arrowheads*). *B,* MR (proton density) imaging of this patient reveals a large, well-defined, ovoid, radiopaque mass in the left antrum (*ar-rowheads*) consistent with a mucous retention cyst. (*B,* From Pollei, S., and Harnsberger, H.R.: The radiologic evaluation of the sinonasal region. Postgrad. Radiol. 9[4]:242, 1989.)

Illustration continued on following page

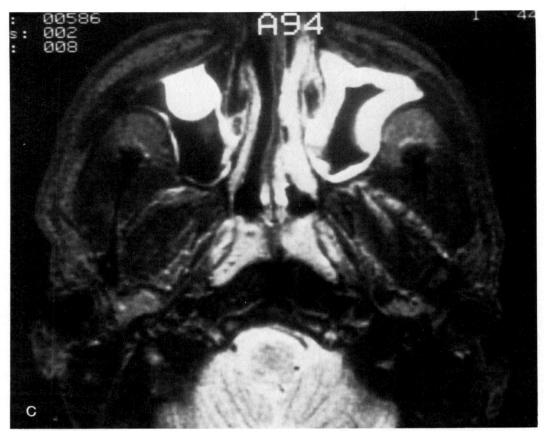

Figure 9–27 *Continued C,* Another MR image of a mucous retention cyst in the left antrum. Note also here as well as in *B* the bright signal of the right sinus representing a uniform thickening of the antral mucosa. (From Pollei, S., and Harnsberger, H.R.: The radiologic evaluation of the sinonasal region. Postgrad. Radiol. 9[4]:242, 1989.)

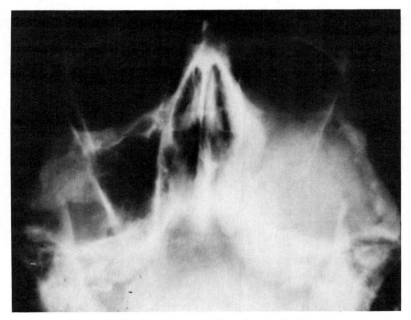

Figure 9–28. A squamous cell carcinoma that has destroyed much of the patient's left maxilla, maxillary antrum, orbital rim, and zygomatic arch.

tooth into the antrum, or the creation of an antral-oral fistula following extraction of a maxillary posterior tooth. Figure 9–29 A reveals the changes brought about in the maxillary sinus by a longstanding antral-oral fistula. The entrance was a small opening beneath a complete denture (Fig. 9–29 B–C). The patient had had multiple courses of antibiotics for "sinus infections" over a period of 7 to 8 years. The chronic, longstanding inflammatory changes induced the lining mucosa to undergo transformation to a squamous papilloma (Fig. 9–29 D).

Confirmation of a suspected antral-oral fistula can also be performed by placing a sterile gutta percha point into the suspected fistular orifice and confirming its presence by a periapical radiograph (Fig. 9–29 E–F).

More severe trauma may produce fluid levels in the sinus, inflammatory responses, or fractures. Accumulation of fluid in the sinus after trauma is frequently due to blood products. There may be soft tissue swelling over the area, or there may be thickening of the lining due to submucosal hemorrhage. Fractures of the maxillofacial complex frequently affect the sinus walls. The "blow-out" fracture was caused by trauma in the area of the orbit. The result is an isolated depressed fracture of the floor of the orbit, which is the roof of the maxillary sinus. The "blow-out" fracture is frequently accompanied by fracture of the anterior wall of the maxillary sinus. A tripod fracture involves the zygomatic arch, inferior orbital rim, and lateral wall of the sinus.

Radiographic Appearance

Displaced root tips are frequently detected with periapical or panoramic films. A Waters view may provide additional information about its exact location. Occasionally the antral-oral defect is large enough to be seen on films (Fig 9–30 A–D), but sometimes the only sign of the fistula is a thickening of the mucosa in the area of the defect.

Evidence of fracture may include "dark lines" (separated fragments), "bright lines" (superimposed fragments), and "stepped lines" (displaced fragments) on plain films. Tomographs provide additional information, and CT has become a standard procedure for the evaluation of maxillofacial trauma owing to the ease of detection of both bony and soft tissue injuries (Johnson, 1984). Magnetic resonance imaging is less able to detect fractures than CT but may prove superior for the evaluation of accompanying soft tissue trauma (Gentry, 1989).

Radiographic signs of a "blow-out" fracture on a Waters view include separation of the lines representing the rim of the orbit and the floor of the orbit and the presence of a soft tissue mass in the superior portion of the antrum. The soft tissue mass represents displacement of the tissue from the floor of the orbit. Any fracture involving the antra may give rise to radiographic signs of sinus opacity, localized thickening of the mucosa, or a fluid level seen on plain films. These changes are depicted well on CT scans. CT studies for trauma are often done in two planes to better demonstrate the displacement of fragments (Johnson, 1984).

References

Gentry, L.R.: Facial trauma and associated brain damage. Radiol. Clin. North Am., 27:435–446, 1989.

Johnson, D.H.: CT of maxillofacial trauma. Radiol. Clin. North Am., 22:131–144, 1984.

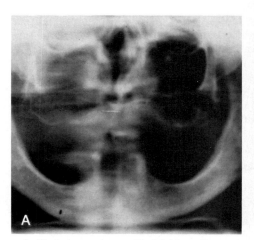

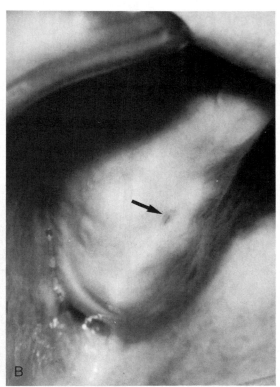

Figure 9–29. *A*, A grossly opacified right maxillary antrum due to a longstanding infection. *B*, A small opening for a fistulous tract (*arrow*) in the maxillary alveolar ridge area. Note also the expansion of the mucobuccal fold area.

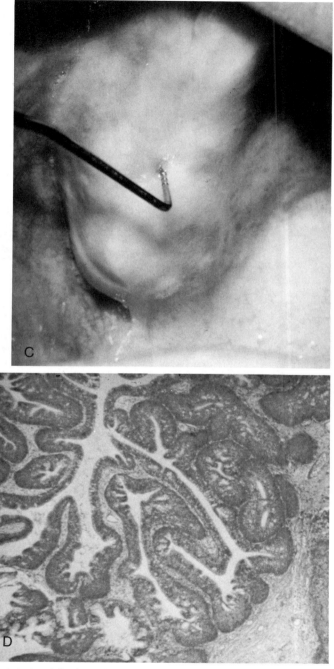

Figure 9–29 *Continued C,* Antral-oral fistula probed with a periodontal probe. *D,* Proliferation of epithelium along the lining of the antral mucosa. The gross infolding suggests a papilloma. A thick fibrous connective tissue stroma is seen between islands of this epithelium. The lesion was diagnosed as a squamous papilloma, a lesion that can undergo malignant transformation.

Illustration continued on following page

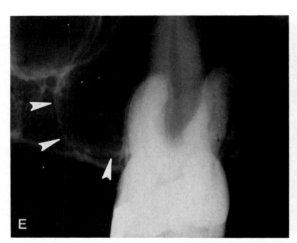

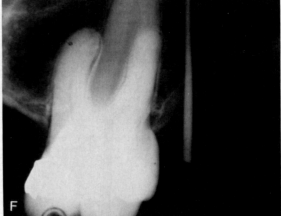

Figure 9–29 *Continued E*, A single molar in the posterior region in close proximity to the maxillary sinus. Note the pneumatization of an antral loculus into the tuberosity region (*arrowheads*). *F*, Introduction of a gutta percha point into a defect in the overlying mucosa that shows extension into the maxillary sinus.

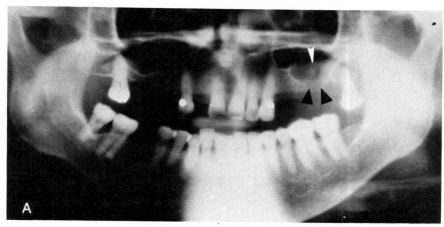

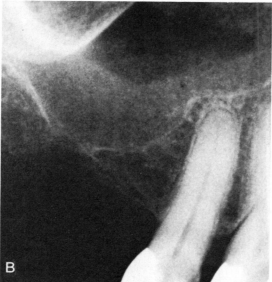

Figure 9–30. *A*, Opacification of the left maxillary sinus in the inferior region. Note the interruption of the cortical border (*black arrowheads*). A small opacity within the inferior portion of the sinus is a root tip in the antrum (*white arrowhead*). *B*, Evidence of the interruption of the antral floor is obvious distal to the premolars. Note also the thickening of the lining mucosa in response to the antral-oral fistula.

Illustration continued on following page

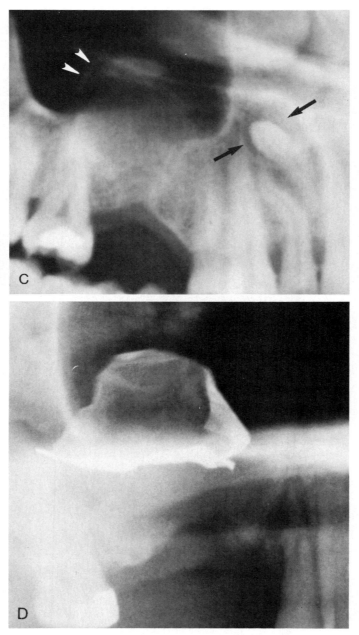

Figure 9–30 *Continued C,* Antral-oral or oral-antral fistula that is continuous with the alveolar tissues. The lesion extends up into the sinus and shows evidence of a slight cortical rim (*white arrowheads*). This was actually an odontogenic cyst that proliferated down into the socket following extraction. Note also the supernumerary tooth between the roots of the central and lateral incisors (*black arrows*). *D,* This large radiopacity in the posterior maxilla actually represents a thin piece of platinum foil placed over the oral-antral defect to assist in repair of the fistula. This platinum foil will be removed later when the tissues have regenerated.

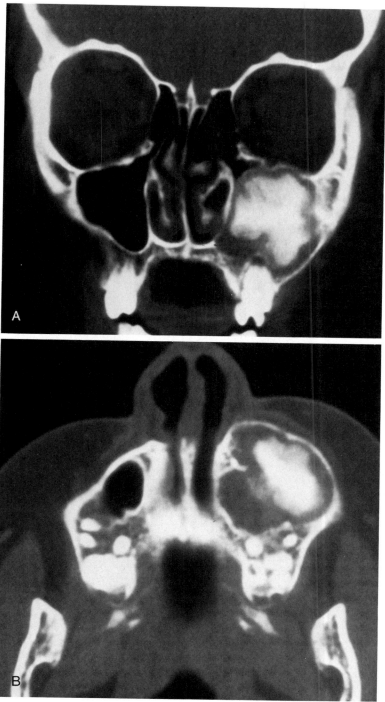

Figure 9–31. *A*, Coronal section CT scan through the midface region shows an opacified mass in the left antrum. Note the radiolucent rimming. This was a ce-mento-ossifying fibroma. *B*, Axial CT section of the patient shown in *A* through the midroot region shows the expan-sile nature of the cemento-ossifying fibroma. The multiple small opacities seen posterior to the sinus spaces are roots of molars. (From Pollei, S., and Harnsberger, H.R.: The radiologic evaluation of the sinonasal region. Post-grad. Radiol., *9*[4]:242, 1989.)

MAXILLOFACIAL RADIOGRAPHIC MANIFESTATIONS OF SYSTEMIC DISEASES

M. VAN DIS

METABOLIC BONE DISEASES
HYPERPARATHYROIDISM
HYPOPARATHYROIDISM
OSTEOMALACIA
OSTEOPOROSIS

DIABETES MELLITUS

INHERITED ANEMIAS
SICKLE CELL ANEMIA
THALASSEMIA

IDIOPATHIC HISTIOCYTOSIS

PROGRESSIVE SYSTEMIC SCLEROSIS

There are several systemic diseases that may affect the maxillofacial complex in such a way that changes in the jaws, teeth, and skull may be seen on dental radiographs. It is important to remember, however, that a significant amount of hard tissue must be altered in order to be detected on radiographic film. Therefore, not all patients with systemic disease will have obvious radiographic abnormalities. Other imaging modalities such as computed tomography (CT) or radionuclide scans may provide more information about bony involvement than do plain films. However, the dental clinician must be aware of any radiographic signs of systemic disease to be able to provide appropriate diagnoses and management strategies for all patients.

METABOLIC BONE DISEASES

HYPERPARATHYROIDISM

One of the primary functions of parathyroid hormone (PTH) is the regulation of proper concentrations of calcium ions in the blood. PTH affects the movement of calcium into and out of bone and also its reabsorption from the kidneys. Elevated levels of PTH, or **hyperparathyroidism**, may be of a primary or secondary nature.

Clinical Features

In most cases (approximately 80%), **primary hyperparathyroidism** is due to a functional adenoma of the parathyroid glands. It may also be related to hyperplasia of the parathyroid glands, but this is a less common cause (Grech et al, 1985).

Primary hyperparathyroidism is most likely to occur in women in the fourth to seventh decades of life. It has been suggested that diminished estrogen levels may be implicated in the disorder (Regezi and Sciubba, 1989). Patients with hyperparathyroidism may be asymptomatic, and hypercalcemia discovered during biochemical profiles is often the first clue to diagnosis. Because levels of serum calcium ions may vary, hypercalcemia should be confirmed on at least two separate occasions with measurements of fasting serum calcium. When symptoms of hypercalcemia do occur, they may include general malaise, loss of appetite, nausea, vomiting, and polydipsia. Pancreatitis, peptic ulcers, recurrent renal stones, muscle weakness, and psychological problems such as memory loss or depression may also be associated with the disorder. Severe bone pain may occur in advanced cases (Regezi and Sciubba, 1989; Goaz and White, 1987). These signs and symptoms may be summarized as "bones, stones, abdominal groans, and psychic moans."

Secondary hyperparathyroidism results from excessive PTH secretion as a compensatory response to persistently low levels of serum calcium. The underlying hypocalcemia may be related to inadequate intake of calcium, malabsorption of calcium, or impaired vitamin D processing due to renal disorders. The kidneys in patients with renal failure do not form 1,25-dihydroxy vitamin D (1,25[OH]$_2$ vitamin D), which in turn impairs the intestinal absorption of calcium. The various bone abnormalities that may result from impaired renal function are termed **renal osteodystrophy**.

Radiographic Appearance

The diagnosis of hyperparathyroidism is usually made through biochemical tests. However, advances in sonography (ultrasound) and scintigraphy (nuclear scan) with technetium-99m and thallium-201 have resulted in sensitive methods that allow early diagnosis of hyperplastic parathyroid glands (Winzelberg and Hydovitz, 1985).

The radiographic changes that occur in more advanced stages of the disorder have been seen much less frequently in recent years owing to improvements in early diagnosis. Skeletal manifestations of primary hyperparathyroidism are evident at the time of diagnosis in only about 5 to 15% of patients (Grech et al, 1985). The classic plain film radiographic features of hyperparathyroidism include:

1. Subperiosteal resorption of bone, commonly seen at the medial aspect of the middle phalanges and distal tufts of the hands.

2. Intracortical resorption, which gives rise to linear striations or a honeycomb or basketweave appearance in the cortices.

3. Endosteal resorption.

4. Trabecular resorption (Stulberg et al, 1984).

Trabecular resorption within medullary bone occurs throughout the skeleton, including the maxillofacial complex. This type of remodeling in the cranium may give rise to a speckled radiographic appearance that has been referred to as a "salt-and-pepper skull." Resorption of bone in the jaws may result in a finer and lacier trabecular pattern, leading to a decrease in overall bone density. Individual trabeculae may become indistinct on the film, giving rise to a ground-glass appearance. Thinning or a partially absent lamina dura or outlines of the dental follicle walls, and thinning of the maxillary sinus floor, nasal fossa walls, inferior alveolar canal, and cortical border of the mandible may also be seen (Stulberg et al, 1984; Goaz and White, 1987; Langland et al, 1989).

Patients with longstanding hyperparathyroidism may develop brown tumors in the bones, including the jaws. These lesions result in significant loss of mineralized tissue and appear as "cyst-like" radiolucencies with ill-defined borders. They may appear unilocular or multilocular, may displace teeth, resorb teeth, or cause cortical expansion (Goaz and White, 1987; Langland et al, 1989). The radiographic features of brown tumors gave rise to the traditional description of hyperparathyroidism as *osteitis fibrosa cystica*.

On CT scans, brown tumors appear as lytic lesions with poorly defined edges (Lee and Rao, 1983). Radionuclide scans of bone in patients with hyperparathyroidism show increased uptake of radionuclide in the skull and facial bones, particularly the mandible (Citrin and McKillop, 1978).

Extraskeletal mineralization may also occur in patients with primary hyperparathyroisim. In fact, most patients with mild primary hyperparathyroidism have no significant metabolic bone disease but are more likely to have renal calculi (Burtis and Lang, 1984). Intraarticular joint cartilage is another tissue commonly affected by dystrophic calcification in primary hyperparathyroidism (Murray, 1989). Ectopic soft tissue calcifications of the lungs and stomach may be seen as dense spots on radionuclide scans of patients with secondary hyperparathyroidism due to renal failure (Citrin and McKillop, 1978).

The severity of bone involvement is often greater in patients with secondary hyperparathyroidism because of the added effects of the underlying disease on bone metabolism (Stulberg et al, 1984). Lesions of renal osteodystrophy include the formation of brown tumors; any combination of osteomalacia, osteosclerosis, and osteoporosis; and extraskeletal calcifications, especially in the kidneys, arteries, periarticular structures, and other soft tissues (Grech et al, 1985). On occasion, the combination of sclerotic trabecular bone and osteoporotic bone in patients with secondary hyperparathyroidism may result in increased radiodensities on films (Stulberg et al, 1984).

Finally, as described in Chapter 8, patients with hyperparathyroidism secondary to renal problems may also have calcifications in the medial layer of various arteries of the head and neck as well as in other vessels, which appear to outline the vessels along their length (Fig. 8–1 *A–C*).

Histopathologic Findings

Although bone biopsy is rarely needed to confirm the diagnosis of hyperparathyroidism, it is a sensitive indicator of the current status of the disorder. Histologic evidence of hyper-

parathyroidism includes osteoclastic resorption, formation of osteoid trabeculae, and peritrabecular fibrosis (Regezi and Sciubba, 1989; Stulberg et al, 1984). Brown tumors, which have been given that description grossly because of the hemosiderin and extravasated red blood cells seen in the lesions, may be found in the bones of patients with hyperparathyroidism. Osteoclastic multinucleated giant cells, large numbers of capillaries, and endothelium-lined spaces are also seen in these lesions. Because the brown tumor is identical histologically to a central giant cell granuloma, hyperparathyroidism must always be ruled out when the histologic diagnosis of a patient's lesions is a central giant cell granuloma (see Chapter 7).

Treatment

Treatment of primary hyperparathyroidism usually consists of surgical removal of the offending adenoma or adenocarcinoma or **subtotal** parathyroidectomy of the hyperplastic parathyroid glands. The patient may experience postsurgical hypocalcemia following the surgery. Brown tumors regress spontaneously without surgical intervention following correction of the calcium imbalance (Stulberg et al, 1984).

Patients with secondary hyperparathyroidism should be treated for the underlying renal or gastrointestinal disorder. However, the hemodialysis that helps to correct uremia in patients with chronic renal failure does not help in correcting serum calcium levels. Calcium and vitamin D supplements are often prescribed, as they are for patients with hypoparathyroidism (Burtis and Lang, 1984).

HYPOPARATHYROIDISM

Decreased levels of PTH, or **hypoparathyroidism**, may occur idiopathically or may follow surgical damage or removal of the parathyroid glands during thyroidectomy. In **pseudohypoparathyroidism**, PTH levels are normal, but the target tissues (renal tubules and osteoclasts) are unresponsive to any level of the hormone.

Clinical Features

Both hypoparathyroidism and pseudohypoparathyroidism may produce clinical manifestations of hypocalcemia, which include muscle spasms, paresthesia in the extremities or perioral regions, and psychological anxiety or depression. Patients with pseudohypoparathyroidism may have short stature due to early closure of the epiphyses. Hypoparathyroidism does occur in young individuals, and their teeth may show evidence of enamel hypoplasia. Teeth that are fully developed are not susceptible to altered levels of circulating PTH (Goaz and White, 1987).

Radiographic Appearance

Patients with hypoparathyroidism may exhibit an increased density of bone on radiographs. There may also be ectopic soft tissue calcification, especially in periarticular structures. The brain may also develop areas of mineralization; the basal ganglia are frequently affected, and the cerebellum has been involved in some patients as well (Grech et al, 1985). The patient may also exhibit enamel hypoplasia, short roots, and enlarged pulps (Goaz and White, 1987; Langland et al, 1989).

OSTEOMALACIA

Osteomalacia results from the replacement of normal adult trabecular bone by unmineralized osteoid due to a defect in bone mineralization. The anatomic bone volume is unchanged, but the mineral content is decreased and the proportion of organic material is increased (Wahner, 1987). Should such a defect occur in newly forming bone or in growth plate cartilage in children, the defect is referred to as **rickets**.

Osteomalacia may be caused by a variety of disturbances in calcium and vitamin D metabolism. Inadequate dietary intake of calcium or vitamin D and malabsorption disorders (especially those affecting the proximal portion of the small intestine, the primary site of vitamin D absorption) may lead to osteomalacia. Renal failure may also contribute to osteomalacia because it results in impaired $1,25(OH)_2$ vitamin D formation and metabolic acidosis. Excess hydrogen ions that are retained in metabolic acidosis are balanced by increased excretion of calcium in the urine, which in turn leads to increased release of calcium from the stores in the bones (Grech et al, 1985; Klein and Maxwell, 1984). Inborn errors of calcium and phosphorus metabolism such as **hypophosphatasia** or **hypophosphatemia** may also play

a role in the development of osteomalacia. Prolonged therapy with drugs that disrupt vitamin D homeostasis such as phenytoin and heparin may contribute to the condition as well.

Clinical Features

Signs and symptoms of osteomalacia frequently include bone pain, which may be severe at times, fractures, and muscle weakness (Liberman and Marx, 1989).

Radiographic Appearance

The bone changes seen in osteomalacia are nonspecific. They relate to the generalized demineralization in the bone. The cortical and trabecular bone of the skull and jaws may appear less dense on plain films. Individual trabeculae may be sparse or coarse. Patients may show signs of fractures or pseudofractures. Pseudofractures are sites of previous fracture that have healed with organic material only and have a radiolucent radiographic appearance (Grech et al, 1984). Bone scans often show a generalized increased uptake of the radionuclide without any specific features (Citrin and McKillop, 1978).

No radiographic change in osteomalacia is specific for the maxillofacial complex. However, there has been a report of multiple sites of internal resorption in the teeth of a patient with end-stage renal disease. These lesions were reported to diminish when the patient was placed on hemodialysis (Hutton, 1985). It must be remembered, however, that many patients with osteomalacia show no radiographic evidence of altered bone metabolism (Wahner, 1987).

Histopathologic Findings

Rickets and osteomalacia are characterized by a lack of mineralization of the organic matrix of bone, usually seen in the form of excess osteoid. Rickets mainly affects the growing skeleton, especially the regions of endochondral ossification. Differentiation between an increase in osteoid due to a mineralization defect, as seen in osteomalacia, and an increase in organic matrix deposition seen in hyperparathyroidism requires dynamic measurements with tetracycline labeling (Liberman and Marx, 1989).

OSTEOPOROSIS

Osteoporosis is a general term denoting loss of bone mass. This loss may be due to defects in collagen or mineral metabolism, proliferative diseases of the marrow, or an alteration in osteoblastic or osteoclastic activity. Prolonged therapy with certain drugs such as corticosteroids and certain disease states such as Cushing's disease are also associated with the development of osteoporosis. However, osteoporosis is a poorly understood phenomenon of older adults and is often termed idiopathic.

Clinical Features

Osteoporosis occurs primarily in postmenopausal white women over 65 years of age. There appear to be contributory or modifying genetic and environmental factors including estrogen deficiency, slender build, alcohol intake, and inactivity (Table 10–1). However, the precise etiology remains obscure. The condition may affect both men and women, including those in younger age groups.

Hypercortisolism, often the result of prolonged corticosteroid therapy for diseases such as rheumatoid arthritis or asthma, has been linked to the development of osteoporosis. The mechanism appears to be a decreased formation of and increased resorption of trabecular bone (Woolf and Dixon, 1988). Corticosteroids also reduce intestinal calcium absorption and increase urinary calcium excretion. Patients with excess endogenous glucocorticoids (**Cushing's disease**) or excess thyroid hormone are also plagued with the condition.

The diagnosis of osteoporosis may not be made until the patient suffers a fracture, commonly of the wrist, rib, spinal column, or hip. Early diagnosis is difficult. Loss of as much as 30% of the bone mass from a vertebral body must occur before it can be detected radiographically on the plain films. Although biochemical profiles may provide information about endocrine dysfunctions, calcium balance, and renal and marrow status, many patients with osteoporosis have no detectable serum or urine abnormalities. A transiliac bone biopsy is the most accurate means of clarifying whether the condition is osteomalacia or osteoporosis (Lane and Vigorita, 1984).

However, special radiographic measurements or tests are often used in the diagnosis of osteoporosis. Radiogrammetry involves measurements of the cortical thickness of metacarpal bones seen on hand films. The Singh index catalogs the order of loss of trabecular bone spicules as seen on a film of the head of the femur. Photon absorptiometry and single-beam absorptiometry are methods that use a beam from a single radioisotope source (iodine-125) passing through an extremity to quantify bone mineral loss. A scintillation counter records the intensity of the beam after it passes through an extremity, giving an estimate of the bone mineral content per unit length of bone. Dual photon absorptiometry allows measurements from deep sites surrounded by soft tissue such as the femoral neck or lumbar vertebrae. Dual photon absorptiometry uses a radioisotope source, gadolinium-153, that emits at both 42 KeV and 100 KeV and measures the mineral content of both cortical and trabecular bone (Woolf and Dixon, 1988). However, absorptiometry may not be able to distinguish osteomalacia from osteoporosis (Wahner, 1987).

Quantitative computed tomography can be used to measure the bone mineral content in a vertebral body, but it may be affected by the amount of fatty marrow present. This may lead to an underestimation of the amount of bone present by as much as 10% (Goodwin, 1987). Bone scans alone are relatively nonspecific for differentiating between osteoporosis and osteomalacia but are useful in monitoring the progress of the diseases (Wahner, 1987).

Radiographic Appearance

Osteoporosis may present on radiographs as an overall decrease in bone density. However, a substantial amount of hard tissue must be lost before the loss can be detected on a plain film. Films of the maxillofacial complex do not provide much diagnostic information about the presence or absence of osteoporosis (Kribbs et al, 1983; Mercier and Inoue, 1981; Mohajery, 1988).

Histopathologic Findings

The transiliac bone biopsy provides a tissue specimen on which histomorphometric meas-

Table 10–1. RISK FACTORS FOR OSTEOPOROSIS

Increasing age	Physical inactivity
Female gender	Smoking
Caucasian race	Alcoholism
Estrogen deficiency	Inadequate calcium intake
Small stature	

urements can be made. The specimen is usually divided into two sections, one of which is decalcified. Useful measurements include the amount of mineralized cortical and trabecular bone present, the relative amount of osteoid present, and the rates of bone formation and resorption (Woolf and Dixon, 1989).

Treatment

There is no established treatment to date for osteoporosis. Effort is usually directed toward prevention, which may include weight-bearing exercises, adequate calcium intake, and estrogen supplements when indicated (Wasserman and Barzel, 1987).

References

Burtis, W.J., and Lang, R.: Chemical abnormalities. Orthop. Clin. North Am., 15:653–669, 1984.

Citrin, D.L., and McKillop, J.H.: Atlas of Technetium Bone Scans. Philadelphia: W.B. Saunders, 1978, pp. 165, 176–178.

Goaz, P.W., and White, S.C.: Oral Radiology: Principles and Interpretation, 2nd ed. St. Louis: C.V. Mosby, 1987, pp. 629–632.

Goodwin, P.N.: Methodologies for the measurement of bone density and their precision and accuracy. Sem. Nuc. Med., 17:293–304, 1987.

Grech, P., Martin, T.J., Barrington, N.A., and Ell, P.J.: Diagnosis of Metabolic Bone Disease. Philadelphia: W.B. Saunders, 1985, pp. 62–67, 85–95.

Hutton, C.E.: Intradental lesions and their reversal in a patient being treated for end-stage renal disease. Oral Surg. Oral Med. Oral Pathol., 60:258–261, 1985.

Klein, K.L., and Maxwell, M.H.: Renal osteodystrophy. Orthop. Clin. North Am., 15:687–695, 1984.

Kribbs, P.J., Smith D.E., and Chesnut, C.H.: Oral findings in osteoporosis. Part II.. Relationship between residual ridge and alveolar bone resorption and generalized skeletal osteopenia. J. Pros. Dent., 50:719–724, 1983.

Lane, J.M., and Vigorita, V.J.: Osteoporosis. Orthop. Clin. North Am., 15:711–729, 1984.

Langland, O.E., Langlais, R.P., McDavid, W.D., and DelBalso, A.M.: Panoramic Radiology, 2nd ed. Philadelphia: Lea & Febiger, 1989, pp. 301–304.

Liberman, U.A., and Marx, S.J.: Disorders of vitamin D metabolism. In Tam, C.S., Heersche, J.N.M. and Murray, T.M. (eds.): Metabolic Bone Disease: Cellular and Tissue Mechanisms. Boca Raton: CRC Press, 1989, pp. 174–179.

Lee, S.H., and Rao, K.C.V.G.: Cranial Computed Tomography. New York: McGraw-Hill, 1983, pp. 375, 379.

Mercier, P., and Inove, S.: Bone density and serum minerals in cases of residual alveolar ridge atrophy. J. Pros. Dent., 46:250–255, 1981.

Mohajery, M.: Oral findings of osteoporosis and its relation with normal bone density (Abstract). American Academy of Dental Radiology, Annual Meeting, Silver Spring, MD, 1988.

Murray, T.M.: Parathyroid hormone and hyperparathyroidism. In Tam, C.S., Heersche, J.N.M., and Murray, T.M. (eds.): Metabolic Bone Disease: Cellular and Tissue Mechanisms. Boca Raton: CRC Press, 1989, pp. 118–122.

Regezi, J.A., and Sciubba, J.J.: Oral Pathology: Clinical-Pathologic Correlations. Philadelphia: W.B. Saunders, 1989, pp. 383–386, 431–433.

Stulberg, B.N., Licata, A.A., Bauer, T.W., and Belhobek, G.H.: Hyperparathyroidism, hyperthyroidism and Cushing's disease. Orthop. Clin. North Am., 15:697–710, 1984.

Wahner, H.W.: Single- and dual-photon absorptiometry in osteoporosis and osteomalacia. Sem. Nucl. Med., 17:305–315, 1987.

Wasserman, S.H.S., and Barzel, U.S.: Osteoporosis: The state of the art in 1987: A review. Sem. Nucl. Med., 17:283–292, 1987. Winzelberg, G.G., and Hydovitz, J.D.: Radionuclide imaging of parathyroid tumors: Historical perspectives and newer techniques. Sem. Nucl. Med., 15:161–164, 1985.

Woolf, A.D., and Dixon, A.S.: Osteoporosis: A Clinical Guide. Philadelphia: J.B. Lippincott, 1988, pp. 57–58, 63, 104.

DIABETES MELLITUS

Diabetes mellitus is a metabolic disorder of glucose intolerance and is a major chronic health problem. It can be classified into two basic types: type I, also known as insulin-dependent diabetes mellitus, and type II, known as non–insulin-dependent diabetes mellitus. The terms juvenile diabetes and adult-onset diabetes have been abandoned because either type of diabetes may occur in any age group.

Clinical Features

The oral effects of diabetes mellitus may include xerostomia and an increased level of glucose in the serous saliva of the parotid glands (Murrah, 1985). There may be a slight acceleration in dental development up in to age 10, possibly due to stimulation of the pituitary gland in the initial stages of diabetes (Bohatka et al, 1973). Because of the decreased salivary flow and increased salivary carbohydrates, diabetic patients are very susceptible to dental caries and periodontal disease, especially those in whom the disease is undiagnosed or poorly controlled. It is felt that diabetes does not cause the caries or periodontal disease directly; however, the diabetic patient's immunologic response to the challenge of carcinogenic bacteria, plaque, and calculus may be altered or impaired. Angiopathy, abnormal collagen metabolism, and abnormal polymorphonuclear white blood cell function are some of the complications found in diabetic patients that may contribute to the patient's compromised response to disease (Manouchehr-Pour and Bissada, 1983).

Radiographic Appearance

The loss of supporting alveolar bone seen in periodontal disease of diabetic patients cannot be differentiated on radiographs from advanced periodontal bone loss in patients who do not have diabetes. However, the severity of periodontal bone loss can be extreme in patients with undiagnosed or uncontrolled diabetes mellitus. Accelerated changes in horizontal bone loss in patients should alert the clinician to an underlying systemic problem such as diabetes.

References

Bohatka, L., Wegener, H., and Adler, P.: Parameters of the transitional dentition in diabetic children. J. Dent. Res., 52:131–135, 1973.

Manouchehr-Pour, M., and Bissada, N.F.: Periodontal disease in juvenile and adult diabetic patients: A review of the literature. J. Am. Dent. Assoc., 107:766–770, 1983.

Murrah, V.A.: Diabetes mellitus and associated oral manifestations: A review. J. Oral Pathol., 14:271–281, 1985.

INHERITED ANEMIAS

SICKLE CELL ANEMIA

Sickle cell anemia is a hereditary hemolytic blood disorder that most commonly affects blacks and people of Mediterranean heritage. The disease is the result of a defective hemoglobin chain that distorts the shape of erythrocytes into crescents or "sickles." In the homozygous form of the disease, a majority of the erythrocytes are affected, but in a patient who is heterozygous only a portion of the red blood cells may be involved. Sickling generally becomes more severe in states of hypoxia in both types of disease. The distorted shape of the erythrocytes leads to stasis of blood flow, and tissue infarction is a potential complication.

Clinical Features

Signs and symptoms of sickle cell anemia are the same as those of most anemias: pallor, weakness, fatigue, and shortness of breath. Patients with the more severe form of the disease may also experience pain in the joints, limbs, and abdomen (Shafer et al, 1983). Sensitivity, swelling, or pain in the oral-maxillofacial complex has been reported in homozygous patients, particularly during times of acute hemolytic crises (Cox, 1984).

THALASSEMIA

The thalassemias are a group of hereditary anemias resulting from reduced synthesis of one or more of the hemoglobin chains. Thalassemias are classified according to the type of globin chain involved, either alpha or beta. The disorder is most common among individuals of Mediterranean descent. As with sickle cell anemia, homozygotes are usually more severely affected; some homozygous forms of the disease are fatal at young ages. Heterozygotes generally experience a milder form of disease, sometimes referred to as thalassemia minor.

Clinical Features

Patients with thalassemia minor may have no clinical evidence of disease or they may have general signs and symptoms of anemia.

Radiographic Appearance

Both sickle cell anemia and thalassemia may affect the bone marrow in that it may proliferate in an attempt to generate more erythrocytes to carry oxygen to the tissues. The proliferation of marrow may or may not be visible on plain radiographs. Skull films may show thickening of the diploë, and the inner and outer tables of the cranium may be thin or ill-defined. Trabeculae may radiate perpendicularly from the inner table, giving the classic "hair-on-end" radiographic appearance (Shafer et al, 1983).

Panoramic or intraoral films may show a generalized loss of bone density similar to that seen in osteomalacia or osteoporosis. Trabeculae of the jaws may appear in a coarse pattern, sometimes described as "chicken-wire," and there may be loss of lamina dura (Poyton, 1982). Plain films of long bones may show evidence of cortical erosions or rarefactions (Van Dis and Langlais, 1986). Bone scans are useful for differentiating between osteomyelitis and bone infarction in patients with sickle cell anemia. Both conditions commonly occur in these patients (Citrin and McKillop, 1978).

References

Citrin, D.L., and McKillop, J.H.: Atlas of Technetium Bone Scans. Philadelphia. W.B Saunders, 1978, pp. 165, 176–178.

Cox, G.M.: A study of oral pain experience in sickle cell patients. Oral Surg. Oral Med. Oral Pathol., 58:39–41, 1984.

Poyton, H.G.: Oral Radiology. Baltimore: Williams & Wilkins, 1982, pp. 230–232.

Shafer, W.G., Hine, L.K., and Levy, B.M.: A Textbook of Oral Pathology, 4th ed. Philadelphia: W.B Saunders, 1983, pp. 727–728, 847.

Van Dis, M.L., and Langlais, R.P.: The thalassemias: Oral manifestations and complications. Oral Surg. Oral Med. Oral Pathol., 62:229–233, 1986.

IDIOPATHIC HISTIOCYTOSIS

Idiopathic histiocytosis (also known as Langerhans cell disease and histiocytosis X) is a disease characterized by proliferation of Langerhans cells or histiocytes. These cells are normally present in the mucosa and are involved in the processing and presentation of antigens to T lymphocytes (Regezi and Sciubba, 1989).

Clinical Features

Idiopathic histiocytosis has traditionally been divided into three disorders: **Letterer-Siwe disease**, **Hand-Schüller-Christian disease**, and **eosinophilic granuloma**.

Letterer-Siwe disease represents a malignant neoplastic process and is referred to as the **acute disseminated form** of idiopathic histiocytosis. This form commonly presents in infants as a widespread proliferative process involving many organs, bones, and skin. The child may demonstrate intermittent fever, hepatomegaly, splenomegaly, lymphadenopathy, and anemia. The process is rapidly progressive and usually fatal.

Hand-Schüller-Christian disease has traditionally represented a specific triad of bone lesions, exophthalmos, and diabetes insipidus;

however, few patients actually present with this classic form. Many patients with the **chronic disseminated form** of the disorder present with a variety of lymph node, visceral, and bone lesions. This form of the disease tends to occur in young people and has a slight male predilection (Regezi and Sciubba, 1989). Oral manifestations may include hyperplastic gingival lesions, gingival hemorrhage, tenderness and swelling in the alveolar process, and painful, loose teeth.

Eosinophilic granuloma most likely represents the least severe form of the disorder and may be referred to as the **chronic localized form**. Single or multiple lesions of bone may occur in one or more bones. The skull, mandible, ribs, vertebrae, and long bones are common sites (Regezi and Sciubba, 1989). Lesions that affect the jaws may lead to painful, mobile teeth and gingival lesions similar to those found in the chronic disseminated form.

Radiographic Appearance

Lesions of the skull and jaws are relatively common in this disorder. Lesions of the jaws tend to occur more often in the mandible than in the maxilla, and more often in the posterior areas of the jaws than in the anterior. The lesions are osteolytic with relatively well-defined borders; they may, however, be irregular in shape. The lesions involving alveolar bone do not resorb roots of adjacent teeth; the teeth appear to lose all bone support and "float" in space. On occasion, lesions of eosinophilic granuloma produce an "onion-skin" appearance like that of proliferative periostitis (Poyton, 1982).

The appearance of the bone lesions on CT scans is similar in all forms of the disorder. They appear as purely lytic lesions with lobulated or scalloped borders. Bony sequestra may be seen in the lytic areas. Any extraosseous soft tissue mass associated with the bone lesions is also be seen on CT scans (Lee and Rao, 1983). Bone scans demonstrate intense increased uptake of radionuclide in the area of the bone lesions (Domboski, 1980).

Histopathologic Findings

The lesions are characterized by a proliferation of Langerhans-type cells with abundant cytoplasm, indistinct cell borders, and ovoid nuclei. These cells are often seen in sheets, and there may be eosinophils or other inflammatory cells mixed in with the Langerhans-type cells. Multinucleated giant cells and foci of necrosis may also be present (Regezi and Sciubba, 1989).

Treatment

The treatment for Letterer-Siwe and Hand-Schüller-Christian disease usually involves radiation therapy (whole body). Lesions of eosinophilic granuloma may be readily excised surgically and rarely recur. Periodic radiographic follow-up would be prudent following excision of a lesion of eosinophilic granuloma.

References

Domboski, M.: Eosinophilic granuloma of bone manifesting mandibular involvement. Oral Surg. Oral Med. Oral Pathol., 50:116–123, 1980.

Lee, S.H., and Rao, K.C.V.G.: Cranial Computed Tomography. New York: McGraw-Hill, 1983, pp. 375, 379.

Regezi, J.A., and Sciubba, J.J.: Oral Pathology: Clinical-Pathologic Correlations. Philadelphia: W.B. Saunders, 1989, pp. 383–386, 431–433.

Poyton, H.G.: Oral Radiology. Baltimore: Williams & Wilkins, 1982, pp. 238–241.

PROGRESSIVE SYSTEMIC SCLEROSIS

Progressive systemic sclerosis (or scleroderma) is a disease characterized by progressive fibrosis and sclerosis of multiple organ systems, including the skin, gastrointestinal system, lungs, cardiovascular system, kidneys, musculoskeletal system, and central nervous system. The precise etiology of the disorder is unknown, but vasculitis and fibrosis in small arteries appear to be involved (Ramon et al, 1987).

Clinical Features

This is a disease of adults, generally striking between the ages of 30 and 50 years. There is a distinct female predilection, women being affected two to three times as often as men. Sclerosis often begins in the face, hands, or trunk. Mild edema is an early sign, and erythema, neuralgia, paresthesia, and joint pain may be present. Eventually, the epithelium undergoes atrophy, induration, and fixation to underlying subcutaneous tissues. The skin becomes waxy in appearance and may be so hardened that the patient's face may resemble a mask, and the hands may be malformed into a claw-like position. The patient may experience difficulty in opening the mouth, swallowing, or breathing as the tongue, lips, and soft palate become involved. Xerostomia, Sjögren's syndrome, and an increased incidence of caries and periodontal disease have also been reported in patients with progressive systemic sclerosis (Wood and Lee, 1988; Ramon et al, 1987).

Radiographic Appearance

One of the radiographic signs of progressive systemic sclerosis is widening of the periodontal ligament space, often to at least twice the normal width. Multiple teeth are usually involved. Anterior and posterior areas are affected with equal frequency. There is no apparent predilection for the maxillary or mandibular area. However, not all patients with the disorder demonstrate this periodontal ligament space widening (Wood and Lee, 1988).

Resorption of the mandibular angles and coronoid processes has also been reported. Most of the mandibular angle erosions are bilateral, symmetric, and have smooth, well-defined edges (White et al, 1977). Ramon and his associates attribute this appearance to vasculitis of the internal maxillary artery (1987). Erosions in the area of insertion of the digastric muscle and condylar head may also be seen (Wood and Lee, 1988). Bilateral condylosis may result in the relatively sudden onset of an open bite in an adult (Ramon et al, 1987).

Histopathologic Findings

Systemic sclerosis is characterized by thickened and hyalinized collagen fibers and atrophy of the epithelium with loss of rete ridges. Blood vessel walls become thickened and sclerotic as well, and subcutaneous fat disappears (Shafer et al, 1983).

Treatment

Partial remission may be obtained for these patients with the use of systemic corticosteroids, but immunosuppressive therapy is generally ineffective (Ramon et al, 1987). Patients demonstrating erosions of the mandible should be followed carefully to avoid pathologic fractures.

References

Ramon, Y., Samra, H., and Oberman, M.: Mandibular condylosis and apertognathia as presenting symptoms in progressive systemic sclerosis (scleroderma). Oral Surg. and Oral. Med. Oral Pathol., 63:269–274, 1987.

Shafer, W.G., Hine, L.K., and Levy, B.M.: A Textbook of Oral Pathology, 4th ed. Philadelphia: W.B. Saunders, 1983, pp. 727–728, 847.

White, S.C., Frey, N.W., Blaschke, D.D., Ross, M.D., Clements, P.J., and Furst, E.D.: Oral radiographic changes in patients with progressive systemic sclerosis (scleroderma). J. Am. Dent. Assoc., 94:1178–1182, 1977.

Wood, R.E., and Lee, P.: Analysis of the oral manifestations of systemic sclerosis (scleroderma). Oral Surg. Oral Med. Oral Pathol., 65:172–178, 1988.

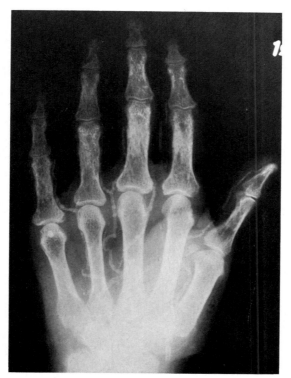

Figure 10–1. Subperiosteal resorption, resorption at the terminal tufts, and loss of cortical bone can be seen in the hand of this patient with secondary hyperparathyroid-ism. Also note the calcifications present in the vessels, another radiographic finding in hyperparathyroidism.

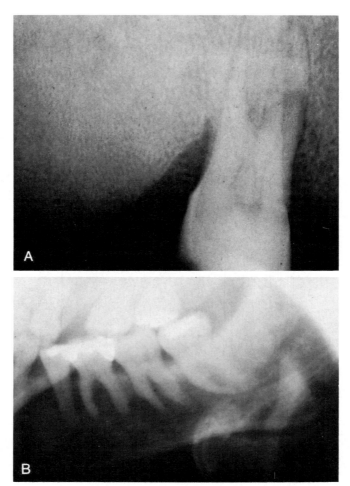

Figure 10–2. *A,* These intraoral films show the loss of lamina dura and alteration of the trabecular bone to a ground-glass appearance. This patient suffered from chronic renal insufficiency. *B,* A lateral oblique jaw film shows loss of radiographic density, loss of lamina dura, and a ground-glass appearance in the trabecular bone. This patient also had a chronic kidney disease.

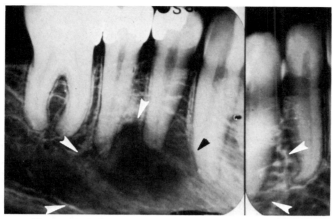

Figure 10–3. Radiograph of brown tumor in bone (*arrowheads*).

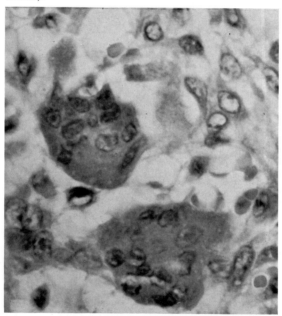

Figure 10–4. Photomicrograph of brown tumor/central giant cell granuloma. Note multinucleated giant cells.

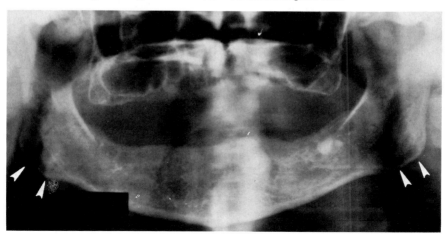

Figure 10–5. This patient was diagnosed as having osteoporosis following a stress fracture in a vertebra. Note the general loss of bone density in this panoramic film. There is also a decrease in the amount of cortical bone present around the angles of the mandible (*arrowheads*).

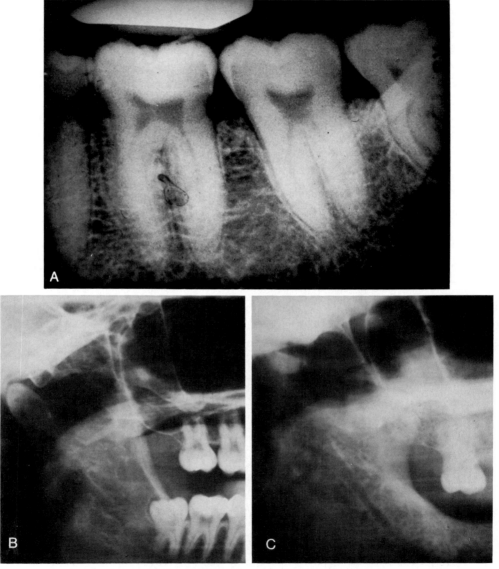

Figure 10–6. *A*, Coarse trabeculae of sickle cell anemia. *B* and *C*, Sickle cell anemia. Note coarse trabecular pattern and large narrow spaces.

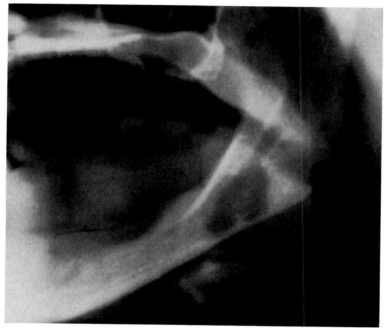

Figure 10–7. This panoramic film shows the irregularly shaped radiolucency of an eosinophilic granuloma. This case is quite unusual in that the patient was a 56-year-old woman when the lesion was found and diagnosed.

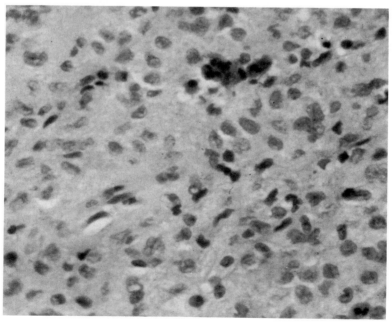

Figure 10–8. This photomicrograph illustrates the sheets of Langerhans-type cells typically seen in idiopathic histiocytosis. This lesion also contains numerous eosinophils.

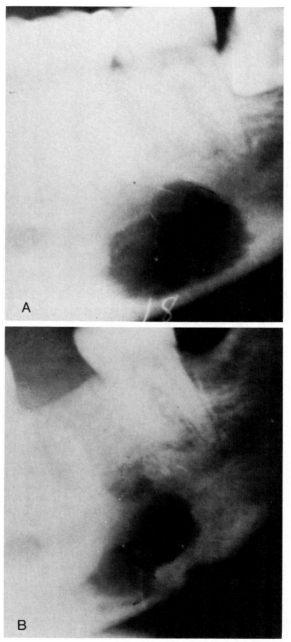

Figure 10–9. *A*, Unilocular radiolucency in left mandible with ragged border. Lesion has eroded the lower cortex. The lesion was diagnosed as eosinophilic granuloma. (Courtesy of Dr. C. Tomich, Indiana University School of Dentistry.) *B*, Follow-up radiograph taken 6 months later after biopsy. Note cortical defect.

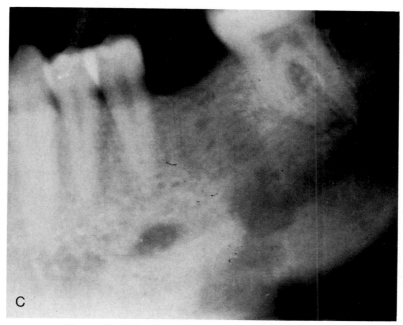

Figure 10–9 *Continued C*, Radiograph taken 13 months after diagnosis. Persistent bony changes are evident. Cortical area has still not completely healed.

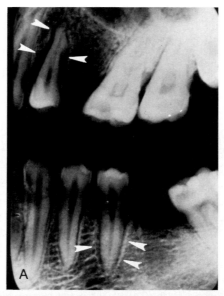

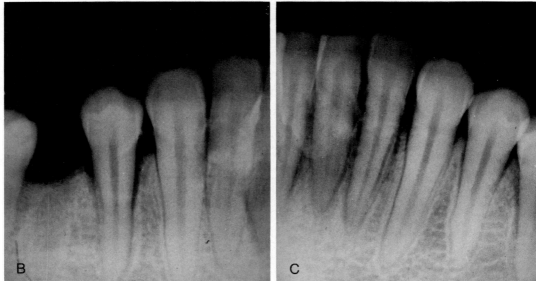

Figure 10–10. *A*, Radiograph of widened pdl spaces (*arrowheads*). The patient also has some periodontal disease. Similar changes are seen in *B* and *C*.

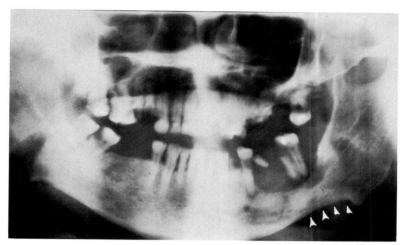

Figure 10–11. Radiograph of mandibular erosion in scleroderma *(arrows)*. The patient also had a squamous cell carcinoma of the mandible involving the molar.

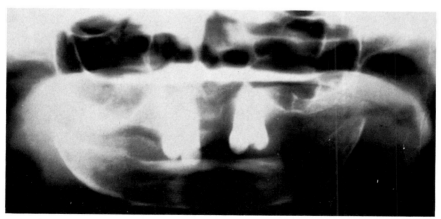

Figure 10–12. Severe osteolysis due to muscle pull problems in patient with scleroderma. (Courtesy of Dr. R. P. Langlais, University of Texas, Health Science Center at San Antonio.)

DISORDERS OF THE TEMPOROMANDIBULAR JOINT

D. MILES

MYOFASCIAL PAIN DYSFUNCTION SYNDROME

DISC DISPLACEMENT

RHEUMATOID ARTHRITIS

DEGENERATIVE JOINT DISEASE

OTHER ARTHRITIDES
SJÖGREN'S SYNDROME
PROGRESSIVE SYSTEMIC SCLEROSIS
SYSTEMIC LUPUS ERYTHEMATOSUS
MIXED CONNECTIVE TISSUE DISEASE
REITER'S SYNDROME
PSORIATIC ARTHRITIS

GOUT

From the chapter outline it is clear that a vast array of conditions or disorders affects the temporomandibular joint (TMJ). Reports of tumors, benign or malignant, are somewhat rare; however, certain arthritides, especially degenerative joint disease (DJD) and rheumatoid arthritis (RA), are quite common. In other disorders such as progressive systemic sclerosis (PSS), systemic lupus erythematosus (SLE), and mixed connective tissue disease (MCTD) the associated arthropathy is rheumatoid arthritis as part of a mixed syndrome of symptoms and complaints. If the dentist has a sound knowledge of the radiographic changes and symptomatology of RA and DJD, this knowledge can be readily applied to other arthritides. Knowledge of these conditions, coupled with the specific signs and symptoms of the patient and the historical and clinical information, allows the rarer diagnoses to be made.

Traumatic changes of the TMJ region are quite specific and usually are easily identified by multiple radiographic views of the involved joint. Tumors also are usually discerned easily, but their diagnosis must be confirmed by histopathologic examination. Crystal-producing or crystal-induced arthritis is uncommon in the TMJ region but should be easily diagnosed by means of historical and radiographic correlation with other joints in the body.

Two of the most common disorders of the TMJ that are seen and often treated by the dentist are myofascial pain dysfunction syndrome (MPDS) and disc displacement problems. Although there are no direct radiographic changes in MPDS, certain joint films are usually taken in the diagnostic work-up. Their usefulness and indirect interpretive findings will be discussed. Disc displacement problems, formerly called internal derangements, are more common than reported earlier and can be readily investigated by advanced imaging modalities such as computed tomography (CT) and magnetic resonance imaging (MRI). There are also tomographic and arthographic radiologic features that can confirm the dentist's diagnostic impression.

The clinician cannot hope to master the diagnosis and treatment of TMJ disorders without a thorough understanding of the unique anatomy of the TMJ complex. Such a discussion is beyond the scope of this textbook. However, several excellent articles and textbooks are recommended for obtaining this information (Okeson, 1985; Worth, 1979).

References

Okeson, J.P.: Fundamentals of Occlusion and Temporomandibular Disorders. St. Louis. C.V. Mosby, 1985, pp. 2–52.
Worth, H.M.: Temporomandibular Joint Function and Dysfunction. St. Louis. C.V. Mosby, 1979, pp. 321–329.

MYOFASCIAL PAIN DYSFUNCTION SYNDROME

Clinical Findings

Among the various disorders affecting the TMJ, MPDS is probably the most common. The diagnostic features of MPDS involve multiple complaints. These are outlined in Table 11–1.

The dentist should realize that with this wide array of signs and symptoms, many of which are not specific—that is, they may be associated with a myriad of other orofacial pain problems or lesions—the diagnosis of MPDS is at best very exacting and very time-consuming. In addition, MPDS may be associated secondarily with disc displacement (internal derangement) problems. If the patient's pri-

Table 11–1. SIGNS AND SYMPTOMS OF MYOFASCIAL PAIN DYSFUNCTION SYNDROME

1. Pain on opening the jaws or with function of the TMJ
2. Restricted opening of the TMJ
3. Unilateral or bilateral facial pain, often preauricular, often referred
4. Headaches in various locations
5. Tired or fatigued muscles of mastication
6. Wear facets on teeth
7. Occlusal problems such as nonworking interferences, premature contacts, or loss of vertical dimension
8. Tinnitus (ringing) in the ears
9. Vertigo
10. Noises in the TMJ such as "clicking"
11. Parafunctional (abnormal) habits

mary problem is an anteriorly displaced disc with pain and restriction of opening, then a "secondary" MPDS complaint may follow. Muscles working in abnormal patterns to compensate for or avoid the pain of dysfunction will themselves become problematic. By the same token, a longstanding MPD problem, may give rise to a secondary disc problem. In any event, it is the responsibility of the dentist to ensure that the MPD problem has not resulted from a mechanical or lesional problem of the TMJ joint itself. In many instances, this is done on a clinical basis, and no radiographs are indicated. In some cases there may be a positive historical or clinical feature that mandates the use of a radiographic examination to rule out a disease process as the cause of the patient's myogenic (muscular origin) pain. Because the treatment of MPDS is both variable and controversial, we will not discuss in detail the various methods used to control the patient's pain. It is enough to say that treatment modalities may involve physiotherapy, pharmacotherapy (muscle relaxants, analgesics, and occasionally antianxiety agents), occlusal equilibration, restorative procedures, psychological counselling, and occlusal splint therapy, either separately or in various combinations. The clinician who uses one therapy to "cure" all of his or her patients is probably *not* meeting the needs of these patients and may wonder sometimes why the patient is not responding to the treatment.

Radiographic Appearance

As might be realized from the previous discussion, there are *no* distinctive radiographic features of MPDS. Some clinicians place a great deal of emphasis on the "joint space" (Fig. 11–1). However, concentricity of the condyle in its fossa is quite variable (Heffez and Blaustein, 1987). When it appears displaced on radiographic examination such as tomography, arthrography, or magnetic resonance imaging (MRI) the diagnosis is usually related to a disc displacement problem, and the clinical features are more consistent with that diagnosis than with MPDS (see next section on disc displacement). Nevertheless, a "scout" film is often necessary to rule out gross pathology such as arthritic conditions, hyperplasia of the condylar or coronoid processes, and neoplasms in MPDS patients. Several plain film techniques are useful in these cases, including:

1. Transcranial films
2. Transpharyngeal films
3. Transorbital films
4. Panoramic films
5. Specialized panoramic films
6. Tomography

Typical images are seen in Figures 11–2 to 11–7, the legends of which outline the advantages and shortcomings of these techniques. Descriptions of the techniques appear in other textbooks (Miles et al, 1989a; Goaz and White, 1987). It must also be cautioned that most of these techniques, even when used in combination, probably underestimate the presence of disease. The dentist *must* determine the clinical and historic information of the patient precisely, and order films accordingly if he or she expects to obtain a positive radiographic finding. If such selection criteria are not employed, the dentist will be exposing patients to an unnecessary radiation burden and exposing himself or herself to possible litigation (Miles et al, 1989b).

References

Goaz, P.W., and White, S.C.: Oral Radiology. Principles and Interpretation, 2nd ed. St. Louis. C.V. Mosby, 1987, pp. 654–670.

Heffez, L., and Blaustein, D.: Diagnostic arthroscopy of the temporomandibular joint. Part I: Normal arthroscopic findings. Oral Surg., 64(6):653–670, 1987.

Miles, D.A., Van Dis, M.L., Jensen, C.W., and Ferretti, A.: Radiographic Imaging for Dental Auxiliaries. Philadelphia. W.B. Saunders, 1989a, pp. 158–163.

Miles, D.A., Lovas, J.G.L., and Loyens, S.: Radiographs and the responsible dentist. Gen. Dent., 37(3):201–206, 1989b.

DISC DISPLACEMENT

Classifications of disc displacements (internal derangements) most commonly include three general variations. These are

1. Anterior displacement with reduction
2. Anterior displacement without reduction ("closed-lock")
3. Disc perforation

Diagnosis of these problems, like MPDS, can usually be made on the basis of the history and clinical findings. However, because treatment of a small percentage of these patients involves surgery, the dentist and the oral surgeon often require radiographic confirmation of the displaced disc. Indirect information can be obtained by tomography and arthrography, but direct visualization of the soft tissues of the disc and its attachments is obtainable only through MRI and, more recently, TMJ arthroscopy. Arthroscopy of the joint will be discussed in the treatment section.

Until very recently the most exact, exacting, and appropriate radiologic evaluation of disc problems was obtained by arthrographic examination. Contrast material, usually a water-soluble agent containing iodine, was injected into the lower joint space or sometimes the upper and lower joint spaces (Fig. 11–8). Although the disc was outlined, the information about its exact position still had to be inferred. The tissues themselves were not directly visible. Also, the technique was successful in the hands of some radiologists or oral surgeons but not others, and often the patient experienced pain and other sequelae postoperatively. Hence, the technique, although useful, is still not widely practiced except in regional areas. Furthermore, many surgeons do not feel the need for radiographic confirmation in many cases because they are able to assess the most symptomatic joints at the time of surgery. Currently, there seems to be growing acceptance and use of arthroscopy (Blaustein and Heffez, 1988; Moses and Poker, 1989)—direct visualization of the tissues by means of fiberoptics—and of MRI (Kreipke et al, 1986; Schellhas et al, 1988; Otis and Aberle, 1988). MRI uses no radiation at all to generate the image. The information is obtained by placing the patient in a strong magnetic field and "capturing" a radiofrequency signal by processing hydrogen protons in various tissues and converting that signal electronically to an image on a videomonitor. The advantages of

MRI are that both hard and soft tissues can be demonstrated, and no radiation is used, so that the patient does not receive any absorbed dose of x radiation. Disadvantages include cost (although at some centers it is not much more expensive than arthrographic examination) and availability or accessibility of MR units in some locales. Despite the current cost and limitations of availability, the future of TMJ imaging appears to include both MRI and arthroscopic examination.

Clinical Features

Patients with disc displacement problems usually have significant pain during and after functional use of the joints. Eating, talking, or even yawning can be traumatic. A "clicking" joint usually indicates disc reduction—that is, the patient is able to manipulate or move his or her jaw sufficiently to enable the anteriorly displaced disc to resume its customary position atop the condyle. The patient can open to a point just before the click, frequently with pain; further opening produces the click as the disc reduces. Closure often produces the same sound, termed a reciprocal click, which may also be accompanied by pain. This abnormal function alone can produce pain, noises, and sometimes heat and swelling over the joint. In some cases, the patient acquires other signs and symptoms of an MPD problem secondary to the disc problem and concomitant protective mechanisms to minimize the pain such as abnormal deviations on opening the joint or chewing on the unaffected side. Disc displacement problems, like MPD, may be unilateral or bilateral. Often the disc problems are preceded by a traumatic event such as direct injury to the condylar area or trauma to the mandible, or even some simple event such as yawning too wide or opening abnormally. Surgery, prolonged dental treatment with wide opening, and improper splint or orthodontic therapy have also been implicated in disc displacement problems. The pain felt by the patient with displacement problems in which the disc reduces is usually less intense than the no-reduction or "closed-lock" variant.

Anterior disc displacement without reduction is manifest by severe pain with limited opening and few or no joint sounds. Because the disc does not reduce, there is no click. In these patients the disc is locked ahead of or anterior to the condyle, and opening produces severe pain, usually in the preauricular region. These patients are frequently very debilitated owing to poor nutrition because eating almost anything is too painful for many to tolerate. The intense pain may even make some patients suicidal. These patients will try any treatment offered by any clinician or medical specialist as well as any home remedy that they think may help. Treatment and evaluation of these patients must be immediate and based on a sound diagnosis.

Patients with perforations of the disc or disc attachments may or may not have symptoms. These perforations are found on arthrographic examination, during which filling of the superior joint space occurs when only the inferior has been injected. They are also identified during surgical evaluation and treatment. Loss of synovial fluid and mechanical "wear and tear" are blamed for the perforations.

Radiographic Appearance

In patients with disc displacements there are radiographic changes. Tomography of the joints demonstrates displacement of the condyle, usually posteriorly but sometimes both inferiorly and posteriorly (Fig. 11–9). Plain films do not contribute much information in these cases and should be used only to rule out gross pathologic change. A submentovertex (SMV), basilar, or occipitomental view is required to calculate the depth for the tomographic "cuts" and to determine the long axis of the condyle to correct for condylar angulation. Figures 11–10 to 11–14 show a typical series. Arthrography will outline the suspected position of the condylar disc and reveal any disc perforation. Figures 11–15 to 11–19 show typical images and outline the information obtainable. Currently, MRI is probably the most reasonable and noninvasive technique used for examination of disc displacement. The soft tissue of the disc and its attachments are revealed in a standard lateral view. Figures 11–20 to 11–23 show a typical case of anterior disc displacement with reduction. Arthroscopy and arthroscopic surgery may someday reduce the necessity for some types of plain film radiography and even tomography, because treatment such as lysis of adhesions can be rendered directly through the arthroscopic cannula. It must be remembered, however, that not all displacement disorders can be managed by arthroscopic surgery. Open surgery of the TMJ region is still required in many cases, mandating presurgical evaluation by some imaging technique.

Text continued on page 275

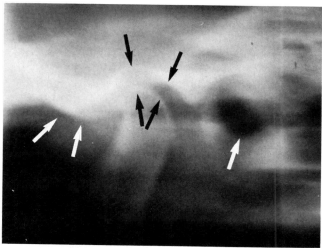

Figure 11–1. Tomographic view of mandible in closed position. *Double white arrows* represent articular eminence. *Single white arrow* represents the external audi- tory meatus. Area between *black arrows* represents "joint space."

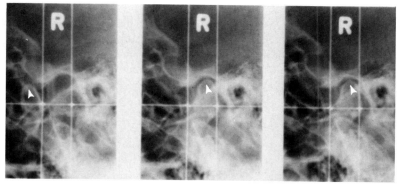

Figure 11–2. Typical transcranial image taken using the Updegrave angle board. From right to left the views represent the closed, rest, and open positions of the temporomandibular joint condyle (*arrowheads*).

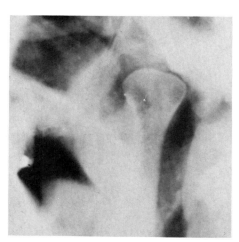

Figure 11–3. A transpharyngeal radiograph. Note how the condylar head is superimposed over the nasopharyngeal airway. There is no superimposition of osseous structures in this view.

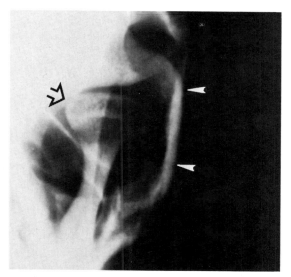

Figure 11–4. A transorbital view of the left condyle. *Open arrow* represents medial pole. *White arrowheads* delineate the orbital rim. The lateral pole of the condyle would be visible if the film were "hot-lighted."

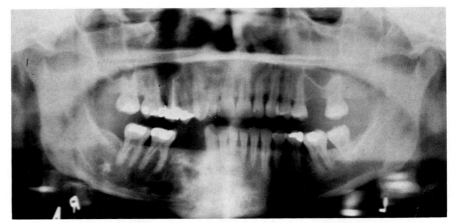

Figure 11–5. A typical panoramic image in which the gross outline of the condyles is usually well depicted.

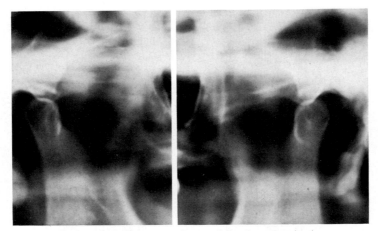

Figure 11–6. Close-ups of a specialized panoramic view of the temporomandibular joint condyles. The radiograph was taken with the patient's mouth open.

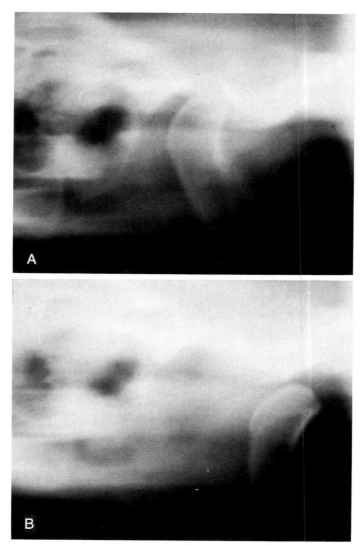

Figure 11–7. *A*, A tomographic view of the "center cut" of the temporomandibular joint condyle in the closed position. *B*, The same condyle seen following translation (full opening) in the open position.

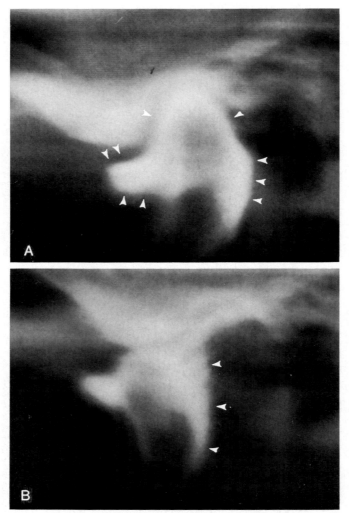

Figure 11–8. *A,* Radiographic contrast material is seen outlining the condyle as a white "shadow" (*arrowheads*). *B,* Condyle in open position outlined by contrast material. Note that more of the dye has flowed into the region posterior to the condylar head (*arrowheads*).

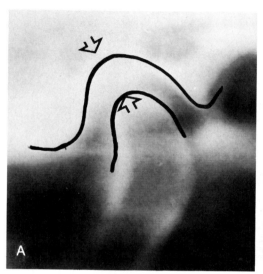

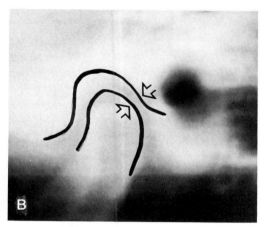

Figure 11–9. *A*, The "joint space" (*arrows*) between the condylar head and the floor of the glenoid fossa appears widened in this view. *B*, The joint space between these *arrows* appears more normal, although it may be narrowed in the posterior region.

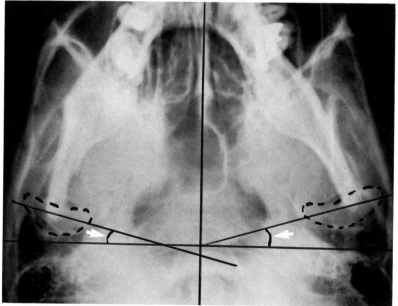

Figure 11–10. A submentovertex view is used to help determine the long axis of the condylar head. The patient's head position can be corrected by using the angles shown by the *arrowheads*.

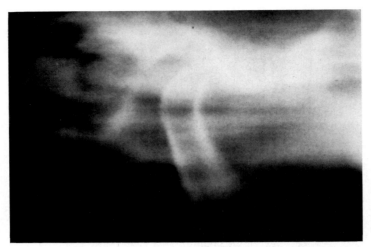

Figure 11–11. Tomograph of temporomandibular joint. Condyle seen in the closed position.

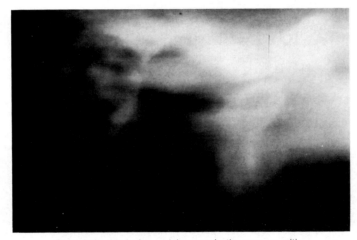

Figure 11–12. Left condyle seen in the open position.

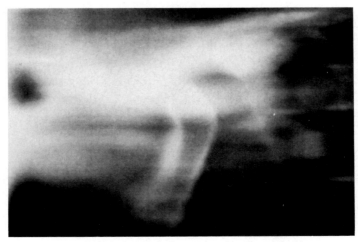

Figure 11–13. Patient's right condyle in closed position. Note the anterior displacement.

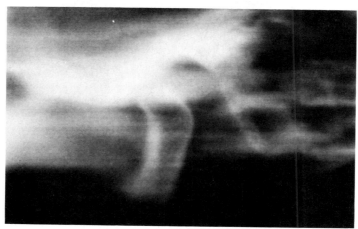

Figure 11–14. Open position of right condyle. In this case the patient could not translate from the fossa to the normal region of the articular eminence or beyond. This most likely represents a disc displacement without reduction.

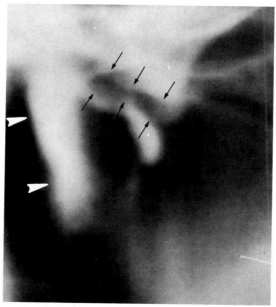

Figure 11–15. Arthrogram of the left temporomandibular joint space. *White arrowheads* represent contrast material in the posterior recess. *Black arrows* outline position of the disc over the condyle in the closed position.

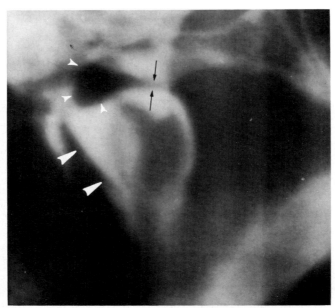

Figure 11–16. Condyle in open position. Area between *black arrows* probably represents the meniscus of the disc (the thinnest portion). *Small white arrowheads* probably represent the region of the posterior attachments of the temporomandibular joint disc. *Large white arrowheads* represent contrast material flowing into posterior recess.

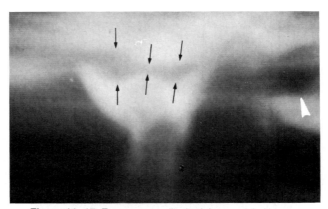

Figure 11–17. Temporomandibular joint condyle in open position. *Black arrows* outline the disc. *White arrowhead* is pointing to the external auditory meatus.

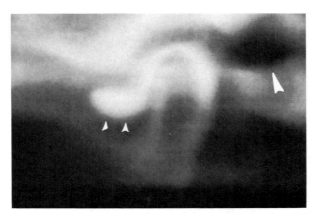

Figure 11–18. Abnormal flow of contrast material in patient with restricted opening. *Large white arrowhead* represents external auditory meatus. *Small white arrow-heads* represent pooling of the dye in the anterior tissue space due to anteriorly displaced discs.

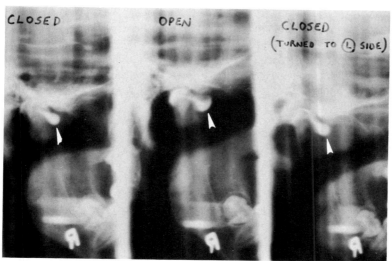

Figure 11–19. The contrast material *(arrowheads)* over the condylar head in these views was imaged using a panoramic machine. The view of the material over the condyle on the far right side represents an attempt to correct the condylar position by rotating the patient's head. (Courtesy of Dr. K. Abramovitch, Houston, Texas.)

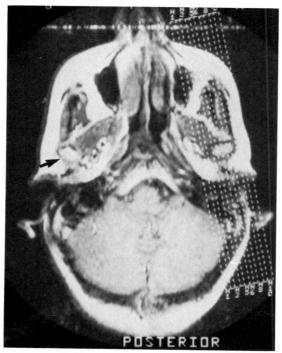

Figure 11–20. Preliminary view of magnetic resonance imaging technique for the temporomandibular joint disc. *Arrow* points to fatty marrow within the condylar head. The cortical rim of the condyle shows as a hypo-intense (black) area surrounding the marrow component.

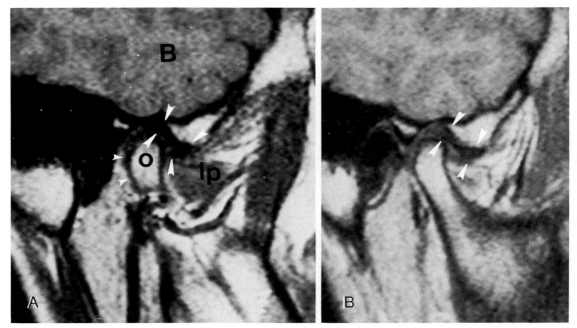

Figure 11–21. *A, Large white arrowheads* outline temporomandibular joint disc in closed position. *Black circle* represents center of condylar head. *Small white arrowheads* outline the mandibular condyle cortex, which has a low-intensity (black) signal. B = brain tissue; lp = lateral pterygoid muscle. *B, Arrowheads* outline the disc in a normal patient, taken in the closed position.

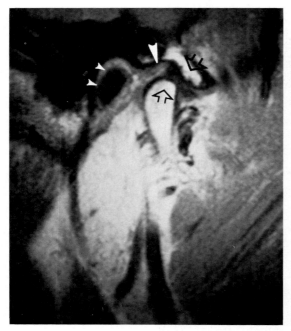

Figure 11–22. *Small open arrow* indicates the temporomandibular joint condyle. *Large open arrow* points to fatty marrow of the articular eminence. *Small white arrowheads* show the external auditory meatus, and the *large white arrowhead* shows the retrodiscal tissue attachments. This view of the temporomandibular joint complex was taken in the closed position.

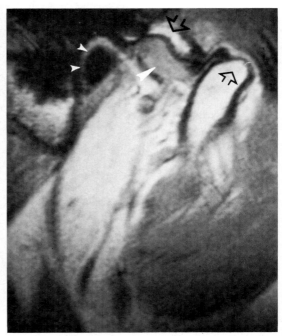

Figure 11–23. This view of the same patient reveals the condyle in an open position. Note the change in position of the structures outlined in Figure 11–22. (The *arrows* show the same features as in Fig. 11–22.)

References

Blaustein, D., and Heffez, L.: Diagnostic arthroscopy of the temporomandibular joint. Part II: Arthroscopic findings of arthrographically diagnosed disc displacements. Oral Surg., 65(2):135–141, 1988.

Kreipke, D.L., Conces, D.J., Jr., Sondhi, A., et al: Normal and abnormal tempromandibular joints as demonstrated by magnetic resonance imaging. Acta Radiol. Diagn., 27(Fase.3):331–333, 1986.

Moses, J.J., and Poker, I.D.: TMJ arthroscopic surgery: An analysis of 237 patients. J. Oral Maxillofac. Surg., 47: 790–794, 1989.

Otis, L.L., and Aberle, A.M.: An expanding technology. CDA J., 8:25–28, 1988.

Schellhas, K.P., Wilkes, C.H., Omlie, M.R., et al: The diagnosis of temporomandibular joint disease: Two-compartment arthrography and MR. Am. J. Roentgenol., 9:579–588, 1988.

RHEUMATOID ARTHRITIS

Rheumatoid arthritis is a systemic disease of unknown origin that affects women twice as often as men in 2 to 3% of the population. Although the disorder can affect any individual from infancy to old age (Zide et al, 1986), the usual age range is from 20 to 60 years. Typically, the disease begins in early adulthood (second decade of life) and can result in crippling deformity of the hands and feet. The chronic inflammatory reaction characteristic of RA occurs in the synovial membrane and results in erosion and destruction of cartilage and surrounding structures, leading to osteolytic changes in the affected joint. Although the disease sometimes goes into total remission, it frequently pursues a rapid or aggressive course causing severe crippling. RA is frequently associated with other so-called connective tissue disorders such as Reiter's syndrome, Sjögrens syndrome, SLE, PSS, and MCTD. Serologic tests such as that determining the presence of rheumatoid factor (RF) or high titers of antinuclear antibodies (ANAs), although not specific, can help the clinician determine the exact nature of the connective tissue problem. Of course, the clinical features of the disorder and the patient's history, coupled with the radiographic and serologic features, are essential to make the correct diagnosis. Consultation with an internist or rheumatologist is mandatory in the management of these patients.

Clinical Features

Early clinical signs of RA include low-grade fever, weight loss, and an elevated erythrocyte sedimentation rate (ESR). Symptoms of the initial onset may include the gelling phenomenon (morning stiffness), fatigue, and muscle soreness. Because these are nonspecific signs and symptoms, early diagnosis is difficult. Later involvement produces complaints such as articular swelling, pain, and restriction of movement of joints, muscle weakness, and contracture of muscles of the hands and feet. When the disease is full-blown (late stage), the patient may have Raynaud's phenomenon, characterized by vasospasm and paresthesia of the digits, peripheral vasoconstriction, rheumatoid nodules on the extensor surface of the ulnar aspect of the wrist, Bouchard's nodes (Fig. 11–24), and cold, clammy skin, often with pallor. The swelling and nodal involvement appear primarily in the proximal interphalangeal joints (PIP) and metacarpophalangeal joints (MCP) of the hands. Systemic lupus erythematosus is found in 20 to 25% of patients with severe RA. In contrast to DJD and psoriatic arthritis (PA), RA is both polyarticular (DJD frequently is not) and bilateral (PA is often polyarticular but asymmetric). The clinical course of RA follows one of three paths:

1. A sporadic or intermittent pattern with long periods of remission.

2. A chronic, insidious path with periodic, debilitating flares.

3. A rapid or aggressive course, sometimes with extra-articular involvement.

Radiographic Appearance

Table 11–2 outlines the early radiographic changes that may be seen by the dentist in RA. These changes are seen in approximately two-thirds of patients who have had clinical symptoms for more than 3 months, and in 85% of those who have had signs and symptoms for more than 6 months. Obviously, some of these changes may not be as discernible in the TMJ region as they would in the PIP or MCP joints. Erosions on the superior surface of the condylar head may be the earliest radiographically

Table 11–2. EARLY RADIOGRAPHIC CHANGES IN RHEUMATOID ARTHRITIS

Periarticular soft tissue swelling
Pseudocysts in bones
Osteolysis of adjacent bones
Periosteal elevation
Widened (or narrowed) joint space
Subluxations
Erosions of articular bone

detectable change on plain films (Fig. 11–25). However, the clinician should consider taking or ordering a correlational hand film if the index of suspicion of TMJ involvement is high. The small joints of the hands are the first to become involved (Fig. 11–26). TMJ changes may not be evident radiographically until later in the course of the disease. Recently, investigators have been searching for more subtle condylar and disc changes using more advanced imaging method such as arthrography, arthrotomography, CT, and MRI. Perhaps TMJ involvement has been grossly underestimated in the past because most radiography such as transcranial, transpharyngeal, and even panoramic techniques demonstrates only a small portion of the articular surface of the condyle. At the very least, tomography of the TMJ region should be ordered if early rheumatic involvement of that joint is suspected.

Later radiographic changes of RA are much easier to detect. The cortices of the marginal bones are thinned or eroded, and recurrences usually produce a periosteal reaction leading to a thickened cortex termed subchondral sclerosis. The margins may become quite irregular in appearance, and in late stages there can be gross reduction of the size and shape of the bone (Figs. 11–27 and, 11–28). In the TMJ region the condylar head is often reduced in size and loses its round or ovoid outline. As the destruction continues, the neck of the condyle also appears shorter. Various muscles of mastication pull the mandible superiorly and posteriorly and may result in a progressive anterior open bite, which is also seen clinically. Nickerson and Moystad (1983) have outlined the radiographic information that can be found with several radiographic techniques including arthrography.

Histopathologic Findings

One of the first reports of the histopathologic changes observed in the TMJ in patients with RA was published by Blackwood (1963). Nowadays, problems of the TMJ rarely involve condylectomies, and thus, tissue changes are not routinely observed and reported by oral pathologists. From Blackwood's article it appears that the initial changes begin in the synovial tissues of the lower joint compartment. The joint capsule is invaded by a dense lymphocytic infiltrate along with vascular granulation tissue (pannus), which results in small adhesions and eventually in destruction of the articulating surface. Resorption of the subarticular bone ensues and, if not arrested, leads to gross bony remodeling of the surface. In the most advanced stages a fibrous ankylosis may occur. These histopathologic changes—articular erosions, periarticular deossification, and subchondral bone destruction—may be the first changes to be detected radiographically, but by this stage the symptoms have often abated, the pain and swelling having occurred months earlier. Recently, it has been demonstrated that arthrography reveals very early changes in the rheumatoid arthritic patient, suggesting that plain films might underestimate the presence of the disease and that earlier radiographic detection of subtle changes might be enhanced by arthrographic examination of the TMJ (Larheim and Bjørnland, 1989).

Treatment

Nonsurgical treatment of RA in patients with TMJ involvement is no different than that given for RA other joints. Symptomatic patients who have intermittent flares of the disease or chronic low-grade involvement are given aspirin (ASA) or other nonsteroidal anti-inflammatory drugs (NSAIDs) for relief of pain and swelling. If gastric complaints or tinnitus accompany ASA therapy, NSAIDs are implemented. Patients who are unresponsive to these agents may be placed on systemic steroid therapy or may be given steroid injections into the involved joints. Other chemical agents used to produce remittance of the disease include hydrochlorquinone, D-penicillamine, and injectable gold salts. Some chemotherapeutic agents such as methotrexate have been used effectively in patients with rapidly progressing RA.

Surgical treatment of the joints of the hands and feet involves reconstruction of the joints with various metals and other implant materials. A good review of the surgical treatment that is available specifically for the TMJ region has been reported by Kent et al (1986). They have also classified the various TMJ involvements of patients so afflicted in an attempt to suggest the most suitable recommended treatment in each instance.

References

Blackwood, M.J.J.: Arthritis of the mandibular joint. Br. Dent. J., 115(8):317–326, 1963.

Kent, J.N., Carlton, D.M., and Zide, M.F.: Rheumatoid disease and related arthropathies. II. Surgical rehabilitation of the temporomandibular joint. Oral Surg., 61(5):423–439, 1986.

Larheim, T.A., and Bjørnland, T.: Arthrographic findings in the temporomandibular joint in patients with rheumatic disease. J. Oral Maxillofac. Surg., 47(8):780–784, 1989.

Nickerson, J.W., Jr., and Moystad, A.: Observations on individuals with radiographic bilateral condylar remodelling. J. Craniomandib. Pract., 1(1):20–37, 1983.

Zide, M.F., Carlton, D.M., Kent, J.M.: Rheumatoid disease and related arthropathies. I. Systemic findings, medical therapy, and peripheral joint surgery. Oral Surg., 61(2):119–125, 1986.

DEGENERATIVE JOINT DISEASE
(Osteoarthritis)

Degenerative joint disease (DJD) is the most common disorder affecting the TMJ. It is a disease of articular cartilage and subchondral bone. Unlike RA, DJD often affects only one of the TMJs; that is, it is primarily a unilateral problem. Mechanical wear and tear of one or both joints because of senescence (aging), trauma, or some other degrading process leads to destruction of the articular hyalin cartilage independent of systemic disease or infection. Cartilage over the condylar surface becomes disorganized and deteriorates with age. It responds by stimulating osseous remodeling of the condyle accordingly. Changes in environment, nutrition, or functional activity occur throughout life and can secondarily affect the TMJ cartilage. It should be pointed out, however, that unlike other disorders of the TMJs, DJD can produce grossly remodeled or deformed-looking condyles that are totally free of associated symptoms (Fig. 11–29). Stress trauma, previous infections, endocrine imbalance, or changes in vertical dimension can initiate DJD of the TMJ. DJD begins as the superficial layers of cartilage split along the the fibrillatory planes, a process called fibrillation. There is a subsequent vascular response in which vessels grow into the subchondral bone. This increased vascularity initiates ossification in the form of new osteophytic bone. The new bone is eventually remodeled by persistent wear and tear until it appears sclerotic or flattened.

Clinical Features

Although young individuals may have DJD, it is much more common in adults in the fifth decade of life or older, and its incidence progresses with age. Unlike RA, degenerative joint changes of the hands usually involve the terminal or distal interphalangeal joints (TIP or DIP); clinically, the individual has swellings in those joints termed Heberden's nodes. Joint pain may be present but often is not severe. The patient complains of pain elsewhere such as the knee, hip, or lower spine—that is, the larger weight-bearing joints. The incidence of DJD is greater in women than in men. All involved joints, including the TMJs, may become stiff with inactivity. Pain, swelling, and tenderness may be present over the joint area. The pain is diffuse and feels like a dull ache. Joint sounds are primarily grating or grinding sounds known as crepitus. Loss of synovial fluid and joint remodeling so that "bone works against bone" lead to these sounds. Kreutziger and Mahan (1975ab) have reviewed the clinical changes that occur in DJD involvement of the TMJ quite thoroughly. Patients often are already taking anti-inflammatory medications such as aspirin and other nonsteroidal agents at their initial evaluation for joint pain elsewhere. Despite the gross remodeling and bone proliferation that occur in DJD, it is rarely debilitating like RA or psoriatic arthritis.

Radiographic Appearance

One of the best reviews of the radiographic changes associated with DJD of the TMJs was written by Worth in 1974. Although he noted that Blackwood (1963) described the earliest changes of DJD of the TMJ on the posterior aspect of the condyle, Worth asserted that the superior and anterior surfaces of the condyle are the best locations in which to observe the changes radiologically. The curved condylar head becomes flattened or faceted, often with a concomitant thickening of the cortex (Fig. 11–30). The new bone laid down and observed radiographically is termed subchondral sclerosis. It may be localized on the surface or may cover the entire condylar head. In addition, cyst-like cavities (pseudocysts) may be seen just below the articular surface. Erosions of the joint surface may also be present. Gross deformity of the entire condylar head is not uncommon in advanced cases of DJD. Another hallmark of DJD is the formation of osteophytes or spurs that extend from the periphery of the condylar head. Osteophytes are usually seen on the anterior aspect of the condyle and may give rise to a "bird's beak" appearance (Fig. 11–32). Again, as in RA, a correlational hand film may be warranted in some patients to confirm the presence of degenerative joint changes.

Histopathologic Findings

At birth the entire TMJ complex is surrounded by a synovial membrane. With aging and function most of this membrane is lost except for that on the inner aspect of the capsule. With abnormal function, trauma, or other problems the loose vascular synovial tissue undergoes degenerative changes. Remodeling of the condylar surface is a normal physiologic process. However, regressive remodeling due to stresses beyond normal physiologic function results in fibrillation—splitting of the articular cartilage, vascular proliferation (granulation tissue), and osteoblastic activity with sclerosis of the subchondral bone and subsequent morphologic changes. Cartilaginous cells undergo necrosis, and fibrous connective tissue proliferates in an attempt to maintain a regular articular surface. Osteoclastic activity also occurs, resulting in the pseudocysts of the bone that are observed radiographically. These changes may elicit an inflammatory response in the joint compartment in which chronic lymphocytic and plasma cell infiltrates are seen. Because surgical intervention is very rare in patients with most of the arthritides, there is little demand for histopathologic interpretation of the changes.

Treatment

Nonsurgical treatment of DJD usually involves physiotherapy and nonsteroidal anti-inflammatory medications. Patients rarely have pain severe enough to warrant steroid injections or surgical intervention. Jaw exercises and restoration of occlusion and the lost vertical dimension will reduce the symptoms in many instances. Concomitant use of analgesics and anti-inflammatory medications is a useful adjunct in controlling the patient's complaints. Condylectomies are rarely performed today and are probably contraindicated.

References

Edeiken, J: Roentgen Diagnosis of Disease of Bone, 3rd ed., Vol. 1. Baltimore: Williams & Wilkins, 1983, pp. 1983, 608–622.

Kreutziger, K.L., and Mahan, P.E.: Temporomandibular degenerative joint disease, Part I. Anatomy, pathophysiology, and clinical description. Oral Surg., 40(2):165–182, 1975a.

Kreutziger, K.L., and Mahan, P.E.: Temporomandibular degenerative joint disease, Part II. Diagnostic procedure and comprehensive management. Oral Surg., 40(3): 297–319, 1975b.

Worth, H.M.: Temporomandibular joint—Function and dysfunction, II. Oral Sci. Rev., 6:3–51, 1974.

OTHER ARTHRITIDES

SJÖGREN'S SYNDROME

Sjögren's syndrome (SS) is characterized by a triad of clinical problems termed the sicca syndrome that include (1) dry eyes (xerophthalmia) and (2) dry mouth (xerostomia). Because the vaginal and oral mucosa are similar, the patient may also have associated (3) vaginal dryness and related yeast (usually candidal) infections. Xerophthalmia produces a condition termed keratoconjunctivitis sicca in which the corneal epithelium is desiccated and sloughs. The diagnostic criteria for SS include keratoconjunctivitis sicca, a labial minor salivary lip gland biopsy with a lymphocytic inflammatory infiltrate, and a related connective tissue or lymphoproliferative disorder. Salivary scintigraphy (radionuclide scan) is also helpful in determining gland function, especially of the parotid and submandibular glands. The most commonly associated (50%) connective tissue disorder is RA.

The RA changes associated with SS are those identified earlier in the chapter. Early erosive changes in the axial skeleton include involvement of the PIP and MCP joints, especially on the radial aspects of the fingers, and similar manifestations on the toes. The TMJs of these patients must be carefully evaluated by several radiographic modalities in order not to underestimate possible arthritic changes. Treatment of these patients with splints or reconstructive procedures may accelerate the RA changes if the procedures are incorrectly employed. Figure 11–34 reveals the consequences of failure to diagnose early RA changes.

PROGRESSIVE SYSTEMIC SCLEROSIS

Formerly termed scleroderma, PSS is another connective tissue disorder in which joint changes do occur. Interestingly enough, the TMJ region is one of the few joints to be involved. However, the changes that become manifest in that region are secondary to extreme muscle pull due to fibrosis and calcification of the muscles themselves. Figure 11–35 reveals an extreme case of condylar and mandibular remodeling resulting from this phenomenon. The hand changes in this disorder are sclerodactyly (spider fingers) and dissolution of the terminal tufts of the distal phalanges. Other clinical features are best summarized by the **CREST** syndrome (a variant of PSS):

C—Calcinosis of the subcutaneous skin.
R—Raynaud's phenomenon—vasospasm and pain of the extremities.
E—Esophageal dysfunction, manifested as dysphagia, esophagitis, or gastric reflux.
S—Sclerodactyly.
T—Telangiectasia—increased surface vascularity of the fingers, lips, hands, and face.

Besides the extensive gastrointestinal involvement, fibrosis of the various organ systems can eventually lead to renal problems, resulting in hypertension, renal failure, and death. Other clinical signs in patients with PSS include taut, shiny skin, especially of the molar region and forehead, and loss of skin folds and creases. Dentally, there is often a generalized widening of the periodontal ligament spaces of the teeth, especially in the anterior segments (Fig. 11–36).

SYSTEMIC LUPUS ERYTHEMATOSUS

SLE is an inflammatory disease that is both acute and chronic. It affects primarily women, involves multiple organ systems, and has a wide array of clinical signs and symptoms. The course can be insidious, presenting sometimes with a single problem, or it can be rapidly progressive and debilitating. Arthritic involvement is polyarticular as in RA but is not deforming. The hands and wrists as well as the small joints of the feet are often involved, thus mimicking changes seen in RA.

A myositis presenting with morning stiffness is often present. Raynaud's phenomenon is present in approximately one-third of afflicted patients. Intraorally, large, asymptomatic ulcers are often present. To date, there has been no published report of SLE arthritic involve-

ment of the TMJs. However, SLE can coexist with PSS, Sjögren's syndrome, and polymyositis in a disorder now termed mixed connective tissue disorder (MCTD) or overlap syndrome. Therefore, the clinician must be aware of possible TMJ involvement because of the RA associated with SS patients and the potential changes of mandibular bone seen in PSS.

MIXED CONNECTIVE TISSUE DISEASE

MCTD, or overlap syndrome, is characterized by the same signs and symptoms seen in SLE, PSS, SS, or polymyositis (Kelley et al, 1985). Table 11–3 describes the most common features. Figs. 11–37 to 11–39 demonstrate some of the clinical and radiographic features necessary to confirm the diagnosis (Lovas and Miles, 1984).

REITER'S SYNDROME

This syndrome consists of conjunctivitis, urethritis, mucocutaneous lesions, and arthritis, either together or in various combinations. The arthritic changes are polyarticular but asymmetric, unlike those seen in RA. However, the syndrome is almost exclusively found in men between 20 and 30 years old. Joints involved include the knees, ankles, and digits of the feet and hands.

Table 11–3. MIXED CONNECTIVE TISSUE DISEASE

Disorder	Clinical Features
Progressive systemic sclerosis	Esophageal dysfunction Raynaud's phenomenon Sclerodactyly Telangiectasia Calcinosis cutis
Rheumatoid arthritis	Swelling of joints Ulnar deviation MCP, PIP involvement Subcutaneous nodules
Polymyositis	Fever, flu-like symptoms Myalgia Muscle weakness
Systemic lupus erythematosus	Sicca syndrome Pericarditis Malar rash Discoid lupus erythematosus Skin ulceration Buccal mucous ulceration Anemia

The oral lesions may appear like those of recurrent aphthous stomatitis, or they may be painless, elevated lesions, often with a granular surface (Shafer et al, 1974). Lesions on the tongue may look like geographic tongue, and similar lesions on the glans penis have been termed circinate balanitis. Arthritic changes of the TMJs would be like those seen in RA but have rarely been reported. The onset of this syndrome frequently follows exposure to a venereal disease, especially urethritis with a chlamydial organism. There is no direct evidence for *Chlamydia* as the etiologic agent; however, chlamydial infections are by far the most common sexually transmitted disease seen today.

PSORIATIC ARTHRITIS

Psoriatic arthritis (PA) is a rare disorder of the TMJ. To date only 28 cases have been reported (Miles et al, 1990). Table 11–4 outlines the "typical" features of the cases reporting TMJ involvement.

PA affects only 5 to 7% of patients with the skin disorder. The joint involvement of affected individuals is polyarticular but can be either asymmetric or symmetric. About 25% of patients with PA have bilateral disease in both the terminal interphalangeal joints and the proximal interphalangeal joints of both hands and both feet. The arthritic damage in

PA can be severely destructive and deforming (Fig. 11–40). Bone resorption, osteolysis, erosions, subluxations, and subchondral cysts may all be present in the affected joints. Most cases of PA of the TMJ have demonstrated erosive changes like those seen in RA. However, several others have produced a florid proliferative osteophytic response in longstanding cases. Clinically, the patient may manifest pitting of the nail beds and "telescoping" fingers termed "doigt en lorguette" (Fig. 11–41).

References

Kelley, W.N., Harris, E.D., Jr., Reiddy, S., and Sledge, C.B.: Textbook of Rheumatology, 2nd ed, Vol. 2. Philadelphia: W.B. Saunders, 1985, pp. 1116–1136.

Lovas, J.G.L., and Miles, D.A.: Abstract: A Case of Lichen Planus/Lupus Erythematosis Overlap in Mixed Connective Tissue Disease. Toronto: American Academy of Oral Pathology, 1986.

Miles, D.A., and Kaugars, G.E.: Psoriatric involvement of the temporomandibular joint: Literature review and report of case (in press 1990).

Shafer, W.G., Hine, M.K., and Levy, B.M.: A Textbook of Oral Pathology, 4th ed. Philadelphia: W.B. Saunders, 1983, pp. 761–763.

GOUT

Gout is a metabolic disorder described as a crystal-induced arthritis. Uric acid crystals

Table 11–4. PSORIATIC INVOLVEMENT OF THE TEMPOROMANDIBULAR JOINT

Author	Age	Race	Sex	Rheumatoid Factor	Unilateral or Bilateral	Ankylosis	Osteolytic/ Osteoblastic	Other Joint Involvement	Skin or Nail Lesions
Franks 1965	40	NS	F	—	Unilateral	Negative	Osteolytic	Feet	Both
Lundberg and Ericsson 1967	17–64	NS	3F 8M	— —	NS NS	NS	17/22—lytic 1/11—blastic	Hands, feet	Both
Blair 1976	28–66	NS	4F 3M	— —	NS NS	NS	2/7—E† 2/7—F† 1/7—O† 1/7—blastic	NS NS NS NS	NS NS NS NS
Lowry 1975	37	C	M	—	Unilateral	Negative	Osteolytic	Hands, feet	Skin
Sanders and Halliday 1979	39	C	M	NS	Bilateral	Positive	Osteoblastic	Spine, hands, feet, hips, knees, shoulders	Both
Rasmussen and Bakke 1982	36	C	M	NS	Unilateral	Positive	Osteoblastic	Spine, knees	Both
	33	C	M	NS	Unilateral	Negative	Osteolytic	Feet	Skin
	24	C	F	NS	Unilateral	Negative	Osteolytic	NS	Skin
	52	C	F	NS	Unilateral*	Negative	None	None	Skin
Larheim and Bjørnland 1989	38	NS	F	NS	Unilateral	NS	Osteolytic	NS	NS
	NS	NS	NS	NS	NS	NS	Osteolytic	NS	NS
Miles and Kaugars 1990	51	C	M	—	Bilateral	Positive	Osteoblastic	Feet, hands, shoulder	Both

Note: Although not specified, the patients are assumed to be Caucasian.
NS = not specified; C = Caucasian.
*The diagnosis was made of psoriatic arthropathy, although no radiographic findings were present.
†E = erosive; F = flattening; O = osteoporosis: All were interpreted in this table as osteolytic.

(monosodium urate) accumulate in tissues such as cartilage or synovial membrane owing to increased production or decreased excretion of uric acid. There is a male predilection.

Gout or gouty arthritis is rare in people under 40 years of age. The underlying cause of primary gout is a defect in purine metabolism. Enzyme defects, blood dyscrasias, multiple myeloma, leukemia, drugs, hyperparathyroidism, and chronic renal insufficiency can lead to secondary gout.

Clinical Features

Onset of gout is often heralded by involvement in a single joint that is acutely painful at night. The joint is frequently tender and swollen, and the skin overlying the joint is warm and dry. Recovery may occur in a few days, and the patient may remain asymptomatic for years following the initial episode. Later episodes tend to involve multiple joints, and pain is less severe but frequently chronic. The small joints of the hands, feet, and wrist are often involved. However, weight-bearing joints such as the knees, hips, shoulders, and spine are affected only occasionally (Gross et al, 1987). TMJ involvement is rare but does occur (Gross et al, 1987; Kleinman and Ewbank, 1969; Fluur et al, 1974).

Pseudogout, also termed calcium pyrophosphate dihydrate arthropathy (CPPD disease), has been described as a separate disorder resembling gout but with a predilection for the knees (DeVos et al, 1981).

Radiographic Appearance

The changes described by various authors include "exostoses" and "spurs" of the condylar head and "condylar remodeling." Three cases reported by Kleinman and Ewbank did not detail any radiographic changes of the TMJ complex. Pseudogout (CPPD) in the literature has been described as a "mass" between the articular eminence and "the leading edge of the left condyle." It is obvious that additional reporting of gouty arthritis of the TMJ will be required before the "typical" radiographic changes can be determined.

Histopathologic Findings

Only the gross histopathologic features of gout of the TMJ have been described. Gross and colleagues (1987) reported severe "osteo-degenerative" changes of the articular cortex with "multiple intracapsular tophi and bizarre exostoses radiating from the cortical surface." Kleinman and Ewbank (1969) described no gross microscopic histopathologic findings in their three cases.

Treatment

Relief of pain caused by gout has been achieved by treatment with colchicine and/or probenecid (Benemid). Local injections of steroids into symptomatic joints may also be helpful.

Diagnosis of gout may be easily made by performing laboratory tests for uric acid concentration. If a patient has a history of gout or clinical features of the disorder such as a tophus of the large toe or other joints, it may be useful to confirm the presence of the disorder by laboratory tests and to use a gout medication as a therapeutic trial to evaluate the effect on suspected TMJ involvement. Consultation with the patient's physician or a rheumatologist would be appropriate in the management of the patient's disease.

References

DeVos, R.A.I., Brants, J., Kusen, G.J. and Becker, A.E.: Calcium pyrophosphate dihydrate arthropathy of the temporomandibular joint. Oral Surg., 5:497–502, 1981.

Fluur, E., Haverling, M., Molin, C.: Gout in the temporomandibular joint: Report on a case. ORL 36:16–20, 1974.

Gross, B.D., Williams, R.B., DiCosimo, C.J., and Williams, S.V.: Gout and pseudogout of the temporomandibular joint. Oral Surg. Oral Med. Oral Pathol., 63:551–554, 1987.

Kleinman, H.Z., and Ewbank, R.L.: Gout of the temporomandibular joint: report of three cases. Oral Surg. Oral Med. Oral Pathol., 2:281–282, 1969.

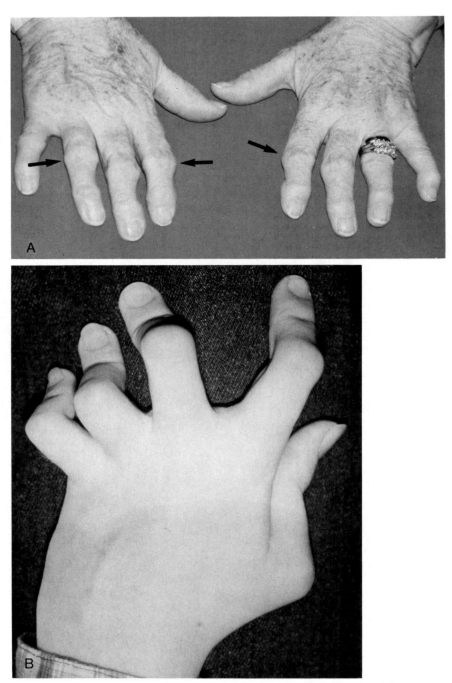

Figure 11–24. *A, Arrows* outline several Bouchard's nodes. This elderly patient had longstanding but mild rheumatoid arthritis. *B,* Joint disfiguration seen in a young patient with juvenile rheumatoid arthritis.

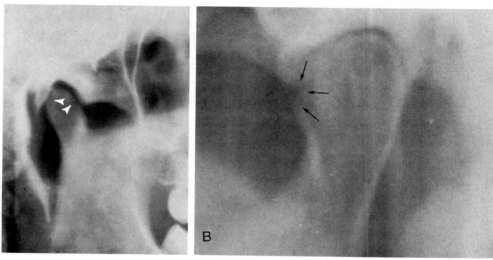

Figure 11–25. *A, Arrowheads* outline small erosions in the articular cortex of the temporomandibular joint con-dyle. *B,* A magnified view of an erosion (*arrows*) involving the articular cortex in a patient with rheumatoid arthritis.

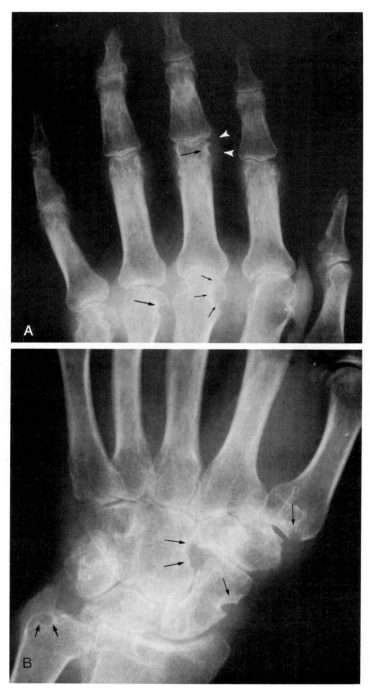

Figure 11–26. *A*, Cortical erosions (*arrows*) on the proximal phalanges and metacarpals in the hands of a patient with rheumatoid arthritis. *White arrowheads* show soft tissue swelling. *B*, More destructive changes (*long arrows*) involving the articular cortices of the carpal and metacarpal bones. *Short arrows* in the lower left represent an erosion and possible disarticulation of the ulnar styloid.

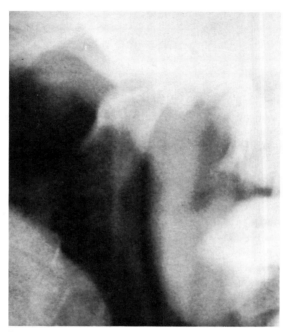

Figure 11–27. Gross destruction of the condylar head in a patient with longstanding rheumatoid arthritis.

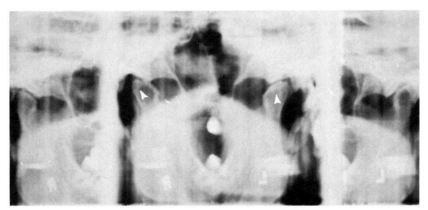

Figure 11–28. Specialized panoramic view in closed and open positions of a patient with longstanding rheumatoid arthritis now arrested. Note the thickened cortical outline *(arrowheads)* termed subchondral sclerosis. These articular changes are also seen in degenerative joint disease; however, they are rarely bilateral.

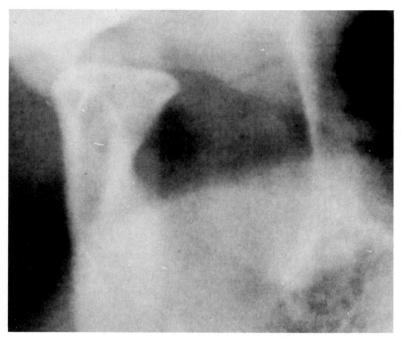

Figure 11–29. Flattening and gross remodeling of the left condylar head of a patient with degenerative joint disease.

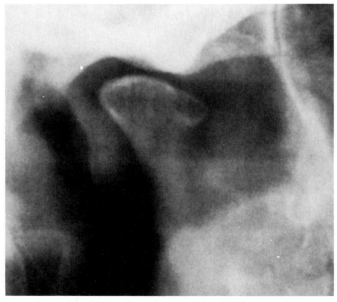

Figure 11–30. Another misshapen condyle in an asymptomatic patient with degenerative joint disease.

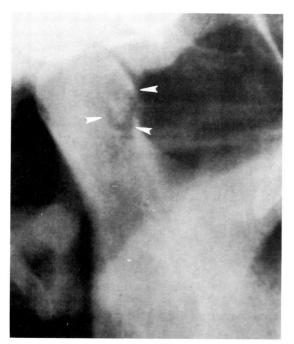

Figure 11–31. *Arrowheads* outline a possible pseudocyst in the anterior region of the condylar head. This region would have to be differentiated from the normal anterior concavity or recess.

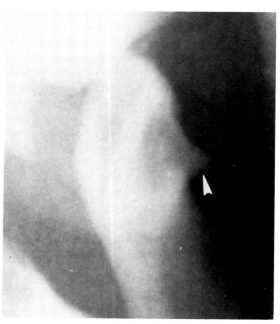

Figure 11–32. Osteophyte on condyle *(arrowhead)* of patient with degenerative joint disease. Note the appearance of a bird's beak.

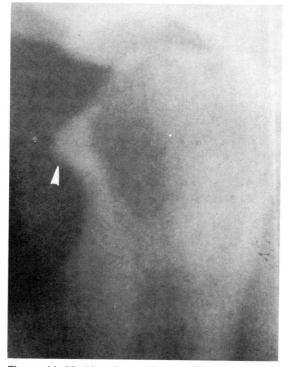

Figure 11–33. Magnified view of another bird's beak *(arrowhead)*.

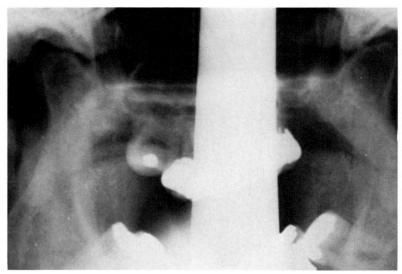

Figure 11–34. Specialized panoramic view of gross structural changes of the temporomandibular joint con- dyles. Note the subchondral sclerosis and flattening of the condylar surfaces.

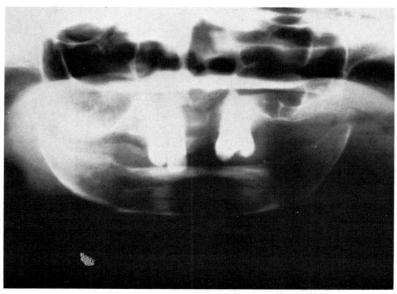

Figure 11–35. Severe osteolysis in a patient with scle- roderma. (Courtesy of Dr. R. P. Langlais, San Antonio.)

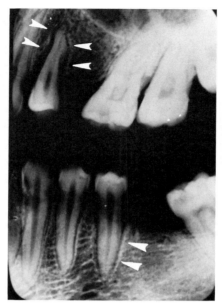

Figure 11–36. *Arrowheads* outline several widened PDL spaces seen in scleroderma.

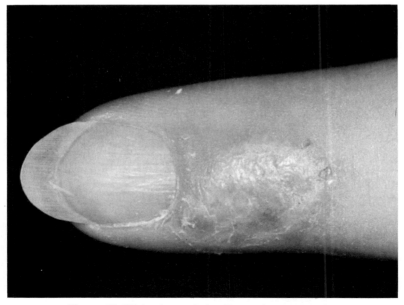

Figure 11–37. Lesion on index finger of young woman with suspected mixed connective tissue disease. The lesion is suggestive of systemic lupus erythematosus.

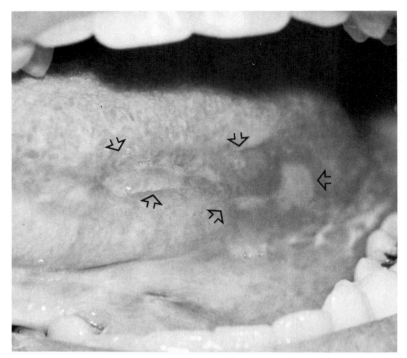

Figure 11–38. An oral lesion (*arrows*) in the same patient as in Figure 11–37, suggestive of systemic lupus erythematosus.

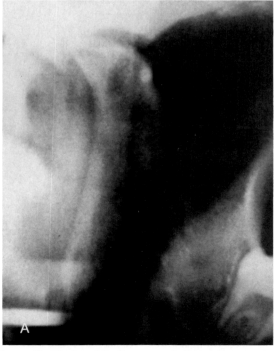

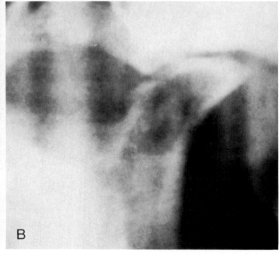

Figure 11–39. *A* and *B*, Gross morphologic changes of the temporomandibular joints bilaterally in a young woman with mixed connective tissue disease. These lesions represent longstanding rheumatoid arthritic changes.

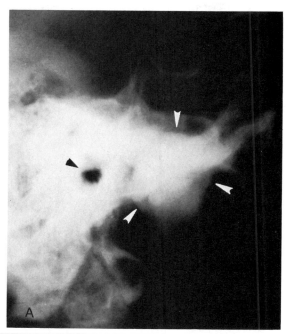

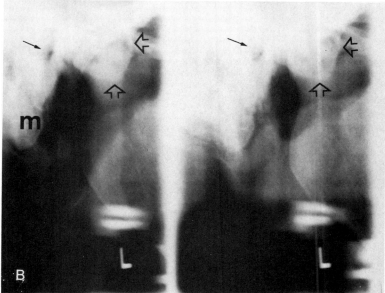

Figure 11–40. *A,* Lateral view of gross proliferative changes in a patient with psoriasis (psoriatic arthritis). Black *arrowhead* points to patient's external auditory meatus. *White arrowheads* outline gross condylar changes. *B,* Specialized panoramic view of the same patient. Note gross condylar changes and lack of translation. *Open arrows* point to condyle, *closed arrows* point to external auditory meatus. Region labeled m is the mastoid air cell area.

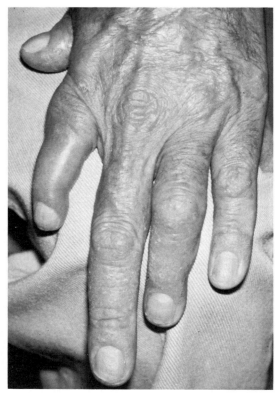

Figure 11–41. Pitting of the nail-bed and "telescoping" of the ring and middle fingers in a patient with psoriasis with joint involvement.

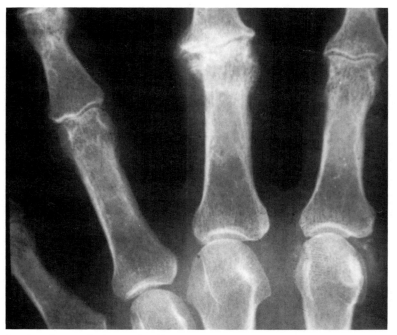

Figure 11–42. Destructive changes in the proximal interphalangeal joint region of the middle finger of a patient with gout. Note the loss of joint space and proliferative "osteoblastic" changes. This patient did not have similar changes in the temporomandibular joint region at this time.

DENTAL ANOMALIES AND INHERITABLE DISORDERS AFFECTING TEETH

G. KAUGARS

DENTAL ANOMALIES

Considering that 52 tooth buds undergo a complex sequence of maturation and growth in close proximity to each other, it is not surprising that anomalies do occur. Although most of the anomalies in this chapter are innocuous clinical findings that may simply stimulate curiosity about tooth development, there are two exceptions. Dens-in-dente usually requires prophylactic restoration, and patients with taurodontic teeth need to be evaluated for the presence of a syndrome. Surprisingly little research has been done in the area of dental anomalies. This explains the paucity of information available concerning incidence, the vague definitions, and the general lack of understanding of the etiology of these entities.

GEMINATION

The terms gemination and twinning are closely related to each other. They imply either partial cleavage (gemination) or complete cleavage (twinning) of a single tooth bud. Clinically, **gemination** produces **a large clinical crown**, whereas **twinning** results in the **formation of two separate teeth**. Numerous descriptive and imaginative synonyms have been used to describe this process; however, gemination and twinning are the most widely accepted terms. Although the cause is unknown, it seems reasonable to assume that twinning is a more severe form of gemination.

Clinical Features

The primary dentition is involved more frequently than the permanent dentition. The clinical crown of a geminated tooth is quite large. It may be difficult if not impossible to distinguish clinically between gemination and fusion because both produce a large tooth. Twinning gives rise to two similar but separate teeth which are indistinguishable from a normal tooth and an adjacent supernumerary tooth. One helpful distinction is that most supernumeraries occur in the permanent dentition and are either mesiodens or maxillary fourth molars (paramolars, distodens).

Radiographic Appearance

Gemination is characterized by a tooth with an enlarged pulp chamber, which may be partially divided, and the presence of only one root. The single enlarged pulp chamber helps differentiate gemination from fusion between a normal tooth and a supernumerary because the supernumerary usually has two pulp chambers.

Treatment

Geminated teeth are unattractive, predisposed to caries, contribute to malocclusion, and are associated with periodontal disease. If possible, the redundant tooth structure should be shaped to approximate a normal tooth, or extraction should be considered.

Reference

Goaz, P.W., and White, S.C.: Oral Radiology: Principles and Interpretation, 2nd ed. St. Louis: C.V. Mosby, 1987, pp. 431–432.

Grover, P.S., and Lorton, L.: Gemination and twinning in the permanent dentition. Oral Surg. Oral Med. Oral Pathol., 59:313–318, 1985.
Tannenbaum, K.A., and Alling, E.E.: Anomalous tooth development: Case reports of gemination and twinning. Oral Surg. Oral Med. Oral Pathol., 16:883–887, 1963.

FUSION

Several theories have been proposed to explain why two separate tooth buds might fuse and develop as a single tooth, but none have been wholly satisfactory. It is attractive to speculate that a physical force pushes two buds together, but it is difficult to identify the origin of the force. Fusion is possible either between two normal teeth or between a normal tooth and a supernumerary.

Clinical Features

In one large study (3557 children) fusion occurred in 0.5% of the patients. The primary dentition is affected more often than the permanent, and anterior teeth are involved more frequently than posterior ones. There is usually an incisal groove oriented in a buccal-lingual direction. This groove may be deep enough to give the clinical crown a bifid appearance.

One method of diagnosing fusion is to consider the fused structure as two teeth and count the remaining teeth. If a normal number is present, the diagnosis is probably fusion. If the count exceeds the normal number of teeth, the diagnosis may be either gemination or fusion between a normal and a supernumerary tooth. Fused teeth can cause obvious cosmetic or periodontal problems. Paradoxically, fusion can cause a loss of space (fusion of two normal teeth) or a lack of space (fusion of a normal and a supernumerary tooth).

Radiographic Appearance

Fused teeth may have a single common pulp chamber or two separate ones. However, there is always a common area of dentin.

Treatment

Extraction should be considered for fused primary teeth. The need for endodontic treatment should be evaluated prior to reshaping any permanent tooth. However, as with many innocuous conditions, the dentist should ascertain the long-range benefits of definitive treatment compared with simply emphasizing good oral hygiene.

References

Clayton, J.M.: Congenital dental anomalies occurring in 3557 children. J. Dent. Child., 23:206–208, 1956.

Goaz, P.W., and White, S.C.: Oral Radiology: Principles and Interpretation, 2nd ed. St. Louis: C.V. Mosby, 1987, pp. 429–430.

Mader, C.L.: Fusion of teeth. J. Am. Dent. Assoc., 98:62–64, 1979.

CONCRESCENCE

Concrescence occurs when two or more teeth are united only by cementum. Although concrescence is generally accepted as being a mild type of fusion, there are some differences between the two conditions. Crowding of teeth and trauma have both been suggested as causative factors, but neither has been proved.

Clinical Features

Concrescence can occur before or after eruption and most commonly affects the permanent maxillary molars. The clinical crowns of the involved teeth appear normal.

Radiographic Appearance

It is hard to differentiate between roots that are very close to each other and true concrescence. Multiple radiographs taken from different angles may be necessary if concrescence is suspected.

Treatment

Extractions of concrescent teeth pose a problem because the unanticipated removal of an additional tooth may be necessary and, in the case of maxillary molars, a portion of the maxillary tuberosity may be involved. Sectioning of the involved teeth should be considered to avoid these potential complications.

References

Goaz, P.W., and White, S.C.: Oral Radiology: Principles and Interpretation, 2nd ed. St. Louis: C.V. Mosby, 1987, pp. 430–431.

Shafer, W.G., Hine, M.K., and Levy, B.M.: A Textbook of Oral Pathology, 4th ed. Philadelphia: W. B. Saunders, 1983, pp. 39–40.

DILACERATION

The diagnosis of dilaceration is typically applied to any tooth that gives radiographically a subjective impression of excessive root angulation. Many teeth have a mild amount of curvature, but there is no clear-cut definition as to when this curvature becomes dilaceration. This subjectivity has hindered epidemiologic studies because of the vagueness of the diagnostic criteria. Trauma has been proposed as a cause of dilaceration, but it is unlikely that this is a factor in all cases. A high incidence of traumatically induced enamel defects has not been reported in dilacerated teeth, and one case has even been discovered in a 6-month-old fetus. Lack of arch space and subsequent difficulty of eruption in the normal expected path of the affected tooth might produce directional changes of root formation.

Clinical Features

If dilaceration is confined to the root and the tooth has erupted, the clinical crown appears normal. However, severe angulation of the root may prevent the tooth from erupting. Dilaceration can affect any tooth but is most common in the permanent maxillary central incisors.

Radiographic Appearance

Mesial or distal curvatures are easier to see on radiographs than buccal or lingual bends because of the geometric relationship between the direction of the x-ray beam and the long axis of the tooth. A buccal or lingual dilaceration is partially obscured by the root, and the apex appears blunted. A severe film bend can give an erroneous impression of dilaceration. Distortion of a tooth image by a film bend is characterized by elongation, lack of clarity in the apical portion, and occurrence at the corner of the radiograph that was bent.

Treatment

Occasionally, a dilaceration may be so severe that the affected tooth does not attain its proper arch position. A combination of surgery and orthodontics may be required to guide the tooth into place. However, the majority of dilacerated teeth are incidental radiographic findings that do not require treatment.

Reference

van Gool, A.V.: Injury to the permanent tooth germ after trauma to the deciduous predecessor. Oral Surg. Oral Med. Oral Pathol., 35:2–12, 1973.

DENS-IN-DENTE

The term dens invaginatus is more appropriate, but the popularity of dens-in-dente has justified continuation of its usage. This anomaly is characterized by an invagination of the outer covering of a tooth into the normal tooth structure. The depth of the invagination ranges from a barely perceptible pit to a direct pulp exposure. As with some other dental anomalies, the lack of a widely accepted definition that can be easily applied explains the wide variability of published findings. Several theories of origin have been proposed, but no one theory is widely accepted.

Clinical Features

Previously published reports are difficult to compare with each other because of the different criteria utilized by the various authors. The reported incidence ranges from 0.04 to 10%, a range that is attributable to whether the authors counted only cases that showed radiographic evidence of invagination or whether they considered clinical evidence of indentation to be adequate. The permanent maxillary lateral incisors are the teeth most commonly affected. Dens-in-dente is rare in primary or mandibular teeth. In the typical case there is a well-defined pit that easily catches the tip of an explorer on the lingual surface of a maxillary lateral incisor. Half of the cases are bilateral. There is a racial predilection because dens-in-dente is more common in Caucasians and mongoloids than in blacks. A rare variant of dens-in-dente affects the root instead of the crown of a tooth. It is presumed that this radicular form is related to the classic type except for its anatomic location.

Radiographic Appearance

Mild cases of dens-in-dente may not demonstrate any radiographic change, but in the more severe ones there is an enamel-lined invagination that can extend to the pulp chamber.

Treatment

Prophylactic restoration of the lingual pit is recommended because the enamel covering is usually very thin and the tooth is predisposed to development of a carious lesion. Conservative acid-etch resin techniques rather than amalgam or gold foil restorations are indicated. Caution should be used during the preparation of the tooth because the underlying pulp chamber can be quite close or even connected to the pit. The more severe forms of dens-in-dente require sophisticated endodontic care. Because of the tendency toward bilateral occurrence, a search for a second affected tooth should be undertaken if a case of dens-in-dente is discovered.

References

Goaz, P.W., and White, S.C.: Oral Radiology: Principles and Interpretation, 2nd ed. St. Louis: C.V. Mosby, 1987, pp. 435–437.

Rotstein, I., Stabholz, A., and Friedman, S.: Endodontic therapy for dens invaginatus in a maxillary second premolar. Oral Surg. Oral Med. Oral Pathol., 63:237–240, 1987.

Shafer, W.G., Hine, M.K., and Levy, B.M.: A Textbook of Oral Pathology, 4th ed. Philadelphia: W. B. Saunders, 1983, pp. 41–42.

ENAMEL PEARL

The enamel pearl is a circular mass of calcified material attached to the external surface of a tooth. Because of its well-defined clinical and radiographic features, the enamel pearl is easily recognized and is seldom confused with any other entity. It probably arises from Hertwig's epithelial root sheath before it loses its enamel-forming potential.

Synonyms: Enamel drop, enamel nodule, and enameloma.

Clinical Features

Enamel pearls are usually associated with the permanent maxillary molars and occasionally the mandibular molars. The incidence of clinically evident enamel pearls is 2.3% on all molars; the maxillary third molar is the one most frequently involved. Enamel pearls are usually less than 3 mm in diameter and are located in the furcation along the CEJ. The patient is unaware of their presence unless there is a secondary periodontal infection.

Radiographic Appearance

Typically, a well-defined, circular radiopacity whose radiodensity is equivalent to enamel is seen in the furcation of a molar. A rare variant, termed the internal enamel pearl, has also been described and is characterized by its occurrence within a tooth and transformation from a well-circumscribed radiolucency to a radiopacity during a period of years.

One potential misinterpretation occurs if there is excessive horizontal angulation during the exposure of a radiograph so that the root structure overlaps. Confirmation of the diagnosis can be achieved by exposing another radiograph from a different angle.

Histopathologic Findings

Microscopically, enamel pearls may consist entirely of enamel but may also contain dentin and pulp tissue. Some of these pearls are covered by a layer of cementum.

Treatment

No treatment is indicated unless a periodontal defect has been created by the presence of the enamel pearl.

Reference

Kaugars, G.E.: Internal enamel pearls: Report of case. J. Am. Dent. Assoc., 107:941–943, 1983.

TAURODONTISM

A taurodont is a tooth that has an enlarged pulp chamber in the apical-occlusal direction and lacks the typical cervical constriction. A considerable amount of information concerning taurodontism has been published because of its role in anthropology and its association with a number of syndromes. Most of the early reports of taurodontism concerned its incidence in our ancestors and how tooth development evolved. The term taurodontism originated because of the radiographic similarity of these teeth to the ones found in ungulates (hoofed animals). No widely accepted defini-

tion of taurodontism exists, which makes comparison of the various studies difficult. Research indicates that taurodontism is related to an unknown type of ectodermal abnormality and in some cases is associated with amelogenesis imperfecta. One popular theory of origin is that the epithelial diaphragm malfunctions in a taurodont, preventing the occurrence of dentinogenesis in the furcation area.

Clinical Features

The clinical crowns of taurodontic teeth are normal. The prevalence in the general population ranges from 0.5 to 5.6%, depending on the criteria used. One reasonable estimate is that at least one taurodont is present in 2.5% of the adult Caucasian population. The permanent mandibular second molar is the tooth most commonly affected, and, in general, permanent teeth are involved more often than primary teeth. Roughly half of all cases are bilateral.

Taurodontism can occur as an isolated finding or as part of a syndrome. Occasionally, a syndrome has been diagnosed initially because of a dentist's recognition of taurodontism. Tables 12–1 and 12–2 list the syndromes and conditions associated with taurodontism.

Radiographic Appearance

The radiographic findings are easier to describe than to measure objectively. Typically, the pulp chamber is elongated in an apical-occlusal direction, and the tooth does not have a discernible cervical constriction. The rectangular shape of the pulp chamber is the feature that prompted the comparison to ungulate teeth. The overall tooth length is normal, but the distance from the CEJ to the furcation is increased, giving the radiographic appearance of very short roots.

Taurodontism has been divided into three subtypes—hypotaurodontism, mesotaurodontism and hypertaurodontism—depending on the severity (longitudinal elongation) of the

Text continued on page 306

Table 12–1. CONDITIONS ASSOCIATED WITH TAURODONTISM

Amelogenesis imperfecta
Ectodermal dysplasia
Oligodontia
Osteoporosis
X-chromosome aneuploidy

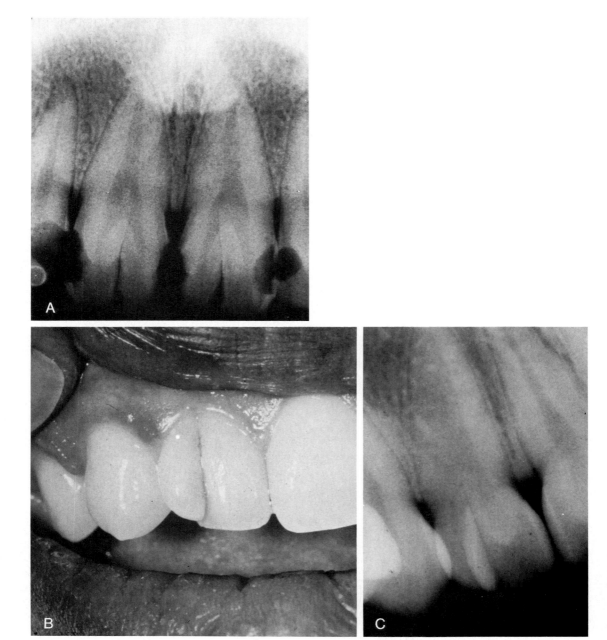

Figure 12–1. *A,* Gemination of both permanent maxillary central incisors is seen in this radiograph. Note the single enlarged pulp chamber and partial cleavage of the crown, which creates a tooth that is wider than normal. *B,* A permanent maxillary lateral incisor shows the typical clinical features of a geminated tooth, which was confirmed by its radiographic appearance (*C*). (Courtesy of Dr. R. Lieb, Richmond, Virginia.)

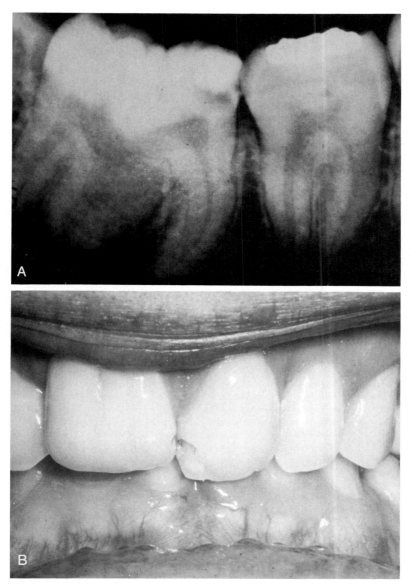

Figure 12–2. *A*, Fusion between a mandibular third molar and a supernumerary fourth molar produced this grossly enlarged tooth with one large pulp chamber and unusual root configuration. *B*, Fusion in a maxillary central incisor. Note groove.

Illustration continued on following page

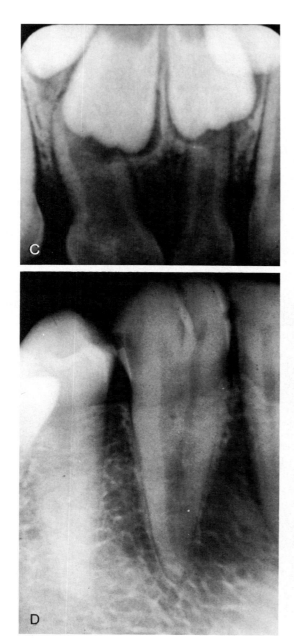

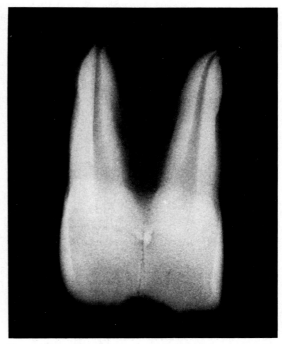

Figure 12–2 *Continued C*, Fusion of primary central and lateral incisor. Note the common pulp chamber. *D*, Fusion or concrescence? A lower lateral and canine appear to have cementum union . . . but do they share the same pulp chamber?

Figure 12–3. Two teeth that are united by cementum appear clinically normal but may be a problem at the time of extraction if the condition is unsuspected. These teeth were extracted simultaneously because of the concrescence.

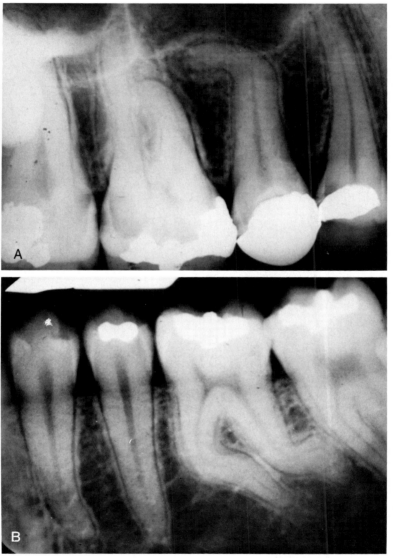

Figure 12–4. *A*, Distal and recurrent caries are seen in this maxillary premolar, whose root has a pronounced distal angulation. Extraction of the root tip in this case would be complicated by the dilaceration. *B*, Severely dilacerated roots of a lower molar.

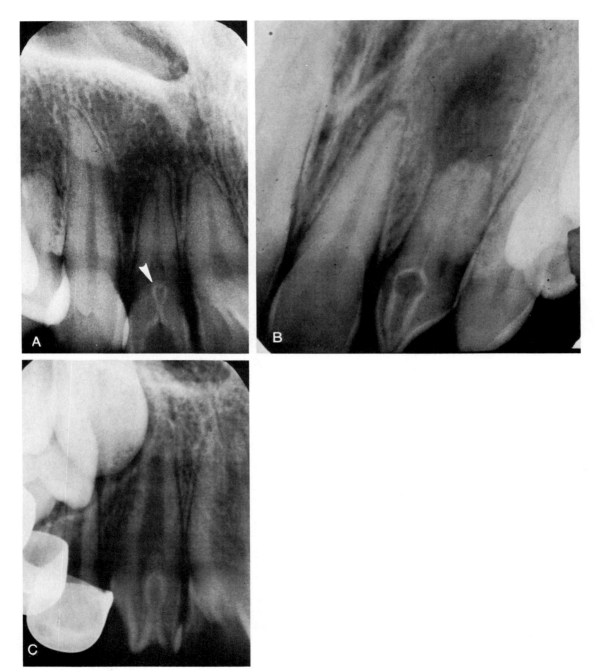

Figure 12–5. *A,* This maxillary lateral incisor has a radiographically visible invagination of the enamel into the underlying tooth at the lingual pit (*arrowhead*). *B,* A more severe variant of dens-in-dente, in which there is a deep invagination resulting in pulp exposure and subsequent periapical pathosis. Some cases of dens-in-dente are so mild that they are difficult to diagnose clinically. *C,* Another case of dens-in-dente.

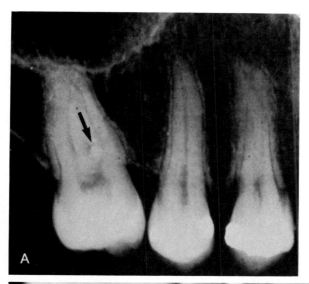

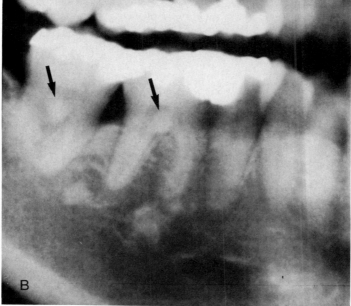

Figure 12–6. *A*, The small, enamel-dense radiopacity (*arrow*) in the furcation of this maxillary first molar is typical of an enamel pearl. *B*, Enamel pearls on lower molars (*arrows*).

Illustration continued on following page

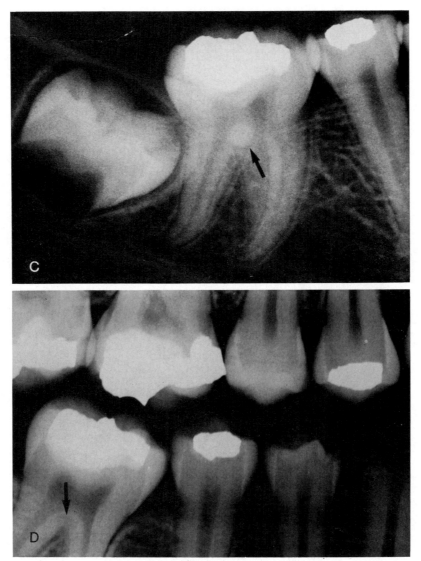

Figure 12–6 *Continued C,* Areas that resemble enamel pearls can be caused by radiographic technique. In this example, a well-defined radiopacity (*arrow*) is seen in the furcation of the mandibular first molar. Note the overlapped contact between the first molar and the second premolar. By simply changing the horizontal angulation of the incoming x-ray beam, it is possible (*D*) to show that the enamel pearl (*arrow*) was an area of overlapped roots. The change in angulation is evident from the open contact between the teeth.

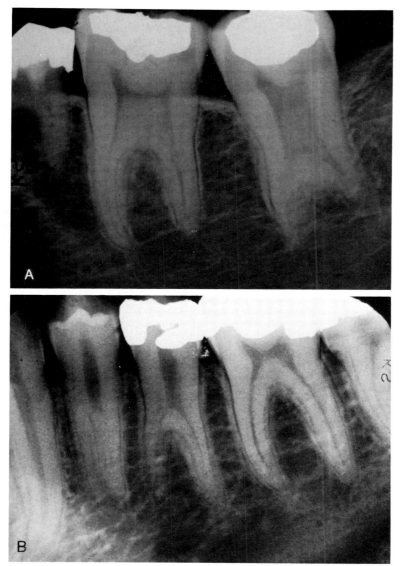

Figure 12–7. *A*, The increased apical-occlusal length of the pulp chamber and its rectangular shape are the radiographic features of taurodontism. In addition, there is a lack of cervical constriction. *B*, Taurodontism of a lower premolar.

Table 12–2. SYNDROMES ASSOCIATED WITH TAURODONTISM

Down's syndrome
Klinefelter syndrome
Microcephalic dwarfism, taurodontism, root resorption
  (Salk syndrome)
Microdontia, taurodontia, dens invaginatus
  (Casamassimo syndrome)
Oral-facial-digital involvement (Mohr syndrome)
Scanty hair, oligodontia, taurodontia
Trichodento-osseous syndrome
Tricho-onychodental syndrome

tooth. The mildest form (hypotaurodontism) is the most common, whereas the most severe (hypertaurodontism) is the rarest.

One potential misinterpretation is the enlarged pulp chambers noted in developing teeth. The open apices of immature teeth should be a diagnostic aid in distinguishing these teeth from taurodonts.

Treatment

No treatment is indicated, but an appropriate work-up should be done to rule out the existence of one of the associated syndromes.

References

Cichon, J.C., and Pack, R.S.: Taurodontism: Review of literature and report of case. J. Am. Dent. Assoc., 111:453–455, 1985.
Darbyshire, P.A., Witkop, C.J., and Cervenka, J.: Prepubertal diagnosis of Klinefelter syndrome in a patient with taurodontic teeth. Pediatr. Dent. 11:224–226, 1989.
Goaz, P.W., and White, S.C.: Oral Radiology: Principles and Interpretation, 2nd ed. St. Louis: C. V. Mosby, 1987, pp. 432–433.
Goldstein, E., and Gottlieb, M.A.: Taurodontism: Familial tendencies demonstrated in eleven of fourteen case reports. Oral Surg. Oral Med. Oral Pathol., 36:131–144, 1973.
Jaspers, M.T., and Witkop, C.J.: Taurodontism, an isolated trait associated with syndromes and x-chromosome aneuploidy. Am. J. Hum. Genet., 32:396–413, 1980.
Jaspers, M.T.: Taurodontism in the Down syndrome. Oral Surg. Oral Med. Oral Pathol., 51:632–636, 1981.
Seow, W.K., and Lai, P.Y.: Association of taurodontism with hypodontia: a controlled study. Pediatr. Dent., 11:214–219, 1989.

INHERITABLE DISORDERS AFFECTING TEETH

A syndrome is a cluster of signs and symptoms that occur in such a unique combination that it characterizes a group of patients. Although syndromes have "classic" lists of features that are typically found in affected patients, it is common for an individual patient to be lacking some of these features, and, in addition, he or she may have some findings that have not previously been reported. This variability is a source of frustration both for the student first learning about syndromes and for the clinician who has to diagnose and treat patients. It should be kept in mind that by necessity this discussion of syndromes is limited to the most prominent features because it is not possible to list all possible manifestations, and that patients with the "classic" syndrome sometimes exist only in textbooks! Because teeth are of both ectodermal and mesodermal origin, the potential exists for dental involvement in almost any syndrome. This involvement is more common than reported because the dental changes may be minor compared with the other stigmas. Considerable variation in the effects of a particular syndrome on the teeth is possible because the degree of penetrance or expressivity is not uniform.

Genetic counseling is a must for any patient in whom these inherited disorders are diagnosed, so that he or she can be apprised of other possible clinical problems and informed about the possibility of transmission to their offspring.

AMELOGENESIS IMPERFECTA

Amelogenesis imperfecta is one of the more common heritable disorders that affects teeth because it is found in approximately 1 in 14,000 people. Amelogenesis imperfecta is an ectodermal disturbance that reduces the quality and strength of the enamel. The clinical changes are classified according to which stage of enamel formation is affected. The **hypoplastic** type of amelogenesis imperfecta indicates a disturbance in formation of the organic matrix, the **hypocalcification** type indicates defective mineralization of the matrix, and the **hypomaturation** type indicates a defect in the maturation of the calcification. Other dental anomalies such as taurodontism have been associated with amelogenesis imperfecta. Determination of the type of amelogenesis imperfecta may require the services of a geneticist or a specialist experienced in this problem.

Enamel defects caused by trauma, malnutrition, metabolic factors, or systemic disease should be separated from hereditary amelogenesis imperfecta so that the patient can receive appropriate treatment and counseling.

Genetic Transmission: Autosomal dominant, autosomal recessive, X-linked dominant, and X-linked recessive. Of the four, autosomal dominant transmission is the most common.

Clinical Features

Both dentitions are equally affected, but if causally examined, the primary teeth seem less involved because their enamel is usually thinner than that of permanent teeth. Typically, the enamel in affected patients wears away quickly, leading to discolored teeth. Mild cases may demonstrate enamel loss with little or no discoloration. In more severe cases the soft enamel can be easily removed with dental instruments or during routine prophylaxis. The softness of the enamel occurs because its organic content is doubled compared with that in normal teeth. Surprisingly, the caries rate is low for affected teeth.

Radiographic Appearance

The enamel is thin, and there is often a loss of normal contact between adjacent teeth. Also, because of the increased organic content of the enamel, it may be difficult to distinguish radiographically between enamel and dentin.

Treatment

The type and extent of dental treatment depends on the clinical severity of the amelogenesis imperfecta. However, rampant caries is rarely a problem.

References

Cameron, I.W., and Bradford, E.W.: Amelogenesis imperfecta: A case report of a family. Br. Dent. J., 102:129–133, 1957.

Congleton, J., and Burkes, E.J.: Amelogenesis imperfecta with taurodontism. Oral Surg. Oral Med. Oral Pathol., 48:540–544, 1979.

Elzay, R.P., and Chamberlain, D.H.: Differential diagnosis of enlarged pulp chambers: A case report of amelogenesis imperfecta with taurodontism. J. Dent. Child., 53:388–390, 1986.

Sedano, H.O., Sauk, J.J., and Gorlin, R.J.: Oral Manifestations of Inherited Disorders. Boston: Butterworths, 1977, p. 16.

Shafer, W.G., Hine, M.K., and Levy, B.M.: A Textbook of Oral Pathology, 4th ed. Philadelphia: W. B. Saunders, 1983, pp. 51–53.

Toller, P.A.: A clinical report on six cases of amelogenesis imperfecta. Oral Surg. Oral Med. Oral Pathol., 12:325–333, 1959.

Winter, G.B., and Brook, A.H.: Enamel hypoplasia and anomalies of the enamel. Dent. Clin. North Am., 19:3–24, 1975.

DENTINOGENESIS IMPERFECTA

In contrast to amelogenesis imperfecta, which is an ectodermal disturbance, dentinogenesis imperfecta is a mesodermal problem. Confusion between these two conditions is understandable because of the similarity in names and clinical appearance. Shields (1973) and colleagues accurately stated that the previous literature concerning dentinogenesis imperfecta was "often confusing, incomplete, and even contradictory." Three types are currently recognized. Dentinogenesis imperfecta type I occurs in conjunction with osteogenesis imperfecta. Type II does not have bone involvement and is a fairly common condition (occurring in 1 in 8000 people), and type III (Brandywine dentinogenesis imperfecta) is found in an inbred isolated population in southern Maryland.

Genetic Transmission: Autosomal dominant.

Synonym: Hereditary opalescent dentin.

Clinical Features

Both dentitions are involved, but the primary teeth are more affected. The color of the teeth ranges from yellow to gray to brown, and they have an opalescent appearance. The tooth color darkens with age. Rapid attrition and dentin exposure occur because of the premature loss of enamel. Patients may suffer a loss of vertical dimension because of the excessive enamel loss. In some cases, the clinical appearance can be confused with amelogenesis imperfecta, but radiographs are diagnostic. Despite the obvious damage to the tooth, a low caries rate has been noted in patients with dentinogenesis imperfecta. The clinical and radiographic features of the inherited dentin disorders (dentinogenesis imperfecta and dentin dysplasia) are summarized in Table 12–3.

Table 12–3. COMPARISON OF INHERITED DENTIN DISORDERS

	Dentinogenesis Imperfecta			Dentin Dysplasia	
	Type I (with osteogenesis imperfecta)	Type II (no osteogenesis imperfecta)	Type III (Brandywine)	Type I (radicular)	Type II (coronal)
Clinically abnormal primary teeth	+	+	+		+
Clinically abnormal permanent teeth	+	+	+		
Pulp obliteration, primary teeth	+	+	+	+	+
Pulp obliteration, permanent teeth	+	+	+	+	
Enlarged pulp, primary teeth			+		
Enlarged pulp, permanent teeth					+
Periapical radiolucencies			+	+	
Short roots	+	+		+	

Radiographic Appearance

Types I and II are characterized by teeth with pulpal obliteration and short roots. Skeletal radiographs and the clinical history identify type I cases because of the effects of osteogenesis imperfecta. The pulpal obliteration can occur prior to eruption.

The radiographic appearance in type III cases is more variable because the pulp chambers in the primary teeth can be either normal, obliterated, or enlarged (shell teeth). The permanent teeth have obliterated pulp chambers, and there is a high incidence of periapical radiolucencies in noncarious teeth.

Histopathologic Findings

The mantle dentin is normal, but the remaining dentin contains unorganized tubules that are irregular in size and shape. In addition, the dentin of affected teeth has an increased content of water and organic matter, a decreased density and number of tubules, and a decreased hardness. The early loss of enamel was previously explained by an absence in the scalloping along the DEJ. However, one study showed that only 1 of 13 teeth that were analyzed had a smooth DEJ, and the remainder had at least some scalloping.

Treatment

Although the caries rate is low, loss of teeth is a major problem, as shown by one survey that found that 60% of patients were wearing dentures before the age of 30 years. The softness of the dentin decreases the longevity of routine restorations.

References

Johnson, O.N., Chaudhry, A.P., and Gorlin, R.J., et al: Hereditary dentinogenesis imperfecta. J. Pediatr., 54:786–792, 1959.

Levin, L.S., Leaf, S.H., and Jelmini, R.J., et al: Dentinogenesis imperfecta in the Brandywine isolate (DI type III): Clinical, radiologic, and scanning electron microscopic studies of the dentition. Oral Surg. Oral Med. Oral Pathol., 56:267–274, 1983.

Sedano, H.O., Sauk, J.J., and Gorlin, R.J.: Oral Manifestations of Inherited Disorders. Boston: Butterworths, 1977, pp. 21–22.

Shields, E.D., Bixler, D., and El-Kafrawy, A.M.: A proposed classification for heritable human dentine defects with a description of a new entity. Arch. Oral. Biol., 18:543–554, 1973.

Sunderland, E.P., and Smith, C.J.: The teeth in osteogenesis and dentinogenesis imperfecta. Br. Dent. J., 149:287–289, 1980.

Witkop, C.J.: Hereditary defects of dentin. Dent. Clin. North Am., 19:33–35, 1975.

DENTIN DYSPLASIA

Dentin dysplasia is separated from dentinogenesis imperfecta by clinical and radiographic differences. See Table 12–3 for a comparison of these conditions. Although the cause is not known with certainty, one plausible theory is that there is a failure in odontoblastic function after interaction with the ameloblastic layer. Two types of dentin dysplasia are recognized; type I (radicular) is more common than type II (coronal).

Genetic Transmission: Autosomal dominant.

Synonym: Rootless teeth.

Clinical Features

Both dentitions are affected in both types, but the teeth in type I are usually normal in clinical appearance, though some teeth exhibit a slight amber color. In type I cases there may be tooth mobility because of the short roots. In type II cases the primary teeth have a brown color, but the permanent teeth are clinically normal.

Radiographic Appearance

Pulpal obliteration, short roots, and periapical radiolucencies are characteristic of type I teeth. Pulpal obliteration is complete in primary teeth, but in permanent teeth there is a residual area of pulp chamber in the shape of a crescent or chevron. Obliteration of the pulp is rapid and can occur prior to eruption. The periapical radiolucencies have been diagnosed as radicular cysts.

Teeth affected by type II dentin dysplasia have a normal root size and shape, but the pulp chambers are obliterated in primary teeth, and the permanent teeth have an unusual "thistle tube" or "flame"-shaped pulp chambers of appearance. This is caused by an enlarged coronal pulp chamber and a normal or restricted radicular pulp canal.

Histopathologic Findings

Foci of calcified tubular dentin and osteodentin are apical to the normal coronal dentin. These histologic findings correspond to the radiographic obliteration of the pulp chamber.

Treatment

Type I teeth are prone to exfoliation because of the short roots, and the need for extraction or endodontic therapy is increased because of the likelihood of periapical pathosis. Pulpal exposure is a greater possibility in permanent teeth in type II cases because of the enlarged pulp chambers.

References

Melnick, M., Levin, L.S., and Brady, J.: Dentin dysplasia type I: A scanning electron microscopic analysis of the primary dentition. Oral Surg. Oral Med. Oral Pathol., 50:335–339, 1980.

Sauk, J.J., Lyon, H.W., Trowbridge, H.O., and Witkop, C.J.: An electron optic analysis and explanation for the etiology of dentinal dysplasia. Oral Surg. Oral Med. Oral Pathol., 33:763–771, 1972.

Shields, E.D., Bixler, D., and El-Kafrawy, A.M: A proposed classification for heritable dentine defects with a description of a new entity. Arch. Oral Biol., 18:543–554, 1973.

Wesley, R.K., Wysocki, G.P., Mintz, S.M., and Jackson, J.: Dentin dysplasia type I. Oral Surg. Oral Med. Oral Pathol., 41:516–524, 1976.

Witkop, C.J.: Hereditary defects of dentin. Dent. Clin. North Am., 19:29–32, 1975.

CHERUBISM

This interesting condition was first described in 1933 and was given the designation cherubism because of the upward gaze of the affected family members in the original report. Cherubism is characterized by a bilateral, symmetric, painless expansion of the mandible or maxilla that begins at a young age and continues to progress until puberty. The radiographic features of this bilateral multilocular lesion are virtually pathognomonic. The predilection for the jawbones has suggested an odontogenic origin, but none has been proved. Another theory is that perivascular fibrosis results in decreased oxygenation that somehow alters the mesenchymal cells.

Genetic Transmission: Autosomal dominant with 100% penetrance in men and 50 to 70% in women. Several cases of spontaneous mutation have also been reported.

Synonym: Hereditary fibrous dysplasia of the jaws.

Clinical Features

Patients are normal at birth, but a painless, bilateral swelling of the mandible or maxilla begins between the ages of 1½ and 4 years. The mandible is involved more often than the maxilla, and the posterior regions of the jawbones are more frequently affected than the anterior. A small number of unilateral cases have been reported. The upward gaze of the eyes occurs only if there is maxillary involvement that causes a superior displacement of the orbital floor so that a rim of the sclera is visible beneath the iris.

Often there is premature exfoliation of the primary teeth, and a number of permanent teeth may be missing or malformed. In particular, the permanent second and third molars are the teeth most likely to be affected. The teeth within the lesion are often mobile.

The expansion will typically continue until puberty, at which time the growth stops. According to a number of case reports, resolution should be complete or almost complete by the age of 30 years, in spite of the impressive size that some of these lesions attain.

Radiographic Appearance

The typical case appears as a bilateral, expansile radiolucency with extensive multiloculation that causes thinning or perforation of the cortex. Involvement of the mandibular condyles is uncommon but does occur occasionally. The first radiographic sign of resolution in the maxilla is the reappearance of the antra. Eventually, the bone returns to a normal radiographic appearance, or there may be residual scattered foci of radiopacities.

Histopathologic Findings

Numerous multinucleated giant cells are found within a vascular connective tissue stroma. The histologic findings are similar to those of central giant cell granuloma and hyperparathyroidism. One possible distinguishing feature is an eosinophilic perivascular band of collagen that is sometimes found in patients with cherubism.

Treatment

The diagnosis of cherubism is often much simpler than deciding how to treat the patient. Any plans for surgery should be tempered by the knowledge that most of these lesions will regress. The temptation to perform curettage or cosmetic recontouring is understandable and is justified in some cases. An impressive amount of bleeding should be anticipated during any surgical procedure because of the vascularity of the lesion.

References

Anderson, D.E., and McClendon, J.L.: Cherubism—hereditary fibrous dysplasia of the jaws. Oral Surg. Oral Med. Oral Pathol., 15(Suppl 2):5–16, 1962.
Regezi, J.A., and Sciubba, J.J.: Oral Pathology: Clinical-Pathologic Correlations. Philadelphia: W. B. Saunders, 1989, pp. 437–439.
Sedano, H.O., Sauk, J.J., and Gorlin, R.J.: Oral Manifestations of Inherited Disorders. Boston: Butterworths, 1977, pp. 93–95.
Thoma, K.H.: Cherubism and other intraosseous giant-cell lesions. Oral Surg. Oral Med. Oral Pathol., 15(Suppl 2):1–4, 1962.

Zachariades, N., Papanicolaou, S., Xypolyta, A., and Constantinidis, I.: Cherubism. Int. J. Oral Surg., 14:138–145, 1985.

CLEIDOCRANIAL DYSPLASIA

Although the prominent feature of this syndrome is the patient's ability to bring the shoulders together, many other osseous and dental changes are noted as well. Typically, the bones that ossify the earliest in the fetus, such as the clavicle, are the ones most affected. The dental changes consist primarily of multiple impacted normal and supernumerary teeth.

Genetic Transmission: Autosomal dominant, autosomal recessive, and spontaneous mutation.

Synonym: Cleidocranial dysostosis.

Clinical Features

Cleidocranial dysplasia affects primarily membranous bones but can involve any part of the skeleton. The skeletal abnormalities include hypoplasia or aplasia of the clavicles and short stature. The numerous skull manifestations are listed in Table 12–4. Patients with cleidocranial dysplasia appear to have a long neck and narrow shoulders because of the clavicular deficiency. In spite of the long list of clinical and radiographic findings, most of these patients live a normal life and can even participate in sports.

Radiographic Appearance

Some of the changes in the skull are listed in Table 12–4. Wormian bones are small ossifications found within suture lines. The unusual

Table 12–4. CLINICAL AND RADIOGRAPHIC CHANGES OF THE SKULL IN CLEIDOCRANIAL DYSPLASIA

Clinical	Radiographic
Brachycephalic skull	Broad cranial sutures
Broad base of nose	Decreased pneumatization of mastoid processes
Depressed nasal bridge	Delayed closure of fontanels
Depressed sagittal suture	Hypoplastic paranasal sinuses
Frontal and biparietal bossing	Multiple unerupted teeth
Hypertelorism	Supernumerary teeth Wormian bones

dental finding is the delayed eruption of both dentitions. In addition, supernumerary teeth are noted in the premolar region.

Histopathologic Findings

The delayed eruption of teeth has been attributed to the lack of cellular cementum. This conclusion may not be valid because erupted teeth that lack cellular cementum have been discovered. The lack of cellular cementum "seems therefore to be neither the cause nor the result of failure of eruption," as noted by Rushton (1956).

Treatment

Extraction of supernumerary teeth and overretained primary teeth is indicated. There is no treatment for the syndrome itself.

References

Goodman, R.M., and Gorlin, R.J.: Atlas of the Face in Genetic Disorders, 2nd ed. St. Louis: C.V. Mosby, 1977, pp. 92–93.
Koch, P.E., and Hammer, W.B.: Cleidocranial dysostosis: Review of the literature and report of case. J. Oral Surg., 36:39–42, 1978.
Regezi, J.A., and Sciubba, J.J.: Oral Pathology: Clinical-Pathologic Correlations. Philadelphia: W.B. Saunders, 1989, pp. 443–445.
Rushton, M.A.: An anomaly of cementum in cleidocranial dysostosis. Br. Dent., J., 100:81–83, 1956.

HYPOHIDROTIC ECTODERMAL DYSPLASIA

This syndrome is characterized by ectodermal changes causing hypodontia (decreased number of teeth), hypotrichosis (decreased amount of hair), and hypohidrosis (diminished perspiration). There are numerous variants of this syndrome, making it difficult to categorize these patients easily. Considerable similarity in facial appearance is seen among many of the patients.

Genetic Transmission: X-linked recessive and some cases of autosomal recessive, which may have been associated with parental consanguinity.

Clinical Features

The facial appearance is distinctive because of the frontal bossing, depressed nasal bridge, protuberant lips, lack of eyebrows, and thin blond hair. The signs may not become noticeable until the second year of life. Patients have normal physical and mental development. Hyperpyrexia (high fever) can be a problem because of the patients' inability to sweat. Hypohidrosis is caused by a generalized aplasia of the eccrine sweat glands. This inability to tolerate elevated temperatures may be the first sign of the syndrome in an infant. A striking dental finding in both dentitions is the presence of only a few teeth or, in some cases, a true anodontia (absence of teeth). The teeth have a conical shape that resembles the shape of teeth in patients with incontinentia pigmenti. Loss of vertical dimension is a natural consequence in the unrestored dentition.

Radiographic Appearance

Dental radiographs confirm the paucity of teeth and the typical cone shape.

Treatment

The longevity of dentures and bridges may be compromised by xerostomia, which predisposes to a higher caries rate and mucositis.

References

Sedano, H.O., Sauk, J.J., and Gorlin, R.J.: Oral Manifestations of Inherited Disorders. Boston: Butterworths, 1977, pp. 159–160.
Shafer, W.G., Hine, M.K., and Levy, B.M.: A Textbook of Oral Pathology, 4th ed. Philadelphia: W.B. Saunders, 1983, pp. 806–808.

GARDNER'S SYNDROME

This syndrome was first described in 1953 in several Utah families that demonstrated an increased incidence of colonic polyposis and subsequent carcinomatous change. The classic triad consists of colorectal polyposis, soft tissue tumors, and skeletal abnormalities. However, the complete triad occurs in less than 10% of affected patients. Of primary importance is the presence of multiple intestinal polyps, which have a very high rate of malignant transformation even at a young age. The soft tissue tumors consist of epidermoid cysts, fibromas, lipomas, desmoid tumors, and fibrosarcomas. Of the skeletal findings, sinus osteomas (50%) are the most common. In addition, impacted teeth, supernumerary teeth, and odontomas have been reported. Early diagnosis of any syndrome is important, but it becomes critical in Gardner's syndrome to prevent a dreadful colorectal malignancy.

Genetic Transmission: Autosomal dominant with variable expressivity and marked penetrance.

Clinical Features

One study evaluated 280 patients in 11 families who were at risk for the syndrome. Of these, 126 (45%) exhibited at least one facet of the syndrome. Not surprisingly, the most common feature among the 126 affected patients was colonic polyposis (67.5%). Next in frequency were soft tissue tumors (59.5%), osteomas (31.7%), and supernumerary or impacted teeth (6.3%). Only 19.8% of the patients had the complete triad at the time of examination. In general, the soft tissue tumors are the first component of the syndrome to be diagnosed because they are discovered before the patients are 20 years of age. Next in order of appearance are osteomas, which are most commonly found in the frontal sinus but may also be attached to the jawbones. Polyps are most frequently found in the colon (88%), but small intestinal involvement (12%) is also noted. There is almost a 100% probability of malignant change within the polyps by the age of 40.

Recently, it has been shown that increased levels of ornithine decarboxylase, an enzyme that has a role in the development of polyps, is a marker for patients with the syndrome.

Radiographic Appearance

Panoramic radiographs may reveal the presence of multiple, well-defined radiopacities, which are the osteomas. In addition, multiple impacted and supernumerary teeth are occasionally present.

Histopathologic Features

Epidermoid cysts are soft, fluctuant lesions that are lined by a thin layer of cystic epithelium and are commonly called sebaceous cysts. Desmoid tumors are aggressive fibromatoses that have some clinical and histologic similarity to low-grade fibrosarcomas but may also behave in a benign fashion. An osteoma is simply a well-defined neoplastic mass of dense viable bone.

Treatment

Total proctocolectomy at the onset of polyposis yields a very high survival rate. The remaining clinical stigmas can be removed as deemed necessary for cosmetic or functional reasons. Routine proctoscopic examinations and genetic counseling must be emphasized for patients at risk.

References

Arendt, D.M., Frost, R., Whitt, J.C., and Palomboro, J.: Multiple radiopaque masses in the jaws. J. Am. Dent. Assoc., 118:349–351, 1989.

Duncan, B.R., Dohner, V.A., and Priest, J.H.: The Gardner syndrome: Need for early diagnosis. J. Pediatr., 72:497–505, 1968.

Fader, M., Kline, S.N., Spatz, S.S., and Zubrow, H.J.: Gardner's syndrome (intestinal polyposis, osteomas, sebaceous cysts) and a new dental discovery. Oral Surg. Oral Med. Oral Pathol., 15:153–172, 1962.

Gardner, E.J.: Follow-up study of a family group exhibiting dominant inheritance for a syndrome including intestinal polyps, osteomas, fibromas and epidermal cysts. Am. J. Hum. Genet., 14:376–390, 1962.

Goodman, R.M., and Gorlin, R.J.: Atlas of the Face in Genetic Disorders, 2nd ed. St. Louis: C.V. Mosby, 1977, pp. 124–125.

Sedano, H.O., Sauk, J.J., and Gorlin, R.J.: Oral Manifestations of Inherited Disorders. Boston: Butterworths, 1977, pp. 135–137.

Watne, A.L., Core, S.K., and Carrier, J.M.: Gardner's syndrome. Surg. Gynecol. Obstet., 141:53–56, 1975.

BASAL CELL NEVUS SYNDROME (Nevoid Basal Cell Carcinoma Syndrome)

Gorlin and Goltz helped to define this syndrome in 1960 and hinted at its potential significance. Since that time its clinical importance has become clear, and dozens of associated findings have been reported. Although the classic triad consists of odontogenic keratocysts, multiple basal cell carcinomas, and bifid ribs, there are so many secondary findings that it is difficult to describe the "typical" patient.

Genetic Transmission: Autosomal dominant with variable expressivity and high penetrance.

Synonyms: Jaw cyst–basal cell nevus–bifid rib syndrome, multiple nevoid basal cell carcinoma syndrome, and Gorlin-Goltz syndrome.

Clinical Features

The more common clinical findings are summarized in Table 12–5. The shortening of the metacarpals has prompted some investigators to assess the relationship of this syndrome to hypoparathyroidism, but the results have been equivocal. Milia, also known as "whiteheads," are small epidermoid cysts that are fairly common in the general population but are found in greater numbers in patients with this syndrome. Basal cell carcinomas are characterized by the large numbers located in nonexposed areas and their occurrence at a young age. In addition, multiple trichoepitheliomas have also been reported. Only a small number of medulloblastomas have been associated with the syndrome, but the incidence is higher than that in the general population.

Radiographic Appearance

Odontogenic keratocysts are one of the most common findings (75%). These are usually discovered in the first or second decade of life and, as such, are often the first sign of the syndrome. The radiographic appearance of these keratocysts is similar to that of nonsyndrome keratocysts except for the presence of multiple lesions in some cases. There is a case report of a patient who had a total of nine keratocysts removed. Unfortunately, the syndrome-associated keratocysts, have a very high recurrence rate (85%), and the average period of time to the first recurrence is 27 months, which is half the time for a recurrence in a nonsyndrome patient. Radiographically, the keratocysts may be multilocular and are often associated with an impacted tooth.

Skull radiographs often reveal calcification of the falx cerebri (80%) or tentorium cerebelli (38%). Rib abnormalities, such as bifid rib, are incidental findings that occur more frequently than in the general population (70% versus 1%).

Histopathologic Findings

Odontogenic keratocysts are lined by a thin layer of parakeratin and are histologically indistinguishable from other keratocysts.

Treatment

Because of their multiplicity, tendency toward recurrence, and aggressive clinical behavior, odontogenic keratocysts can become a surgical nightmare. Adequate surgical margins should be obtained during the initial surgery to reduce the recurrence rate. The patient should be referred for evaluation and removal of the basal cell carcinomas and to rule out any cranial tumors. Genetic counseling is important because the syndrome may become manifest only after a patient starts to have children.

An unusual complication related to anesthesia is that severe bradycardia and hypotension develop after induction of general anesthesia in 8% of the patients.

References

Brannon, R.B.: The odontogenic keratocyst: A clinicopathologic study of 312 cases. Oral Surg. Oral Med. Oral Pathol., 42:54–72, 233–255, 1976.

Donatsky, O., Hjørting-Hansen, E., Philipsen, H.P., and Fejerskov, O.: Clinical, radiologic, and histopathologic aspects of 13 cases of nevoid basal cell carcinoma syndrome. Int. J. Oral. Surg., 5:19–28, 1976.

Gilhuus-Moe, O., Haugen, L.K., and Dee, P.M.: The syndrome of multiple cysts of the jaws, basal cell carcinomata and skeletal anomalies. Br. J. Oral Surg., 5:211–222, 1968.

Gorlin, R.J., Vickers, R.A., Kellen, E., and Williamson, J.J.: The multiple basal-cell nevi syndrome. Cancer 18:89–104, 1965.

Sedano, H.O., Sauk, J.J., and Gorlin, R.J.: Oral Manifestations of Inherited Disorders. Boston: Butterworths, 1977, pp. 139–141.

Southwick, G.J., and Schwartz, R.A.: The basal cell nevus syndrome. Cancer 44:2294–2305, 1979.

Table 12–5. CLINICAL FEATURES OF BASAL CELL NEVUS SYNDROME*

Face	Skeletal
Broad nasal root (25%)	Shortening of third to fifth
Frontal bossing	metacarpals (100%)
Hypertelorism	
Mandibular prognathism	**Central Nervous System**
	Medulloblastomas
Skin	Mental retardation (15%)
Milia	
Multiple basal cell carcinomas (50%)	
Palmar/plantar keratosis and pits (60%)	

*The percentages within the parentheses indicate the percentage of affected patients with the particular findings.

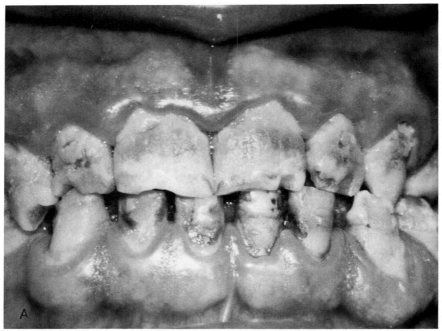

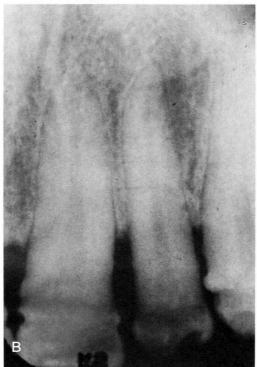

Figure 12–8. *A,* Loss of enamel and unsightly appearance of the teeth are common clinical features of amelogenesis imperfecta. (Courtesy of Dr. C. Kaugars, Richmond, Virginia.) *B,* A periapical radiograph demonstrates a generalized loss of enamel and abnormal contacts between the teeth. (Courtesy of Dr. C. Kaugars, Richmond, Virginia.)

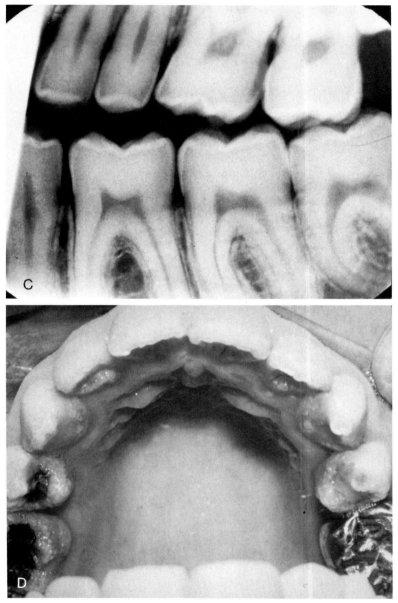

Figure 12–8 *Continued C*, A milder case shows a radiographic layer of enamel that is intact but very thin. *D,* Clinical appearance of amelogenesis imperfecta in a 21-year-old woman.

Illustration continued on following page

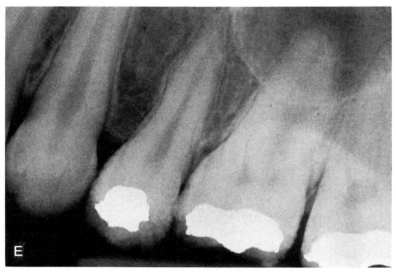

Figure 12–8 *Continued E*, Radiographic appearance of the mottled enamel of the woman shown in *D*.

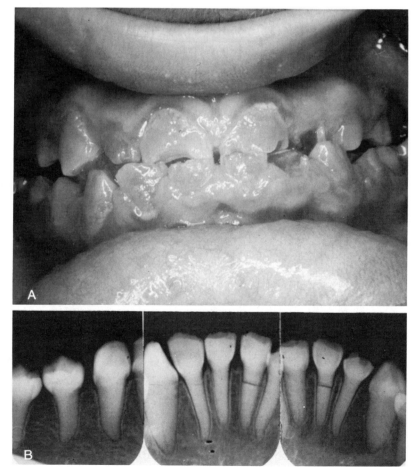

Figure 12–9. *A*, Attrition and associated cosmetic problems are readily seen in this example of type II dentinogenesis imperfecta. (Courtesy of Dr. B. Kemp, Richmond, Virginia.) *B*, Radiographs reveal pulpal obliteration and loss of incisive enamel. Note the horizontal root fracture on one of the mandibular incisors. (Courtesy of Dr. B. Kemp, Richmond, Virginia.)

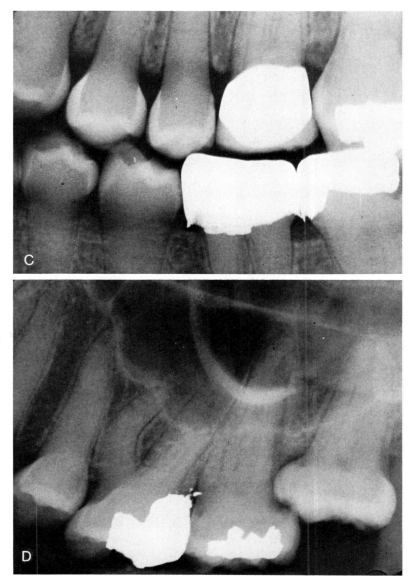

Figure 12–9 *Continued C*, A case of dentinogenesis imperfecta in a 19-year-old woman. Note the absence of pulp chambers and bulbous crowns of the maxillary first premolar and mandibular second molar. *D*, Periapical film of case shown in *C*. Note bulbous crowns.

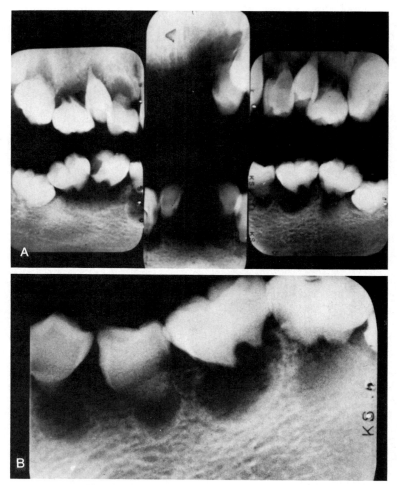

Figure 12–10. *A*, Dentin dysplasia, type I. Note pulpal obliteration. *B*, Close-up of periapical film shown in *A*.

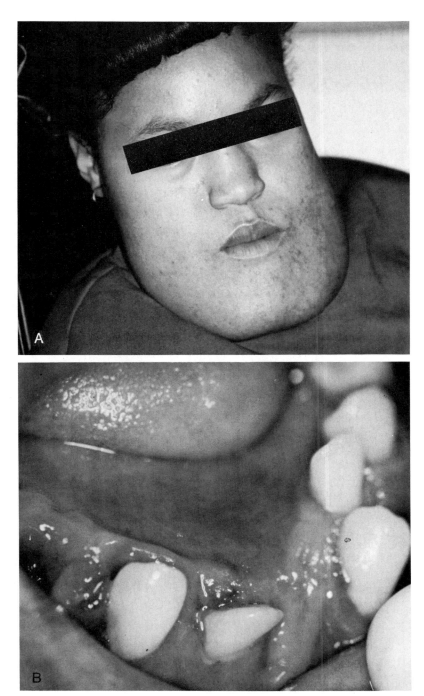

Figure 12–11. *A*, This 16-year-old girl had a severe case of mandibular cherubism. She first noticed an expansion of her lower jaw several years ago, but it became symptomatic only recently. (Courtesy of Dr. J. Naimtu, Richmond, Virginia.) *B*, An intraoral view reveals that the lingual expansion of the mandible has elevated the tongue. Also, premature exfoliation and mobility of the permanent teeth are evident. (Courtesy of Dr. J. Naimtu, Richmond, Virginia.)

Illustration continued on following page

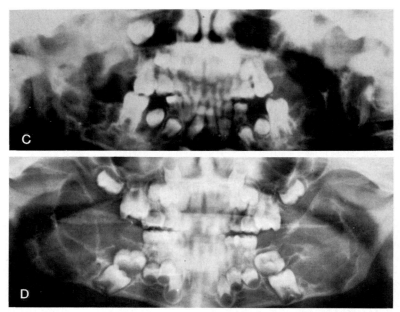

Figure 12–11 *Continued C,* Although the mandibular lesions are prominent, there is also evidence of maxillary involvement in this case. Note the number of impacted teeth as well as the absence of the mandibular second and third molars. Extensive bilateral multiloculation in a young person is virtually diagnostic of cherubism. With time, the radiolucent areas resolve, and the bone appears normal. *D,* Large multilocular, expansile lesions in the mandible. These lesions have displaced teeth.

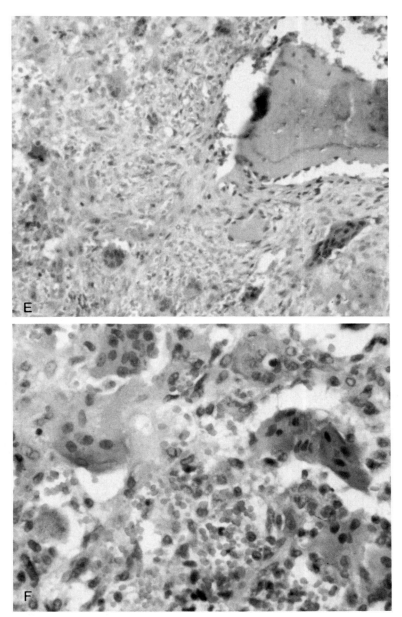

Figure 12–11 *Continued E,* The presence of numerous multinucleated giant cells within a vascular connective tissue stroma is similar to the appearance of central giant cell granuloma and hyperparathyroidism. *F,* A high-power view shows the randomly scattered giant cells and proliferation of vascular spaces. Surgical procedures may result in bleeding problems because of the increased vascularity.

Illustration continued on following page

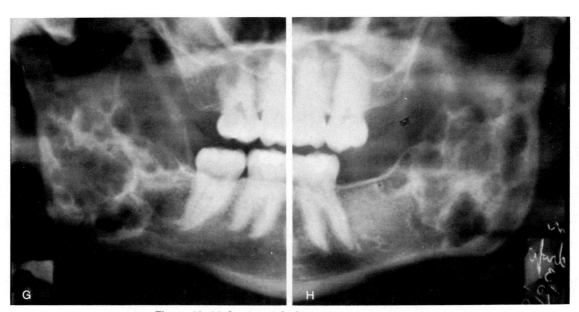

Figure 12–11 *Continued G,* Cherubism: close-up of the patient's right side. *H,* Close-up of the left side of the patient in *G.* Note the remarkable symmetry.

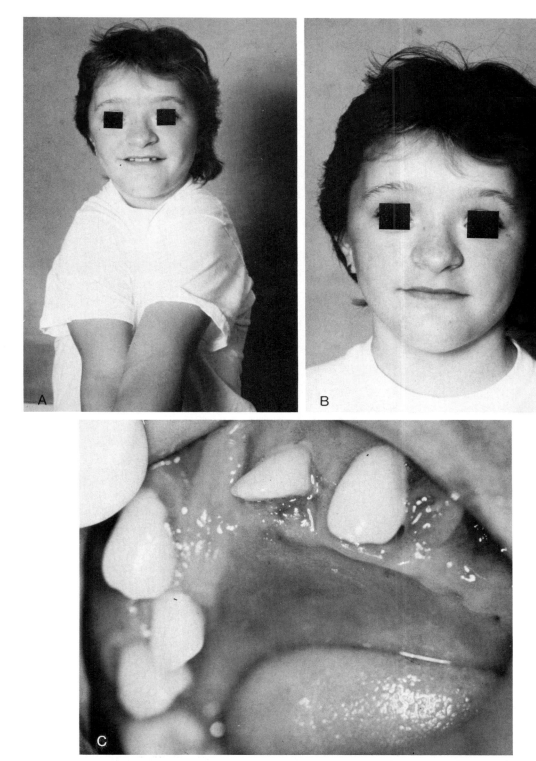

Figure 12–12. *A,* This 14-year-old girl demonstrates her ability to put her shoulders almost together. (Courtesy of Dr. L. Abbey, Richmond, Virginia.) *B,* Typical facial appearance of cleidocranial dysplasia is seen in this patient. (Courtesy of Dr. L. Abbey, Richmond, Virginia.) *C,* Delayed eruption of permanent teeth is readily evident in this patient. (Courtesy of Dr. L. Abbey, Richmond, Virginia.)

Illustration continued on following page

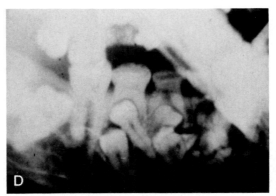

Figure 12–12 *Continued D*, "Tooth factory" characteristic of cleidocranial dysplasia in mandible.

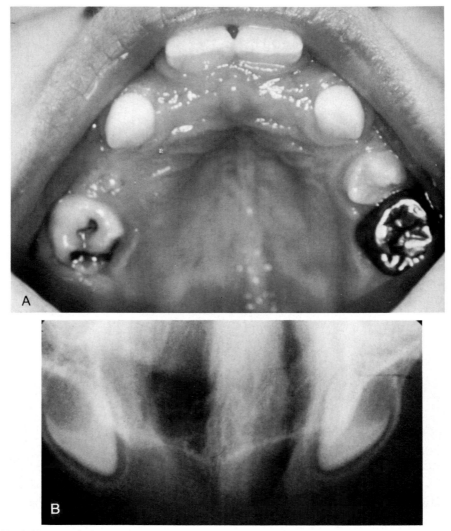

Figure 12–13. *A*, Hypodontia is seen in this 27-year-old woman. Her only permanent maxillary teeth have been restored. *B*, Developing canines were the only anterior teeth that developed in this patient with ectodermal dysplasia.

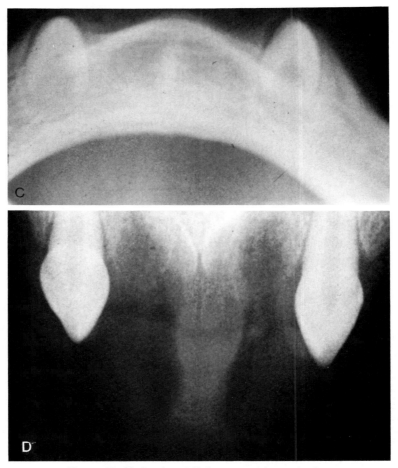

Figure 12–13 *Continued C*, Lower anterior teeth of patient shown in *B. D*, The same patient a few years later as the canines erupt.

Illustration continued on following page

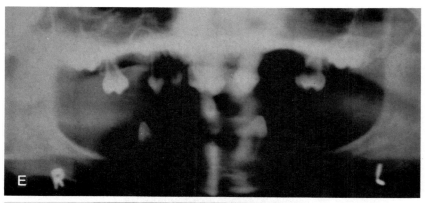

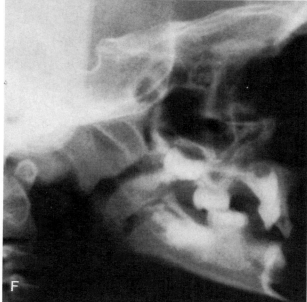

Figure 12–13 *Continued E,* Panoramic view of the "full" dentition that finally developed. *F,* Lateral skull radiograph of a patient with ectodermal dysplasia.

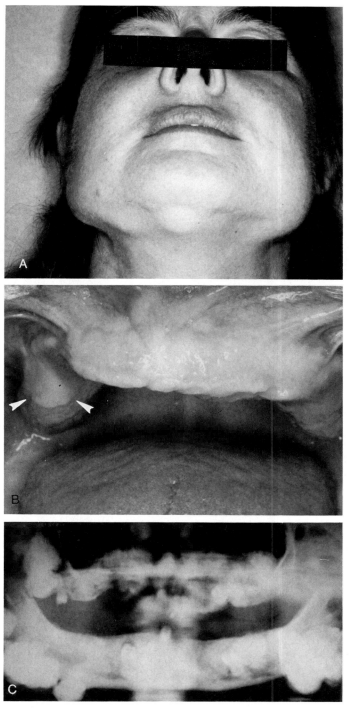

Figure 12–14. *A,* This film was taken in a 42-year-old woman who had noticed these "bumps" for a number of years. The mass in the submental region is an epidermoid cyst, and the swellings on both the right and the left posterior mandible are osteomas. She also has multiple polyps in the colon. (Courtesy of Dr. R. Baker, Lynchburg, Virginia.) *B,* An intraoral view reveals a well-defined hard mass (*arrowheads*) in the edentulous right posterior maxilla that was an osteoma. (Courtesy of Dr. R. Baker, Lynchburg, Virginia.) *C,* Multiple dense osteomas are present throughout the mandible and maxilla. Note the presence of the impacted teeth. (Courtesy of Dr. R. Baker, Lynchburg, Virginia.)

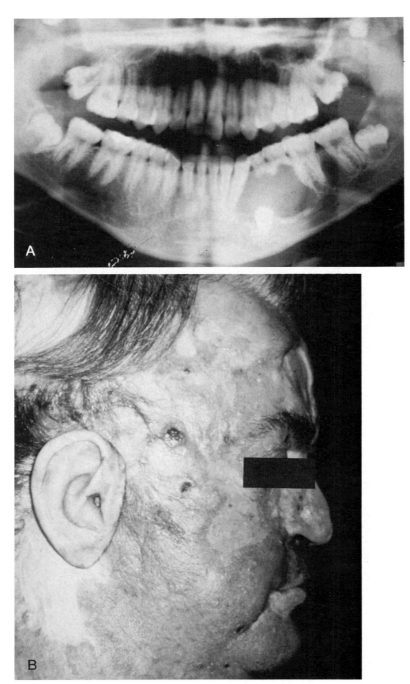

Figure 12–15. *A*, Two large odontogenic keratocysts are seen in the left mandible of this 14-year-old girl. Also, odontogenic keratocysts in the posterior right and left maxillas have prevented eruption of the third molars. *B*, Another patient had had multiple basal cell carcinomas removed. The film demonstrates the extensive scarring that may occur. (Courtesy of Dr. V. Saunders, Richmond, Virginia.)

APPENDIX

PERIAPICAL RADIOLUCENCIES
COMMON
Periapical abscess
Periapical granuloma
Periapical cyst
Fibrous healing defect (surgical scar)
Periapical cemental dysplasia
(cementoma) (early stage)
UNCOMMON
Eosinophilic granuloma (histiocytosis X)
Sarcomas (osteosarcoma, fibrosarcoma,
etc.)
Odontogenic keratocyst

RADIOLUCENCIES WITH DISTINCT BORDERS
COMMON
Incisive canal cyst (nasopalatine duct
cyst)
Residual cyst
Traumatic bone cyst
Median palatal cyst
Fibrous healing defect (surgical scar)
Submandibular salivary gland
depression
UNCOMMON
Primordial cyst
Lateral periodontal cyst
Ameloblastoma (unicystic)
Osteoporotic bone marrow defect
Multiple myeloma
Nevoid basal cell carcinoma syndrome
(Gorlin-Goltz syndrome)
Squamous odontogenic tumor
Plasmacytoma

RADIOLUCENCIES WITH INDISTINCT BORDERS
Chronic osteomyelitis
Osteosarcoma
Chondrosarcoma
Squamous cell carcinoma
Metastatic tumors to the jaws
Histiocytosis X (Letterer-Siwe disease,
Hand-Schüller-Christian disease)
Fibrous dysplasia
Osteoradionecrosis
Malignant salivary gland tumors
Adenocarcinoma
Mucoepidermoid carcinoma
Adenoid cystic carcinoma
Pleomorphic adenoma

PERICORONAL RADIOLUCENCIES *WITHOUT* CALCIFICATIONS
Dentigerous cyst
Ameloblastoma
Odontogenic keratocyst
Mucoepidermoid carcinoma
Ameloblastic fibroma

PERICORONAL RADIOLUCENCIES *WITH* CALCIFICATIONS
Calcifying epithelial odontogenic tumor
(Pindborg tumor)
Adenomatoid odontogenic tumor
Calcifying odontogenic cyst (Gorlin cyst)
Ameloblastic fibro-odontoma
Ameloblastic odontoma

MULTILOCULAR RADIOLUCENCIES
Odontogenic keratocyst
Ameloblastoma
Central giant cell granuloma
Aneurysmal bone cyst
Hemangioma
Fibrous dysplasia
Cherubism (familial fibrous dysplasia)
Odontogenic myxoma

MIXED RADIOLUCENT-RADIOPAQUE LESIONS
Periapical cemental dysplasia (intermediate)
Condensing osteitis
Odontoma (compound and complex)
Florid osseous dysplasia (gigantiform cementoma, sclerosing cemental masses, diffuse sclerosing osteomyelitis)
Cemento-ossifying fibroma
Calcifying odontogenic cyst (Gorlin cyst)
Calcifying epithelial odontogenic tumor (Pindborg tumor)
Adenomatoid odontogenic tumor
Ameloblastic fibro-odontoma
Ameloblastic odontoma

PERIAPICAL RADIOPACITIES THAT MAY CONTACT TEETH
Condensing osteitis
Idiopathic osteosclerosis
Periapical cemental dysplasia (mature)
Hypercementosis
Cementoblastoma
Odontoma (complex or compound)

SOLITARY OR MULTIPLE RADIOPACITIES WITHIN JAWS
Enostosis
Exostosis
Idiopathic osteosclerosis
Periapical cemental dysplasia (mature)
Retained root tip
Odontoma

SOLITARY OR MULTIPLE RADIOPACITIES OUTSIDE JAWS
Sialolith
Antrolith
Phlebolith
Tonsillolith
Calcified lymph node
Calcified stylohyoid ligament
Miliary osteoma
Myositis ossificans
Calcified facial arteries

GENERALIZED RADIOPACITIES
Paget's disease of bone
Hyperparathyroidism
Osteomyelitis
Fibrous dysplasia
Florid osseous dysplasia (gigantiform cementoma, sclerosing cementral masses, diffuse sclerosing osteomyelitis)
Osteopetrosis (Albers-Schönberg disease)

"FLOATING TOOTH"
Severe, localized periodontitis
Juvenile periodontitis
Eosinophilic granuloma
Osteosarcoma
Fibrosarcoma

PERIOSTEAL REACTIONS
Garré's osteomyelitis (proliferative periostitis, juvenile periostitis of the mandible)
Ewing's sarcoma
Caffey's disease (infantile cortical hyperostosis)
Osteogenic sarcoma
Eosinophilic granuloma
Osteomyelitis
Fibrous dysplasia

SUN-RAY APPEARANCE
Osteogenic (classic description) sarcoma
Hemangioma
Chondrosarcoma
Ameloblastomic odontoma
Complex odontoma

INDEX